Are We Pushing Animals to Their Biological Limits?

Are We Pushing Animals to Their Biological Limits?

Welfare and Ethical Implications

Edited by

Temple Grandin
Professor of Livestock Handling and Behavior, Colorado State University, USA

Martin Whiting
Lecturer in Veterinary Ethics and Law, Royal Veterinary College, UK

CABI

CABI is a trading name of CAB International

CABI
Nosworthy Way
Wallingford
Oxfordshire OX10 8DE
UK

Tel: +44 (0)1491 832111
Fax: +44 (0)1491 833508
E-mail: info@cabi.org
Website: www.cabi.org

CABI
745 Atlantic Avenue
8th Floor
Boston, MA 02111
USA

Tel: +1 (617)682-9015
E-mail: cabi-nao@cabi.org

A catalogue record for this book is available from the British Library.

Library of Cangress Cataloging-in-Publication Data

Names: Grandin, Temple, editor.
Title: Are we pushing animals to their biological limits? : welfare and ethical implications / edited by Dr. Temple Grandin, Professor of Livestock Handling and Behavior, Colorado State University, USA, Dr. Martin Whiting, Lecturer in Veterinary Ethics and law, Royal Veterinary College, UK.
Description: Wallingford, Oxfordshire, UK ; Boston, MA : CABI, [2018] | Includes bibliographical references and index.
Identifiers: LCCN 2018014303| ISBN 9781786390547 (pbk) | ISBN 9781786390554 (epdf) | ISBN 9781786390561 (epub)
Subjects: LCSH: Animal welfare--Moral and ethical aspects. | Animals--Effect of human beings on.
Classification: LCC HV4708 .A73 2018 | DDC 179/.3--dc23 LC record available at https://lccn.loc.gov/2018014303

ISBN: 978 1 78639 054 7 (pbk)
978 1 78639 055 4 (e-pdf)
978 1 78639 056 1 (e-pub)

Commissioning editor: Caroline Makepeace
Editorial assistant: Alexandra Lainsbury
Production editor: Shankari Wilford

Typeset by SPi, Pondicherry, India
Printed and bound in the UK by Severn, Gloucester

Contents

Contributors

Donald M. Broom, Centre for Animal Welfare and Anthrozoology, Department of Veterinary Medicine, University of Cambridge, Cambridge, UK. E-mail: dmb16@cam.ac.uk

Sarah Chan, Chancellor's Fellow, Usher Institute for Population Health Sciences and Informatics; Deputy Director, Mason Institute for Medicine, Life Sciences and the Law, University of Edinburgh, Edinburgh, UK. E-mail: Sarah.Chan@ed.ac.uk

Andrew Gardiner, Royal (Dick) School of Veterinary Studies, University of Edinburgh, Edinburgh, UK. E-mail: Andrew.Gardiner@ed.ac.uk

Temple Grandin, Department of Animal Sciences, College of Agricultural Sciences, Colorado State University, Fort Collins, Colorado, USA. E-mail: cheryl.miller@colostate.edu

Stefan Gunnarsson, Associate Professor DVM; Diplomate ECAWBM, Swedish University of Agricultural Sciences, Department of Animal Environment and Health, Skara, Sweden. E-mail: Stefan.Gunnarsson@slu.se

Felicity Huntingford, Institute of Biodiversity, Animal Health and Comparative Medicine, University of Glasgow, Glasgow, UK. E-mail: Felicity.Huntingford@glasgow.ac.uk

Sunil Kadri, Aquaculture Innovation, Edinburgh, UK. E-mail: sunil.kadri@gmail.com

Manuel Magalhães-Sant'Ana, Disciplinary Committee, Ordem dos Médicos Veterinários, Lisbon, Portugal; Research Fellow, Faculdade Medicina Veterinária, Universidade de Lisboa, Lisbon, Portugal. E-mail: manuel.santana@omv.pt

Stephen May, Senior Vice Principal, Royal Veterinary College, University of London. E-mail: smay@rvc.ac.uk

David Morton, University of Birmingham, UK. E-mail: dbmgm2@gmail.com

Elisabeth Ormandy, Animals in Science Policy Institute, Vancouver, Canada. E-mail: elisabeth@animalsinscience.org

Nikki Osborne, Responsible Research in Practice, Horsham, UK. E-mail: nikki@responsibleresearchinpractice.co.uk

Rowena M.A. Packer, Department of Clinical Science and Services, Royal Veterinary College, University of London. E-mail: rpacker@rvc.ac.uk

Jan-Bas Prins, Universiteit Leiden, The Netherlands. E-mail: J.B.Prins@lumc.nl

Bernard Rollin, Department of Philosophy, College of Liberal Arts, Colorado State University, Fort Collins, Colorado, USA. E-mail: bernard.rollin@colostate.edu

Jimmy Turnbull, Institute of Aquaculture, University of Stirling, Stirling, UK. E-mail: J.F.TURNBULL@stir.ac.uk

Melissa Upjohn, Brooke, Action for Working Horses and Donkeys, London. E-mail: melissa.upjohn@dogstrust.org.uk

Kimberly Wells, Brooke, Action for Working Horses and Donkeys, London. E-mail: Kimberly.Wells@thebrooke.org

Martin Whiting, RVC Animal Welfare Science and Ethics, Royal Veterinary College, University of London. E-mail: martinwhiting@mac.com

1 Introduction: Use New Genetic Technologies and Animal Breeding Methods Carefully to Avoid Problems

Temple Grandin

Department of Animal Sciences, Colorado State University, USA

Many authors have contributed to this book to provide an overview of how conventional animal breeding, GMOs, gene editing and performance enhancing pharmaceuticals have been used to produce more productive farm animals. These methods have also been used to change the appearance of dogs and enhance the performance of horses. When used carefully, animal welfare is probably acceptable, but pushing the animal's biology too hard may have detrimental effects. I call this 'biological overload'. If problems gradually become worse, people may not notice them until the animal's welfare is seriously compromised. I call this 'bad becoming normal'. To set the stage, I will describe problems that occurred in pigs produced with conventional breeding.

For over 40 years I have been working with farm animals. During a long career I have observed many changes in animal genetics. Some of the changes have been beneficial and others detrimental. I have had the opportunity to observe cattle and pigs from many different breeders in numerous countries. At the stockyards (lairages) of large meat plants, pigs, cattle and other animals of many different origins were housed in adjacent pens. In this situation, differences in animal temperament (startle response), or problems such as a lack of stamina during handling, became obvious. In the 1980s, a breeder of a new line of rapidly growing lean pigs told me that since I was not a geneticist I was not qualified to have opinions on the behaviour of his pigs. In reply I said that I had one important qualification – I had seen pigs from many different genetic lines housed side-by-side where I could compare them. He had worked exclusively with his own genetic line of pigs and almost never saw pigs from other breeders. The pigs from his new genetic line were more excitable than other pigs.

Do Not Let Bad Become Normal

If the only animals a breeder or producer sees are their own animals, it is really easy to allow bad to become normal. A good example is lameness in dairy cattle. Gradually, over many years, lameness levels slowly increased until a quarter of the dairy cows

E-mail: cheryl.miller@colostate.edu

became lame (Von Keyserlingk *et al.*, 2012). When producers were asked to estimate the percentage of lame cows, their estimates were less than half the actual percentage (Espejo *et al.*, 2006). When lameness is actually measured, people can work to reduce it. In the state of Wisconsin, a successful programme to reduce lameness lowered it to half the national average (Cook *et al.*, 2016). To prevent bad from becoming normal, lameness should be measured on a regular basis. This detrimental change had progressed so slowly that people failed to see it until it got really serious.

Livestock Became Weaker since 1980

When farm animals are selected for increased production, there is often a trade-off. I offer several striking examples that I have observed from the 1970s to the 1990s. In the early 1970s, when my career started, both market weight pigs and old sows were walked up to the third floor of large multilevel meat packing plants. Each plant had a long ramp that led to the third floor. The pigs ran up the ramp and the percentage of dead pigs or those exhausted from climbing the ramp was almost zero.

In 1980, I was hired by an old meat plant where the pigs had to walk up long ramps to reach the stunner. The total vertical rise of the ramp was over 24 ft (7 m). The company was having difficulty getting the pigs to climb the ramp and some pigs were too weak. My assignment was to design a pig race with a conveyor belt in the bottom of it to convey the pigs up to the stunner. In my youthful days, when I thought I could fix everything with engineering, I jumped at this opportunity. My early view was that engineering was the way to fix every problem. I have designed many systems that have worked well (Grandin, 1988, 2003, 2014) but the 'conveyorized' pig ramp was a total failure. The pigs sat down on the conveyor and it flipped them over backwards. I was devastated that my system had failed. Then I had a sudden flash of insight; maybe there were differences between the pigs that had difficulty climbing the ramp and the pigs that could climb it easily.

Always Look at Root Causes of Problems

Today, I know that it is important to fix the root causes of problems and not just the symptoms. The next day, with the conveyor turned off, I watched pigs climb the ramp. When a pig became too fatigued to walk up the ramp, I recorded its ID number. It quickly became obvious that almost all the pigs that were not able to walk up the ramp originated from a single farmer. They all had a genetic condition called splayed leg (Lax, 1971; Macks *et al.*, 2001). Their hindquarters were weak and they had a tendency to fall down and with their hind legs splayed out sideways. They also had overgrown hooves, which were caused by the smooth metal flooring in their barns. This problem could have been fixed easily by purchasing new boars and replacing some of the flooring of the farm. The BIG mistake I had made was to attempt to fix the symptoms of the problem instead of the root cause. These particular pigs were the problem. After I had supervised tearing out the conveyor ramp and moving all the stunning equipment to a lower floor, my approach to solving problems was forever changed. Today, all new swine-handling systems are level; pigs are grown to much heavier weights, and they are too weak to walk up ramps.

Excitable Pigs and Aggression

In the late 1980s and early 1990s, I continued visiting many meat packing plants that were processing pigs from many different farmers. Several additional new genetic lines of rapidly growing hybrids were introduced. They were selected for rapid weight gain, large loin size and thin back fat. When these pigs were housed next to pens containing the older, fatter genotype, the differences in their behaviour were striking. The new lean-line pigs had three times as many bitten tails. They also startled easily. When the pen gate was rattled, they would jump and squeal. The pigs in the adjacent pen, from an older genetic line, would often not move when their gate was rattled. Today, breeders have corrected many of these problems; they are breeding animals in a more holistic way instead of focusing solely on production traits (Canario *et al.*, 2012).

Nobody would deliberately select a pig that is more aggressive or excitable; such characteristics are linked to desirable production traits. One of the reasons why it took time to identify these problems was that the breeders were only looking at their own pigs.

All of the conditions I have described were created with conventional breeding. Now there are new genetic tools that make it possible to create animals with new traits more easily. Genomic tests can be used to choose breeding animals (Bolormaa *et al.*, 2012). These tests are used to select sires that have genes for desirable traits such as improved feed conversion (Pryce *et al.*, 2014). There are always trade-offs. Selection for better feed conversion may be associated with lower fertility in cattle (Pryce *et al.*, 2014). GMO and gene editing methods will also speed up the process of genetic selection. We must be careful to avoid problems. The field of plant science is way ahead of the animal breeders in using new technologies (Lin *et al.*, 2014).

Plant Breeders Lead the Way in Using GMOs and Gene Editing

In the field of plant science, GMO soybeans have been grown for years. One of the early products was soybeans that could be sprayed with glyphosate (Padgette *et al.*, 1995). This would kill all weeds without harming the soybean plant. The benefit of this is that it allowed the use of no-till (no ploughing) farming, which greatly reduces soil erosion. The reduction or elimination of deep ploughing to control weeds is a benefit of which many are not aware. When the public finally found out that plants were being altered with foreign genetic material they became upset. Further problems occurred when the weeds developed resistance to glyphosate and it became less effective.

Another method where plant breeders have made great strides is the use of gene editing methods such as CRISPR or talon. When these methods are used, no new genetic material is added. Existing genetic code is either rearranged or a piece of code may be deleted. This method has already been used to produce corn, soybeans and grapes that have a more healthful composition (Pennisi, 2016). Gene editing has also been used to produce drought tolerant and more disease resistant rice, tomatoes and citrus (Pennisi, 2016). Advances in plant biology are already being developed to reduce the use of nitrogen fertilizer (Jez *et al.*, 2016). This will help reduce problems with nitrogen contamination of water supplies and aquatic ecosystems (Jez *et al.*, 2016). Drought resistant plants will also help reduce the need for water for irrigating crops. Water used for irrigating crops represents a significant percentage of world water usage.

What Could Be the Downsides of these Genetic Advances?

The use of all these new technologies shows great promise for reducing world hunger. When antibiotics and selective herbicides were first introduced, some people predicted that infectious disease would be forever eradicated and that glyphosate would never stop working (Bradshaw *et al.*, 1997). That has not been the case. One of the biggest health concerns today is antibiotic resistance (Laxminarayan *et al.*, 2013). The bacteria developed resistance to antibodies and the weeds stopped being killed with glyphosate (Duke, 2017).

It is important to avoid a single-minded approach. A lesson can be learned from the field of medicine. The use of single molecules to combat health problems has not lived up to expectations. When a new molecule was discovered, such as the hormone leptin to combat obesity, or sirtuin to improve health, they have not performed as promised (Leslie, 2016). Perhaps a single-minded approach on mouse experiments is a mistake. In another set of experiments, changes in the mouse microbiome in their guts caused pharmaceutical experiments to have opposite results (Servich, 2016).

Where Do Animals Fit in?

In many situations, raising animals for food requires more inputs than crops. Pigs and chickens compete directly with people for grain. Chickens convert grain to animal protein more effectively than pigs. Fish, being cold blooded, are the most efficient feed converters. There is one place where animals can provide food for humans and where they are really efficient and sustainable. There are vast tracts of land in the USA, Australia and other countries where it is not possible to grow crops. The land has either a lack of water or it is too rugged. Grazing on the land will provide advantages for food security (Foley *et al.*, 2011). The only way to obtain food from the vast interior of the Australian outback is through grazing animals. One cannot understand the vastness of the outback until you experience it. In 2015, I had the opportunity to fly over a small part of the outback. We took off from Darwin and flew two-and-a-half hours straight south in a small prop plane. Once we got about 30 minutes out of Darwin, I could look out of the window and see no signs of civilization except a single gravel road. There were no houses or electrical lines. Then, all of a sudden, I could see the headquarters of the cattle station, located in the middle of nowhere. They were off the electrical grid and used generators.

All of western Europe will fit inside the Australian outback. In areas where crops can be raised, progressive farmers are integrating grazing animals into their crop rotation systems. Integrating crops and livestock may enhance biodiversity (Lemaire *et al.*, 2014). The animals help replenish soil nutrients. In the right ecosystems, grazing animals can improve biodiversity when they are well managed (Fraser *et al.*, 2014).

Avoiding Problems in the Future

The new tools for gene editing and breeding plants will be increasingly applied to animal breeding (Lu *et al.*, 2013; Thompson *et al.*, 2014, 2016). We must be careful not to repeat the mistakes that were made with conventional breeding where bad traits were linked with desirable traits. One of the best ways to prevent this is for both animal and plant breeders to do what I did in the 1980s and 1990s: I observed many different pigs from many places and the behaviour problems became obvious. This enabled me to compare animals from different lines in the same environment. Today, both animal and plant breeders have 'genomic power tools' for changing an organism's genetics. Power tools are good things, but they must be used carefully because changes can be made more quickly. A circular saw can chop your hand off much more easily than a hand saw. It has to be used with more care.

Problems can sneak up slowly and may not be noticed in the early stages. This was the case with lameness in dairy cows. Up to a quarter of all dairy cows were lame before corrective action was taken. A large review article on the effect of GMO feed on farm animals and fish indicated that most studies showed no effects on an animal's metabolism (Swiatkiewicz *et al.*, 2014). However, a few studies showed slight effects such as lower blood glucose in pigs and changes in metabolism in fish. The present GMO and gene-edited plants used for an animal feed are safe. CRISPR could improve animal welfare by removing horns from dairy cows (Carlson, 2016). We must be careful and make sure that these subtle changes do not slowly increase and allow bad to become normal. Steps must be taken to ensure that CRISPR does not do unintended off-target editing. Sometimes CRISPR will modify the wrong piece of genetic code (Chapman *et al.*, 2016; Tycko *et al.*, 2016). This can be prevented by proofreading the edits with whole genome sequencing (Schaefer *et al.*, 2017).

New technologies, when used carefully, can provide great benefits. One must look at things in perspective. Modern corn (maize) looks completely different to its ancestor teosinte. The ancestor plant looks like wheat with corn kernels. The corn we harvest today was created with natural breeding and it looks like another species. It was not created with either gene editing or a GMO. Conventional plant breeding has created plants that have become totally different.

References

Bolormaa, S., Pryce, J.E., Kemper, K., Savin, K. *et al.* (2012) Accuracy of prediction of genomic breeding values for residual feed intake and carcass and meat quality traits in *Bos taurus*, *Bos indicus* and composite beef cattle. *Journal of Animal Science* 91, 3088–3104.

Bradshaw, L.D., Padgette, S.R., Kimball, S.L. and Wells, B.H. (1997) Perspective on glyphosate resistance. *Weed Technology* 11, 189–198.

Canario, L., Mignon-Grasteau, S., Dupont-Nivet, M. and Phocas, F. (2012) Genetics of behavioral adaptation of livestock to farming conditions. *Animal* 7(3), 357–377.

Carlson, D.F., Laneto, C.A., Zang, B., Kim, E.S. *et al.* (2016) Production of hornless dairy cattle from genome-edited cell lines. *Natural Biotechnology* 34, 479–481.

Chapman, J.E., Gillum, D. and Kiani, S. (2017) Approaches to reduce CRISPR off target effect for safer genome editing. *Applied Biosafety* 22(1), 7–13.

Cook, N.B., Hess, J.P., Foy, M.R., Bennett, T.B. and Grotziman, R.L. (2016) Management characteristics of lameness and body injuries in dairy cattle housed in high performance dairy herds in Wisconsin. *Journal of Dairy Science* 99, 5879–5891.

Duke, S.O. (2017) The history and current status of glyphosate. *Pest Management Science.* DOI: 10.1002/ps.4652.

Espejo, L.A., Endres, M.I. and Saifer, J.A. (2006) Prevalence of lameness in high producing Holstein cows housed in freestall barns in Minnesota. *Journal of Dairy Science* 89, 3052–3058.

Foley, J.A., Ramankutty, N., Bauman, K.A., Cassidy, E.S. *et al.* (2011) Solutions for a cultivated planet. *Nature* 478, 337–341.

Fraser, M.D., Moorby, J.M., Vale, J.E. and Evans, D.M. (2014) Mixed grazing systems benefit both upland biodiversity and livestock production. *PLOS ONE* 9(2), e89054. DOI: 10.137/journalpone0089054.

Grandin, T. (1988) Double rail restrainer for livestock handling. *Journal of Agricultural Engineering Research* 41, 327–338.

Grandin, T. (2003) Transferring results of behavioral research to industry to improve animal welfare on the farm, ranch, and at slaughter plants. *Applied Animal Behavioral Science* 81, 215–228.

Grandin, T. (2014) Behavioral principles of handling cattle and other grazing animals under extensive conditions. In: Grandin, T. (ed.) *Livestock Handling and Transport*. CAB International, Wallingford, UK, pp. 421–450.

Jez, J.M., Lee, S.G. and Sharp, A.M. (2016) The next green movement: plant biology for the environment and sustainability. *Science* 353, 1241–1244.

Lax, T. (1971) Hereditary splaying in pigs. *Journal of Heredity* 62, 250–251.

Laxminarayan, R., Duse, A., Wattal, C., Zaidi, A.K.M. *et al.* (2013) Antibiotic resistance: the need for global solutions. *The Lancet* 13, 1057–1098.

Lemaire, G., Franzluebbers, A., deFacio Carvalho, P.C. and Dedieu, B. (2014) Integrated crop livestock systems: strategies to achieve synergy between agricultural production and environmental quality. *Agriculture Ecosystem and Environment* 190, 4–8.

Leslie, M. (2016) Whatever happened to celebrity molecules promised to transform our health, but haven't lived up to their billing? *Science* 353, 1198–1201.

Lin, Z., Hayes, B.J. and Daetwyles, H.D. (2014) Genomic selection in crops, trees, and forages: a review. *Crop and Pasture Science* 65, 1177–1191.

Lu, D., Sargolzaei, M., Kelly, M., VanderVoor, G. *et al.* (2013) Genome wide association analysis for carcass quality in crossbred beef cattle. *MMC Genetics* 14, 80. DOI:10.1186/1471-2156-14-18

Macks, J.S., Neumann, K. and Yerle, M. (2001) Isolation of expressed sequence tags of skeletal muscle of neonatal healthy and splay leg piglets and mapping by somatic cell hybrid analysis. *Animal Genetics* 32, 303–307.

Padgette, S.R., Kolacz, K.H., Dehannay, X., Rd, D.G. *et al.* (1995) Development identification and characterization of glyphosphate-tolerant soybean line. *Crop Science* 35, 1451–1481.

Pennisi, E. (2016) The plant engineer. *Science* 353, 1220–1224.

Pryce, J.E., Wales, W.J., Haas, Y., deVeerkamp, R.F. and Hayes, B.J. (2014) Genomic selection for feed efficiency in dairy cattle. *Animal* 8, 1–10.

Schaefer, K.A., Wu, W.H., Golgan, D.F., Tsang, S.H. *et al.* (2017) Unexpected mutations after CRISPR Cas9 editing in vivo. *Nature Methods* 14, 547–548.

Servich, K. (2016) Of mice and microbes. *Science* 353, 741–743.

Swiatkiewicz, S., Swiatkiewicz, M., Arczewska-Wiosek, A. and Joseflak, D. (2014) Genetic modified feeds and their effect on the metabolic parameters of food producing animals: a review of recent studies. *Animal Feed Science and Technology* 198, 1–19.

Thompson, N.M., DeVuyst, E.A., Brorsen, B.W. and Lusk, J.L. (2014) Yield and quality grade outcomes as affected by molecular breeding values for commercial beef cattle. *Journal of Animal Science* 93, 2045–2055.

Thompson, N.M., DeVuyst, E.A., Brorsen, B.W. and Lusk, J.L. (2016) Using genetic testing to improve fed cattle marbling. *Journal of Agricultural and Resource Economics* 41, 286–306.

Tycko, J., Myer, V.E. and Hsu, P.D. (2016) Methods for optimizing CRISPR – Cas9 genome editing specificity. *Molecular Cell* 63, 355–370.

Von Keyserlingk, M.A.G., Barrientos, A., Ito, K., Galo, E. and Weary, D.M. (2012) Benchmarking cow comfort of North American freestall dairies, lameness, leg injuries, lying time, facility design, and management of high producing Holstein dairy cows. *Journal of Dairy Science* 95, 7399–7408.

2 Domestication to Dolly and Beyond: A Brief History of Animal Modification

Andrew Gardiner

Royal (Dick) School of Veterinary Studies, University of Edinburgh, Edinburgh, UK

Introduction

The first animal modification involved a dog. In excess of 14,000 years ago, someone noticed something about a friendly grey wolf (*Canis lupis*). Perhaps one of those allowed to lie close to the camp fire was seen to be limping badly. Perhaps this animal was an especially good hunter. Driven by curiosity, perhaps someone – was it a man, a woman, a child? – looked at the animal's paw and noticed a large thorn. Something (empathy?) caused them to remove the thorn, immediately returning the animal to soundness and hunting fitness. The first act of veterinary surgery had taken place (Fig. 2.1).

The dog in our imaginary scenario had already been modified, even before the human did anything to her/his body. Dogs' increasing proximity to humans in hunter-gatherer society can be explained as a behavioural modification of dogs by humans. Alternatively, we can attribute agency to the dogs. Dogs choose or allow proximity to humans, whose hunting behaviour gets modified, which also confers survival advantages on dogs. It depends on who made the first move; did the dog edge towards the human, or vice versa?

> [T]he most likely scenario has wolf wannabe dogs first taking advantage of the calorie bonanzas provided by humans' waste dumps. By their opportunistic moves, those emergent dogs would be behaviorally and genetically adapted for reduced tolerance distances, less hair-trigger flight, puppy developmental timing with longer windows for cross-species socialization, and more confident parallel occupation of areas also occupied by dangerous humans.
>
> (Harraway, 2003)

Early canine domestication may be best understood as a co-evolution (Budiansky, 2000; Jensen *et al*., 2016) – a mutually beneficial arrangement with advantages for both species. Canids changed themselves and became more sociable with humans, and humans did likewise with them; there is evidence that dogs were buried with people in the early Neolithic period (Losey *et al*., 2013; Smith *et al*., 2017). This general pattern was probably replicated with other species, making domestication less anthropocentric than we might think: less 'taming' and more co-evolution. However, at some point, humans' relations with animals began to change. Co-evolution was replaced with artificial selection.

E-mail: Andrew.Gardiner@ed.ac.uk

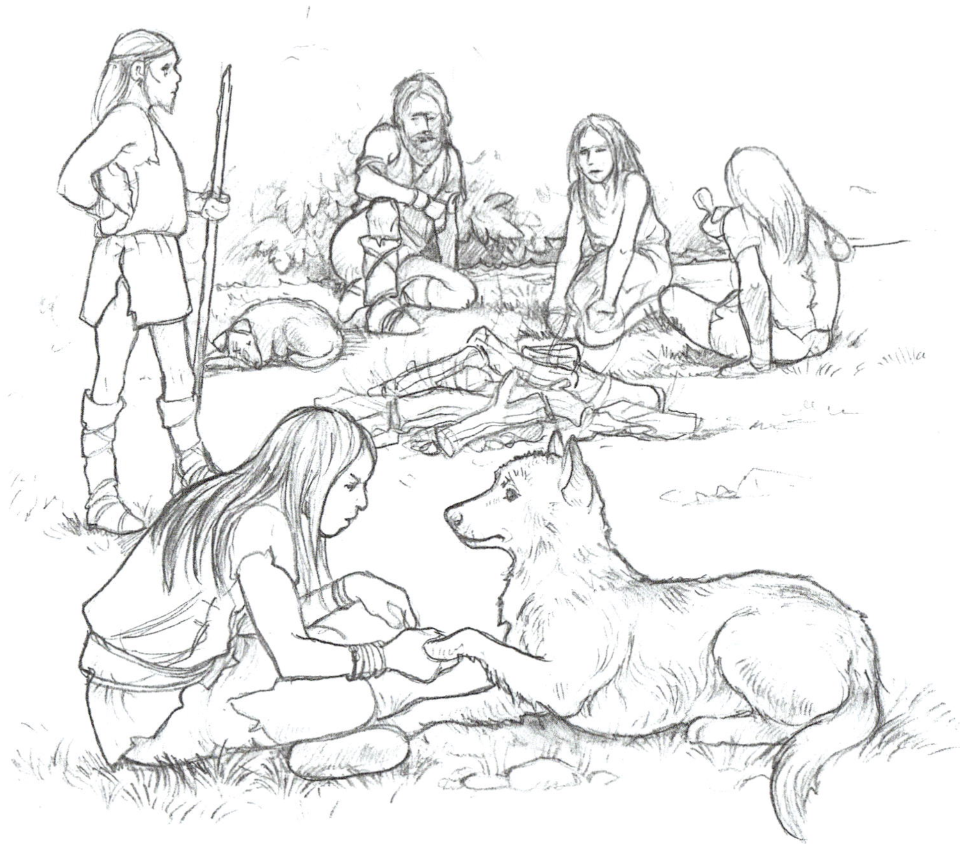

Fig. 2.1. Sometime in prehistory a dog was treated (modified) for the very first time (credit: Maggie Raynor).

Varieties of Modification

In Azerbaijan, in 2011, a horse is seen pulling two men in a cart (Fig. 2.2). We notice obvious and removable modifications to the horse's body – the fact that she wears a harness and probably a metal bit. Closer examination reveals a more invasive modification – a harness strap has been passed through a fold of skin on the horse's right (and, probably, left) flank.

The lame dog and the mutilated draught horse represent different ends of a spectrum of animal modification. At one end there is restoration of body integrity (an act of treatment); at the other end, a purely instrumental modification (making the horse's body fit the harness). Terms such as modification, improvement, treatment and enhancement invite questions such as, 'By what means?', 'For whom?' and 'To what end?'

Modification can be 'built-in' by selective breeding over generations or brought about much more quickly via genetic engineering. Different 'layers' of modification may be seen. The transformation that occurred in the body of the dairy cow between the dual-purpose breeds of the 1930s and the present-day Holstein-Friesian is dramatic. That change sits on top of a gradual enhancement of agriculturally useful attributes, the

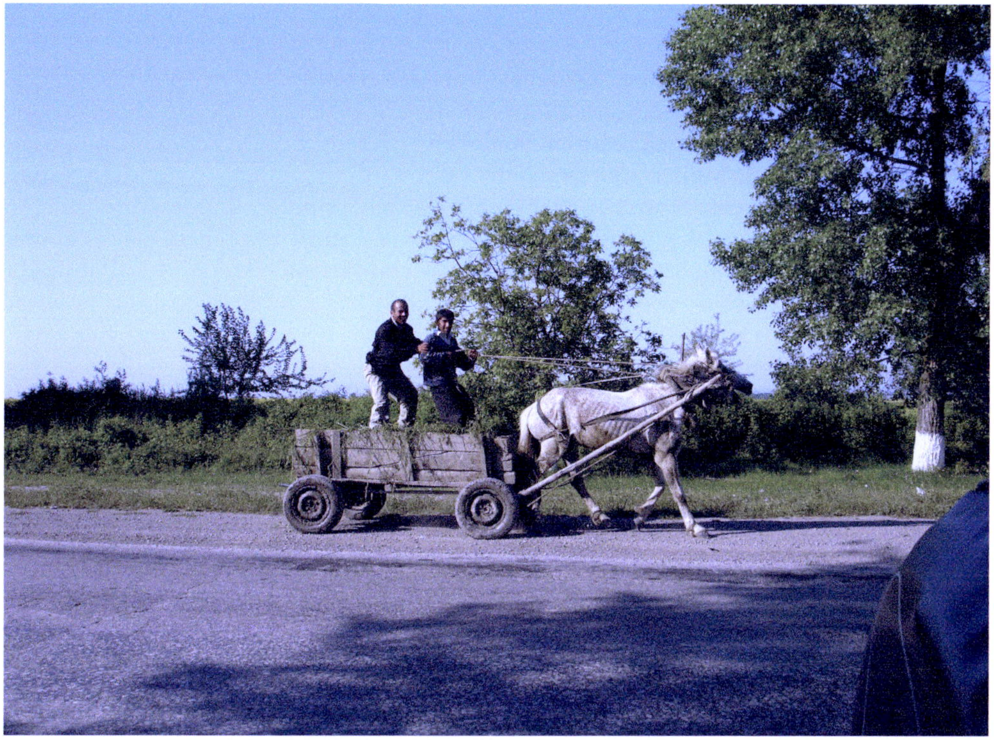

Fig. 2.2. Draught horse in Azerbaijan (photo: Fiona Maclachlan).

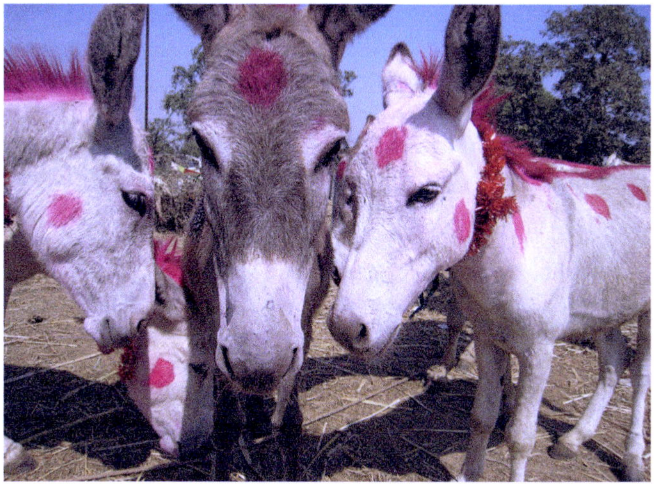

Fig. 2.3. Decorated (modified) donkeys at Vautha Fair, Gujurat, India. They are painted with a non-toxic pink dye as part of a local religious festival (photo: Stephen Blakeway/ The Donkey Sanctuary).

pace of which has, until recently, been determined by bovines' own mating preferences and natural breeding cycles.

Given the variety, it can be useful to try to categorize animal modification into some different types. The categories are not mutually exclusive but they can help us think about historical, contemporary and future examples.

Domestication

Domestication is a modification. There is a question of exactly how to define domestication, but it is generally agreed that settled livestock agriculture began about 10,000 years ago in an area of the near east encompassing present-day Turkey and Iran (Price, 2002). To prehistoric hunter-gatherers and early farmers, animals would have presented as very different entities to the creatures that populate our own world. An important type of animal modification – perhaps *the* most important one – is that which takes place in the human imagination to change our perception of animals' nature of being. In many ways, this facilitates all other modifications and how we think about them. Ontological modifications have occurred throughout the entire history of human–animal relations, and continue.

Modification of behaviour and phenotype

Modification of behaviour and phenotype tend to be linked. However, we can see behavioural modification without much change in phenotype in animals such as the donkey. Unlike most domestic animals, donkeys are not easily distinguished from their main ancestor, the Nubian wild ass (Kimura *et al.*, 2011). From earliest times, donkey-using cultures have made little use of selective breeding (Shackelford *et al.*, 2013; Marshall *et al.*, 2014). Free breeding with wild populations is encouraged to this day. Female donkeys may be tethered overnight in places where wild donkey stallions are known to frequent (Jill Goulder, personal communication). Much like cats, donkeys seem to be an exception to one of the normal 'rules' of domestication – reproductive isolation from the wild relatives.

In *The Variation of Animals and Plants under Domestication*, Darwin noted that, compared to their wild relatives, domestic animals tend to be smaller, with floppier ears, curlier tails and coat colours that are more often two-toned than solid (Darwin, 1868). In the late 1950s, Russian geneticist Dmitry Belyaev selected silver foxes on fur farms for tameness. The foxes were not trained, simply selected for breeding by displayed behaviours. His results showed that, within very few generations, behavioural tendencies of tameness brought with them the characteristic phenotypes of domestication that Darwin had observed (Belyaev, 1979; Trut, 1999). In the long history of domestication, once these tameness-associated variants begin to appear, artificial selection can favour further or exaggerated modifications. For example, a differently coloured animal may be easier to find; or people may just prefer a certain appearance (Linderholm and Larson, 2013). In considering the tiny sleeve cats and dogs belonging to rulers in Renaissance Mantua, historian Sarah Cockram has shown how both physical and behavioural modification were linked to ideas of power, status and ownership, as well as to aesthetics, affection and tactility (Cockram, 2017).

We know that domestic species with extreme phenotype modifications often suffer welfare problems. Frequently cited examples are dogs, dairy cows and broiler chickens. Breeding for improved welfare may be possible except where the reason for the modification is primarily aesthetic, as in the case of the Mantuan sleeve dogs and many modern pedigrees (O'Neill *et al.*, 2014; Oberbauer *et al.*, 2015). In the latter cases, improved welfare requires a change in the aesthetic (Packer *et al.*, 2012). In farm animals, there may be capacity to improve welfare, even within accepted production parameters, by exploiting genetic diversity through careful breeding where welfare itself is given greater prominence (Dawkins and Layton, 2012).

Genetic engineering for extreme behavioural modification – as in the production of 'zombie animals' with reduced sentience and therefore greater tolerance of confinement – was regarded as a fundamentally objectionable modification to the nature of animals and their integrity in early reports examining genetic modification of animals (Banner, 1995; Royal Society, 2001; FAWC, 2004). Ideas of 'naturalness' are therefore seen to be ethically important, even if the concept can be difficult to pin down, given that the history of domestication is one of artificial selection (Rollin, 1990; Sandøe and Holtug, 1996; Verhoog, 2003).

Non-therapeutic modification

Interference with the animal body for non-therapeutic reasons can be termed mutilation. Most non-therapeutic modifications are carried out to make animal identification, control or management easier. Common examples include painting and tattooing, ear notches and tags, tissue-damaging procedures to facilitate tethering or other handling (e.g. nose rings), and castration/neutering. Clearly these modifications are not going to be inherited and need to be repeated in every new generation and every individual. They may also require repetition in the same individual if paint washes out, tags get pulled off or tissues regrow. Selective breeding and/or genetic engineering can reduce the need for certain mutilations, e.g. the production of polled breeds that do not require dehorning.

Treating all non-therapeutic modifications symmetrically raises ethical questions for the veterinary profession as the *Primum non nocere* ('First, do no harm') intent of non-maleficence in medicine is almost always contravened. For example, in the UK, routine docking of horses' tails is now unethical. The British Veterinary Association (BVA) opposes mutilations such as routine tail docking in dogs, as well as ear cropping and devoicing. However, other modifications which disrupt the body integrity of healthy animals to a similar or greater extent, such as neutering and castration, fall within the realm of current practice. Non-therapeutic modification is also heavily 'specied', i.e. mutilations that are unacceptable in some species are routine in others of presumed equal sentience, or else are carried out in very different ways. Non-therapeutic modifications may be ethically problematic even when culturally accepted (Palmer *et al.*, 2012).

Modification by technology

Removable modifications on or in the animal body permit more effective use of animal power. The first working animals were probably draught oxen. Horses were probably initially controlled by a simple rope noose around the muzzle or neck. In some cultures, bridle-less control was achieved by the use of the rider's legs and weight only. There is evidence for this early 'natural horsemanship' in Numidian culture. Passing the noose through the mouth developed into the use of a bit made of various materials, such as hide. Metal ones originated in the near east around 1500 BCE. Evidence of paired stirrups resembling those used today was found in a Jin Dynasty tomb of around 302 CE (Hyland, 2002). This single invention may have changed the course of human civilization because of the advantage it gave mounted soldiers (White, 1962). Hoof protection was known to be employed by migratory Eurasian tribes around 2 BCE, and leather and metal 'hipposandals', precursors of contemporary 'equiboots', have been found in Roman remains.

Animals, especially equids, have frequently been modified for war, for example with body protection and, in World War I, gas masks. The first miniature camera for aerial reconnaissance was fitted to a German pigeon in 1907. Pack mules were routinely devoiced in World War II and trained dolphins were modified into naval 'suicide bombers' by having mines fixed to their bodies. In 2002, scientists at the State University of New York Downstate Medical Center developed remotely guided rats known as 'Roborats' or 'Ratbots'. The rats were controlled via a radio receiver and electrodes implanted into the sensorimotor cortex, to allow a human to remotely control the animal's direction of movement. The modification was said to have applications in search and rescue and bomb disposal but was condemned by animal welfare organizations.

The use of electronic collars and implantable microchips are modifications for identification and are now used very frequently on domestic animals and wildlife. There is great interest in the use of technology to enhance natural human capabilities. In animals, non-therapeutic uses tend to be more utilitarian and are focused on identification and control. There is usually little benefit to the animal per se.

Therapeutic modification

Disease and injury are natural. Treatment is a modification from nature, undertaken to try to restore an animal to health. The World Health Organization defines health as 'a state of complete physical, mental, and social well-being and not merely the absence of disease or infirmity'(WHO, 1948). However, many other definitions of health exist, with biomedical, ethical, socioeconomic and political implications. According to Georges Canguilhem (1991), the French physician and philosopher of medicine, health is a question of philosophy. Perfect health may be an idealized state that can never be attained.

The history of animal modification as treatment predates settled agriculture. However, once people started living with enclosed larger animals, the amount of treatment increased, probably starting with obstetric interventions. Some of earliest written records of animal treatment date from *c.*1800 BCE Egypt and are contained within the Kahun Papyri kept at University College London. Various species are mentioned but most attention is directed towards cattle, reflecting their economic and religious importance in Egyptian society. Cattle husbandry and medicine were also well developed in ancient India around 1500 BCE (Somvanshi, 2006).

The history of animal treatment is clearly much longer than the history of the veterinary profession which, in Europe, only started in the late 18th century. In the early modern period, many individuals undertook animal treatment and were recognized as expert animal doctors and healers (Curth, 2002). Organized farriery was established in London as a Fellowship in 1356 and the modern history of the Worshipful Company of Farriers began with its first Royal Charter in 1674. Farriers carried out much general medical treatment in horses and other species.

Modification for treatment often involves the use of technology, for example:

- setons inserted into the animal body to release fluids;
- bandages, splints and casts;
- prostheses and implants (Fig. 2.4);
- cardiac pacemakers.

Drugs and medicines, similarly, modify animals, even if not visibly. In contrast to the technological modifications described above, the object of therapeutic modification is to improve form and/or function towards normal health. Modifications may also take animals beyond normal health. Preventives, such as vaccines and other prophylactics, e.g. growth-promoting antibiotics, work by modifying the animal to 'more than normal' health. Treatments producing more than normal health or capacity may be ethically dubious, as in performance enhancing drugs and technologies.

Cloning (nuclear transfer) and genetic modification

Dolly, a cloned Finn Dorset lamb, was born to her surrogate mother, a Scottish Blackface ewe, at The Roslin Institute, Edinburgh, in 1996 (Fig. 2.5). Her birth was part of a series of experiments that modified animals to produce therapeutic proteins in their milk. Dolly's place in history is assured because her birth proved that specialized cells could be used to create an exact copy of the donor animal. Previously, sheep had been successfully cloned from undifferentiated embryo and foetal cells. The first such sheep was born in 1984 in Cambridge, UK. Dolly was cloned from an adult mammary gland cell – something which had been thought impossible.

In cloning, a nucleus from a donor animal cell is transferred into an egg cell that has had its own nucleus removed. The modified egg cell is then stimulated to divide by administration of a small electrical charge. If successful, the developing embryo is then transferred into a surrogate mother to grow to term. A clone is derived from a single ancestor by asexual means; there is no mixing of DNA from another individual, as in genetically modified (GM) animals. Cloning occurs naturally in bacteria and plants and in asexual reproduction (parthogenesis) in insects such as aphids, which are clones of their mothers. The first companion animal, a cat called CC, was cloned at Texas

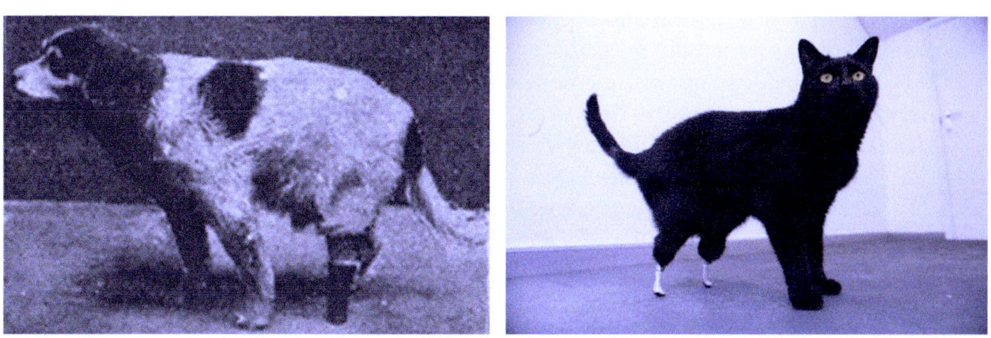

Fig. 2.4. Veterinary prostheses around 1900 (a simple wooden prop) and 2012 (titanium implants) (photos: Balliére Tindall & Cox/Elsevier (wooden prop); Noel Fitzpatrick (titanium implants)).

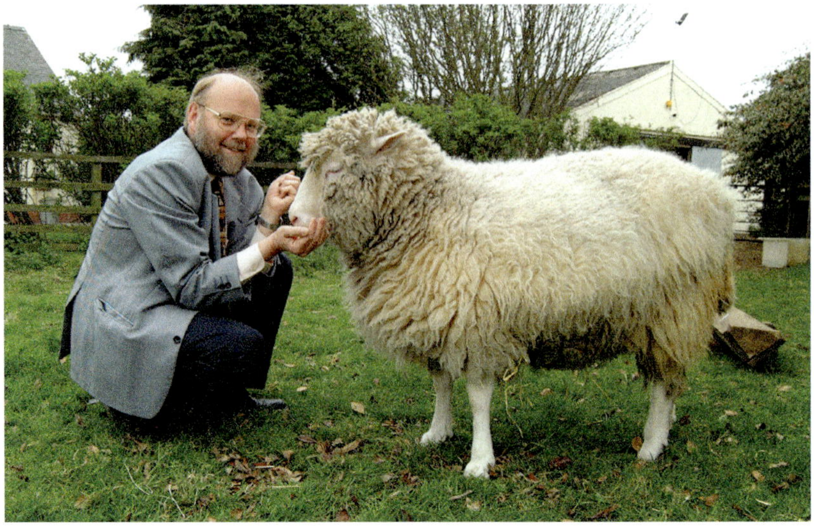

Fig. 2.5. Dolly the sheep with embryologist Ian Wilmut (photo: The Roslin Institute, University of Edinburgh).

A&M University in 2001 (Shin *et al.*, 2002) and many other species have now been cloned. In September 2015, the European Union voted to ban the cloning of animals for non-research purposes.

Genetic modification is the process of modifying the DNA of an organism. The modifications can range from inserting or deleting a few individual DNA bases in an individual's genome, to inserting a new gene comprising hundreds to millions of DNA bases from another individual of the same or a different species. In GM organisms, 'the genetic material has been altered in a way that does not occur by natural breeding or natural recombination' (AEBC, 2002). The first genetically modified animals were transgenic mice, produced in the early 1980s. Transgenesis works by inserting one or more active genes from an individual of the same or different species into a fertilized egg, which is then implanted into a surrogate mother where the transgenic embryo grows to term. By 'knocking in' or 'knocking out' specific gene functions in transgenic animals, individual protein production and regulation can be modified. Between 1990 and 2001, the number of experimental procedures involving transgenic/GM animals rose from 50,000 to over 630,000 as this line of research expanded hugely (Home Office, 2002) and over 500 transgenic mouse lines were in existence by 2013 (Schonig *et al.*, 2013).

Gene editing is a high-fidelity genetic modification of the genome using 'molecular scissors' to insert, replace or delete DNA sequences. The 'scissors' are engineered nucleases of four main classes that can reform DNA structure and so modify, block or add gene expression, with profound applications for agriculture, medicine and human interaction with the living world. The CRISPR method of editing DNA was co-discovered in 2012 by Jennifer Doudna and Emmanuelle Charpentier at the University of California, Berkeley, USA, and is heralding a new era of genetic modification of animals, humans and plants. The technique is relatively easy, fast and cheap to apply.

Taking a historical view, there are some differences between GM and traditional breeding practices, including artificial selection techniques not involving recombinant

DNA, e.g. in vitro fertilization. Compared to conventional breeding, changes occur much faster with GM as there is no need for numerous backcrosses to establish the modification. In addition, GM technologies allow for the mixing of kinds of animals to produce modifications that have not been possible before, some of which can be said to change the fundamental nature and integrity of animals. The speed of change has been such that the regulation of GM animals has had to develop alongside or in response to the technologies themselves.

Conclusion

An Aristotelian or Cartesian view of animals is one of soul-less entities or machines. Such a view has implications for how animals can be treated and modified to satisfy human needs and interests. Historical varieties of utilitarianism from Bentham onwards take some account of animals' own interests and preferences and admit the notion that animals can suffer and that this is morally significant. The 1999 Treaty of Amsterdam recognizes animals as sentient beings. More recent developments claim personhood status for certain species.

We have modified how we regard animals throughout history, and will continue to do so. However there is not a clearly phased narrative of progression in how we do this. Each of the different historical ontologies mentioned above, and others, coexist in the present and are reflected in the varieties of animal modification we see around us. Consideration of animal modification as an ethical issue is a lens for a multifaceted and challenging debate that goes to the heart of the nature of human–animal relations and animal well-being.

References

AEBC (Agriculture and Environment Biotechnology Commission) (2002) *Animals and Biotechnology: A Report by the AEBC*. AEBC, London.

Banner, M. (Chairman) (1995) *Report of the Committee to Consider the Ethical Implications of Emerging Technologies in the Breeding of Farm Animals*. HMSO, London.

Belyaev, D.K. (1979) Destabilizing selection as a factor in domestication. *Journal of Heredity* 70, 301–308.

Budiansky, S. (2000) *The Truth about Dogs*. Penguin, New York.

Canguilhem, G. (1991) *The Normal and the Pathological*. Zone Books, New York.

Cockram, S. (2017) Sleeve cat and lap dog: affection, aesthetics and proximity to companion animals in Renaissance Mantua. In: Cockram, S. and Wells, A. (eds) *Interspecies Interactions: Animals and Humans between the Middle Ages and Modernity*. Routledge, London.

Curth, L.H. (2002) The care of brute beast: animals and the seventeenth century medical marketplace. *Social History of Medicine* 15(3), 375–392.

Darwin, C.R. (1868) *The Variation of Animals and Plants under Domestication*. John Murray, London.

Dawkins, M.S. and Layton, R. (2012) Breeding for better welfare: genetic goals for broiler chickens and their parents. *Animal Welfare* 21, 147–155.

FAWC (Farm Animal Welfare Council) (2004) *Report on the Welfare Implications of Animal Breeding and Breeding Technologies in Commercial Agriculture*. FAWC, London.

Harraway, D. (2003) *The Companion Species Manifesto: Dogs, People and Significant Otherness*. Prickly Paradigm Press, Chicago, Illinois.

Home Office (2002) *Statistics of Scientific Procedures on Living Animals*. 23 July (Cmd 5581).

Hyland, A. (2002) *The Horse in the Ancient World*. Sutton Publishing, Stroud, UK.

Jensen, P., Persson, M.E., Wright, D., Johnsson, M., Sundman, A.-S. and Roth, L.S.V. (2016) The genetics of how dogs became our social allies. *Current Directions in Psychological Science* 25, 334–338.

Kimura, B., Marshall, F.B., Chen, S., Rosenbom, S., Moehlman, D. *et al.* (2011) Ancient DNA from Nubian and Somali wild ass provides insights into donkey ancestry and domestication. *Proceedings in Biological Sciences* 278(1702), 50–57. DOI: 10.1098/rspb.2010.0708.

Linderholm, A. and Larson, G. (2013) The role of humans in facilitating and sustaining coat colour variation in domestic animals. *Seminars in Cell and Developmental Biology* 24, 587–593.

Losey, R.L., Garvie-Lok, S., Leonard, J.A., Katzenberg, M.A., Germonpré, M., Nomokonova, T. *et al.* (2013) Burying dogs in Cis-Balkan Siberia: temporal trends and relationships with human diet and subsistence practices. *PLOS ONE* 8(5), e63740. DOI: 10.1371/journal.pone.0063740.

Marshall, F.B., Dobney, K., Denham, T. and Capriles, J.M. (2014) Evaluating the roles of directed breeding and gene flow in animal domestication. *Proceedings of the National Academy of Sciences USA* 111(17), 6153–6158. DOI: 10.1073/pnas.1312984110.

Oberbauer, A.M., Belanger, J.M., Bellumori, T., Bannasch, D.L. and Famula, T.R. (2015) Ten inherited disorders in purebred dogs by functional breed grouping. *Canine Genetics and Epidemiology* 2, 9. DOI: 10.1186/s40575-015-0021-x.

O'Neill, D.G., Church, D.B., McGreevy, P.D., Thomson, P.C. and Brodbelt, P.C. (2014) Prevalence of disorders recorded in dogs attending primary care practices in England. *PLOS ONE* 9(3), e90501. DOI: 10.1371/journal.pone.0090501.

Packer, R.M.A., Henricks, A. and Burn, C.C. (2012) Do dog owners perceive the clinical signs related to conformational inherited disorders as 'normal for the breed'? A potential constraint to improving canine welfare. *Animal Welfare* 21(Suppl. 1), 81–93.

Palmer, C., Corr, S. and Sandøe, P. (2012) Inconvenient desires: Should we routinely neuter companion animals? *Anthrozoos* 25(Suppl.), S153–S172. DOI: 10.2752/175303712X13353430377255.

Price, E.O. (2002) *Animal Domestication and Behaviour*. CAB International, Wallingford, UK.

Rollin, B.E. (1990) *The Frankenstein Syndrome: Ethical and Social Issues in the Genetic Engineering of Animals*. Cambridge University Press, Cambridge, UK.

Royal Society (2001) *The Use of Genetically Modified Animals*. The Royal Society, London.

Sandøe, P. and Holtug, N. (1996) Ethical limits to domestication. *Journal of Agricultural and Environmental Ethics* 9(2), 114–122.

Schonig, K., Freundlich, S. and Gossen, M. (2013) Tet-transgenic rodents: a comprehensive up-to-date database. *Transgenic Research* 22, 251–254.

Shackelford, L., Marshall F. and Peters, J. (2013) Identifying donkey domestication through changes in cross-sectional geometry of long bones. *Journal of Archaeological Science* 40, 4170–4179. DOI: 10.1016/j.jas.2013.06.006.

Shin, T., Kraemer, D., Pryor, J., Liu, L., Rugila, J. *et al.* (2002) Cell biology: a cat cloned by nuclear transplantation. *Nature* 415, 859. DOI: 10.1038/nature723.

Smith, B.P., Browne, M. and Scupell, J.A. (2017) Owner reported behavioural characteristics of dingos (*Canis dingo*) living as companion animals: a comparison of modern and ancient dog breeds. *Applied Animal Behaviour Science* 187, 77–84.

Somvanshi, R. (2006) Veterinary medicine and animal keeping in ancient India. *Asian Agri-History* 10(2), 133–146.

Trut, L.N. (1999) Early canid domestication: the farm-fox experiment. *American Scientist* 87, 160–169.

Verhoog, H. (2003) Naturalness and the genetic modification of animals. *Trends in Biotechnology* 21(7), 294–296.
White, L. (1962) *Medieval Technology and Social Change*. Oxford University Press, Oxford, UK.
WHO (World Health Organization) (1948) Preamble to the Constitution of the World Health Organization as adopted by the International Health Conference, New York, 19–22 June, 1946; signed on 22 July 1946 by the representatives of 61 States (Official Record of the World Health Organization, no. 2, p. 100) and entered into force on 7 April 1948.

3 Good for Whom? Differences between Human and Animal Enhancement

Sarah Chan

Usher Institute for Population Health Sciences and Informatics; Mason Institute for Medicine, Life Sciences and the Law, University of Edinburgh, Edinburgh, UK

Introduction

Human enhancement has been much discussed in bioethics. The possibility of genetic, pharmaceutical, cybernetic and other interventions to augment human capacities has excited the bioethical as well as the public imagination, provoking optimism and concern in roughly equal measure.

Less attention has been given to the concept of 'animal enhancement', and yet it is something we have been doing for much longer, at least in one sense. Domestication and generations of selective breeding have created cattle that produce higher yields of milk or meat, sheep that produce more fleece, and dogs that fulfil a variety of human purposes. Modern techniques of molecular biology now allow us to accomplish these ends much more directly, as well as introduce properties that could not be achieved merely by selection: rabbits that express fluorescent jellyfish proteins, goats that produce spider silk protein in their milk, and mice with humanized immune systems to act as animal models.

How should we evaluate these interventions from an ethical perspective as forms of animal enhancement? This chapter addresses the concept of animal enhancement with reference to bioethical debates over human enhancement.

Human enhancement

Human enhancement has variously been characterized in terms of technologies aimed at 'improving human performance' (Roco and Bainbridge, 2003); 'enhancing human capacities or traits' such as long life, intellectual and moral development (Parens, 1998); or 'interventions designed to improve human form or function beyond what is necessary to sustain or restore good health' (Juengst, 1998). Frequently discussed examples include 'smart drugs' to enhance cognition; genetic modification to make us less susceptible to disease or to increase our capacities, such as strength or endurance

E-mail: Sarah.Chan@ed.ac.uk

for athletes; and lifespan extension, by whatever means. Common themes in human enhancement, then, include the use of technology to increase or augment capacities beyond the limits of health or nature.

The idea of going 'beyond' requires us to define a limit, most often drawn as a line between 'therapy' and 'enhancement'. Most potential 'enhancement technologies' derive from existing or emerging therapies, the original purpose of which was to treat disease or dysfunction and to restore health, but which when used on 'already healthy' individuals might make us 'better than well' (Elliott, 2004). In most accounts of the therapy–enhancement distinction, therapy is something that restores normal function or cures disease, whereas enhancement seeks to improve on an already normal, already healthy state. This distinction, however, raises problems with respect to the concepts of health, normalcy and disease and how these should be defined, whether in terms of biological nature, 'species-typical function' (Boorse, 1975; Daniels, 2000), or otherwise. Critics of the distinction note that modern medicine encompasses many 'therapies' that, in fact, increase function beyond both the species-typical and the global average (Savulescu, 2006; Harris, 2007).

Furthermore, being able, conceptually, to distinguish between enhancement and therapy does not necessarily mean that this distinction carries moral weight. Even if we are able, consistently, to define normal function, is there anything wrong with going beyond this? While emerging technologies have been the focus of the debate, proponents of enhancement often point to traditional, long-accepted methods of augmenting function, such as spectacles and binoculars to enhance vision, in order to demonstrate the acceptability of enhancement as a concept in itself.

If we take a more general approach to enhancement, then, as 'anything that improves our function: any intervention that increases our general abilities and allows the individual to flourish' (Chan, 2008), another question is: *By whose standards* something should be considered an improvement? In place of a predominantly biomedical model of function and its improvement, an alternative account focuses on the individual and what is in her/his interests, as per John Harris: 'If it wasn't good for you, it wouldn't be enhancement' (Harris, 2007).

Part of the debate over enhancement technologies depends on whether or not they would actually be considered 'good'; for example, smart drugs might impair some aspects of cognition, even while enhancing others. A question arises, however, regarding what is or can be 'good *for* one'. Can, for example, 'extreme' body modification, cutting off one's own leg or being deaf ever be 'good for you'? Auto-amputation might well stretch most people's definition of 'enhancement'. Yet characterizing the expressed desires and preferences of some individuals for such states as irrational or pathological reverts to an underlying biomedical standard to determine which interventions are acceptable. A standing problem for defenders of enhancement is – if we reject the normative significance of biomedical models of function that support a moral distinction between therapy and enhancement – how to evaluate differing states of being with reference to the individual 'good'.

Another prominent concern about human enhancement is its potential effects on fairness, both individually and at a societal level. Is technological enhancement a form of 'cheating', and under what circumstances – for example in competitive sport, or academic performance? More broadly, there are questions about justice in a partly enhanced society: Who will have access, and will it widen existing inequities? (Buchanan *et al.*, 2000; Mehlman, 2003).

A consideration of animal enhancement is ethically necessary in relation to current uses of technology to modify animals, but may also shed some light, from a different angle, on these issues in human enhancement.

Animal Enhancement: Conceptual Issues

What is, or should be, considered 'animal enhancement'? As noted, whether by traditional methods or modern technologies, we have been modifying animals in various ways to suit our needs for centuries. Indeed, a point often cited in support of genetic modification is that it simply enables us to accomplish this end more efficiently, accurately and quickly.

Individuals or species?

This argument regarding the acceptability of technology following tradition might be seen as analogous to the 'spectacles and binoculars' argument in human enhancement. There is, however, an important difference in who or what is the focus of the enhancement. Does selective breeding count as enhancement? Selection involves choosing which animals should reproduce and in what combination. It thus affects which animals are born in subsequent generations, rather than modifying individual animals; the composition of the population and the characteristics of the breed will change over time, but no animal can be said to have been directly 'enhanced'.

The distinction between changing a given individual or choosing which individuals should be born has played a significant part in discussions of human enhancement and reproductive selection (Harris, 1992; Savulescu, 2001). Here, it exposes a potential conceptual fallacy with respect to animal enhancement: we tend to think of animals in terms of species or breeds, rather than as individuals, each with a welfare of their own. Selective breeding may result in changes to the population over time, but it cannot be considered enhancement *of* that particular animal, either from its perspective or ours.

Of course, the characteristics of the breed or species may be what we are interested in, rather than the individual animal's interests. If we are to refer to this as animal enhancement, however, we should be clear that, in so doing, we are not considering humans and animals on like terms.

Whose interests?

This issue also arises when we examine 'animal enhancement' technologies with reference to interests. The idea of human enhancement being 'good for you' may raise questions over what can properly be considered good, but the good itself is evaluated in terms of the enhanced individual's own interests. By contrast, many of what we might term animal enhancements are not in the animal's own interests, but in the interests of humans for whose purposes the animal is made more fit.[1]

Recognizing animals' interests as morally significant requires us to acknowledge that interventions on animals ought, properly speaking, to be termed enhancement only when it is good for *them* in some sense; otherwise 'modification' might be a more appropriate term. For example, the creation of GloFish by insertion of a fluorescence gene is probably neutral in terms of their welfare, but is an enhancement for our purposes, aesthetic and scientific.

The animal identity problem

Another conceptual question in animal enhancement is: How much can we change an animal before it is no longer the same animal, morally speaking? Human cognitive enhancement has been much discussed; methods also exist by which we might increase cognitive performance in animals, such as chimeric or transgenic techniques. Taking this to extremes, would a mouse suddenly invested with human-like intelligence still be 'the same mouse' in a morally meaningful way? Certainly, its range of capacities and interests would have changed and expanded, perhaps unrecognizably. On accounts of identity beyond the mere numerical or biological, this might imply that rather than enhancing the existing animal, we would effectively have created a new entity with a different moral significance.

The problem of identity-altering changes has been raised in relation to extreme forms of human enhancement, or what some have termed post-human enhancement: we might alter our capacities so radically that we would no longer be ourselves, or human (Agar, 2010). Even without transcending species limitations, if indeed this is what post-human enhancement would imply, there are many possibilities for potentially identity-affecting modifications (see, for example, Glannon, 2002).

This raises difficulties regarding the concept of enhancement being in a creature's interests; if the enhancement involves being transformed into a different entity, can we say that it was in the *original* creature's interests? These are difficult philosophical issues to resolve, but we should at least note that problems of identity that have been raised in relation to human enhancement also require consideration with respect to animals.

Animal Enhancement: Ethical Challenges

How should we determine an animal's interests? We cannot simply assume that what is good for us is good for them. Of course, the same goes for humans, although we are better equipped to guess what humans might want. Nevertheless, some degree of uncertainty does not preclude us from making a good guess, nor does it mean that we can abdicate all responsibility for taking care of *any* interests that animals or other humans might have.

Animal de-hancement and creative beneficence

A particular issue in animal enhancement arises when modifying them to suit *our* interests results in harm to *their* interests – what we might call de-hancement. One might think here of pedigree dogs, who often suffer chronic health problems either as a side effect of inbreeding or as a direct result of the physical features for which they have been bred. As argued above, however, breeding pedigree puppies is not really individual modification. We are not taking healthy puppies and inflicting ailments upon them; these are animals that otherwise would not be born at all.

The problem then is not what simply constitutes enhancement or de-hancement for a particular animal, but a much broader issue of ethical versus unethical projects of creation: what sorts of beings it is right or wrong to create. If a pedigree dog will have a life worth living, even with health problems, we cannot say we have harmed that dog by choosing to create it, rather than a healthy crossbreed. From the perspective of the dog, the alternative is non-existence.

This is, of course, an animal version of the well-characterized 'non-identity problem' (Parfit, 1984, Part IV). In human reproduction, this creates a dilemma with respect to the common intuition that it is wrong to create deliberately a child with an impairment or disease rather than a healthy one. If we cannot say who is harmed, is it wrong? Attempts to support this philosophically have resulted in development of concepts such as the 'harmed condition' (Harris, 2000; Harris, 2001) and the 'principle of procreative beneficence' (Savulescu, 2001); that in choosing which possible child to bring into existence we should select the one with the best chance of having the best life. Although intuitively appealing, however, this principle is difficult to justify philosophically (see, for example, Bennett, 2009).

Expanding our horizons to consider projects of not just human procreation but animal creation, we encounter further problems with creative beneficence. It cannot be the case that we are always obliged to create the being with the most potential for a good life, otherwise (at least if we follow Mill in thinking that it is 'better to be a human being dissatisfied than a pig satisfied') we would have to create humans instead of breeding pigs, even when what we want is bacon. Any obligations of creative beneficence that obtain must depend on what *type* of being we aim to create, what particular project of creation we are undertaking. If what you want to create is a German shepherd or a bulldog, even though they may have congenital hip dysplasia or breathing issues, a mongrel dog with healthy hips and unobstructed airway is not necessarily an appropriate replacement.

A full exploration of this problem would also require us to consider, *inter alia*, questions of instrumentalization and whether it is right to want a German shepherd rather than a mongrel as a pet. Without going further, however, we can at least say that *if* we are going to create such beings, we might have a moral obligation to attempt to fix their health problems – an obligation to enhance, as has been argued in relation to humans (Savulescu, 2005; Chan and Harris, 2007; Harris, 2007). We ought also to consider the implications for human enhancement/de-hancement: What can the ethics of choosing to create impaired animals tell us about the ethics of choosing to create impaired humans?

De-hancement and telos

A bigger problem arises when the de-hancement is not a side effect but is the desired aim of the modification, that makes the animal useful for our purposes. Examples include oncomice, genetically programmed to develop cancer, and blind or brain-dead chickens for the food industry. While as for pedigree dogs it is difficult to say whether the animal is harmed in comparison to the alternative of non-existence, in this case enhancing them by curing these problems would make them less fit for our purposes. But can we say that, beyond our failure to cure, creating such animals is wrong?

The brain-dead chicken is not an intrinsic problem from a welfare-focused perspective, though an analogy with creating brain-dead humans for spare organs and the moral unease this invokes, despite posing no direct welfare issues, suggests there is more to be explored here. Being blind or prone to develop cancer, however, would certainly not be considered enhancement for a human. We might instead try to explain these cases in terms of *telos* – that these modifications are wrong because they are somehow against the animal's intrinsic nature.

Many consider that *telos* has normative implications in discussions of animal modification, but are these to do with what sorts of animals are created or how animals are treated? (Rollin, 1995; Rollin, 2015). Is *telos* something that can be changed, or something that we *should not* change; does it require that we refrain from modifying animals in a way that is against *telos*, or that we treat animals according to a *telos* that is itself mutable?

If we see *telos* as alterable without moral consequences, its normative significance collapses to interests: *telos* determines interests – animals have an interest in doing what they are 'meant' to do – and we have an obligation not to violate an animal's *telos* by harming those interests. This is the account adopted by Rollin with respect to genetic modification of animals: 'Telos is not sacred; what is sacred are the interests that flow from it' (Rollin, 1995). On this account, frustrating a chicken's nesting instincts by forcing it to lay eggs in a cage is wrong because it violates the chicken's interests, but changing the chicken's *telos* by engineering it to prefer laying eggs in cages is not. Likewise it would be unproblematic to change a lion's *telos* by engineering it to be herbivorous, unless we were then to force it to eat meat, against its altered *telos*.

Might we thus simply consider it part of an oncomouse's *telos* to be prone to cancer? Insofar as possessing such a *telos* is detrimental to interests, we might see it as morally better to change this. But breeding oncomice that develop cancer and then engineering them not to would be self-defeating in terms of the purpose of the animals' existence. The practical alternative is that these animals would not be created at all. Given that the only way in which these creatures will come into existence is as oncomice, one might say that they fulfil their function by *being* oncomice. Yet it seems instrumentalizing, not to mention illogical, to impose our account of an animal's purpose on their interests. Can we really say they are living a good life by doing what they are meant to do, where what they are meant to do is to develop cancer?[2]

If, on the other hand, we consider an animal's *telos* to be violated by certain changes, we might have reason to consider that engineering oncomice, blind chickens or vegetarian lions is a *telos*-violating, morally impermissible change. We are left, though, with the problem of what determines *telos* and why it is morally significant. Why is carnivory essential to lion-hood, or the ability to see essential to chicken-hood? Why in the case of oncomice is the appropriate reference category 'mouse', for whom cancer is abnormal function, and not 'oncomouse', for whom cancer is typical? Did the dodo's inability to fly violate its *telos* as a bird?

Again, a comparison with human enhancement yields an analogy with species-typical function and biological nature accounts of health and normalcy, and their associated problems. Why, in considering what constitutes enhancement and what disability, should the appropriate reference category for assessments of function and normality be the human species today and not the post-human or prehistoric human, or the human species as a whole rather than, say, elite athletes, deaf humans, university professors or nicotine addicts?

A social model of enhancement?

The case of blind chickens can perhaps be analysed in a different way, drawing upon a social model of function. According to the social model of human disability, 'disability' is not (only) caused by physical impairment, but by the social norms and circumstances that decrease the potential for those with certain physical conditions to participate fully in society or live a 'good life'. On this account, the classification of disability is produced by the intersection of state of being and the world around us. In a similar way, we might propose a social model of enhancement where an enhancement is something that increases potential for a good life *given* existing circumstances.

It is clear that in considering what might be a good life, we cannot completely ignore the environment. For example, it is said that domestication of various species, such as dogs, has resulted in decreased fitness, which might be thought to be a bad thing. While, as noted above, we cannot consider changes in species properties to be an individual enhancement or de-hancement, we can, nevertheless, evaluate the effect on an animal's interests by asking whether it would be an enhancement to restore these properties in a domestic dog of our generation. Certain characteristics that benefit a feral dog or one of its wild ancestors might be decidedly non-beneficial for a domestic dog whose existence depends on living peacefully alongside humans in a built environment.

Then, should we change the environment to suit the individual or the individual to suit the environment? In terms of human enhancement and reproductive selection, disagreement persists over 'disability' and whether, when certain states of being in the world result in being materially worse off, we ought to remedy this by altering the states of being or changing the world. It is clear, however, that in some cases it is the environment that ought to change. For example, current human social structures suggest, for many, that being straight, white, male and cisgender are advantageous properties. These traits, if engineerable, might be considered an enhancement in that they would result in an individual with more opportunities to flourish in this society. Nevertheless, we see this as a reason to change the social norms that disadvantage certain individuals rather than to 'enhance' everyone to possess those traits!

In the same way, a chicken born into a battery-farming society might have a better welfare if it and its companions were blind, but is this a reason to 'enhance' them in this way? Some circumstances we can and ought to try to change, and an environment where chickens are better off blind might be one of these. While there is not scope in this chapter to establish why this might be so, I will briefly sketch a possible reason, based on what we might call interspecies justice.

Justice in Human and Animal Enhancement

Considerations of justice often exclude animals entirely as proper subjects of justice. To the extent that animals do feature, accounts of interspecies justice are often quite narrow, concentrating on animals with quasi-person interests such as great apes (Persson, 1993), or extremely broad, at the level of concern for ecosystems or species rather than animals as individuals (Bosselman, 2006). Moreover, interspecies justice is often raised merely as an antidote to speciesism (McLeod-Kilmurray, 2012), stopping at the recognition that animals have morally relevant interests and without paying attention to the distribution of fulfilment of those interests. Justice between species requires us to consider not just that animal, as well as human, suffering and well-being matter, but whether the suffering or benefit are disproportionately or unjustly allocated.

To illustrate, let us return to the case of domesticated dogs. Living in mixed species social groups results in good lives for both humans and dogs. For the individual dogs concerned, it is better that they have the domestic properties that allow them to do so. It has probably also resulted in the existence of more dogs overall. Whether the lives of those dogs are better than those of the wild dogs who would have lived had domestication never occurred is another question, but without getting into quantity/quality comparisons of potential universes, we can at least say that the combination of environment and capacities enables good lives on both sides. We could perhaps live better and distribute the benefits to dogs more justly, but both humans and dogs benefit from the arrangement.

By contrast, it is difficult to see any way in which blind chickens in a battery farm benefit from their circumstances, except by the mere fact of their existence which, if not worse than death, is still hardly worthwhile. True, they would suffer less than sighted chickens, and humans might benefit from decreased egg production costs (and clearer consciences with respect to animal welfare). If all that is required is to reduce harm and increase benefits, this seems like a win–win situation. Interspecies justice, though, demands more. Chickens as a group are systemically disadvantaged by the social institution of battery farming; engineering them to suffer less under that institution does not mitigate the fact of that disadvantage. It is the system, and not the individuals living under it, that should change.

There is perhaps a temptation to frame issues of justice in animal enhancement by analogy with concerns about fairness in human enhancement: for example whether a genetically enhanced racehorse should be allowed to compete against non-enhanced horses, or whether some farmers having access to 'enhanced' breeds of livestock might produce unfairness in agricultural communities. These concerns, however, focus on human interests and humans as the subjects to which considerations of justice should apply.

Of course, recognizing animals as subjects of justice raises many other problems of defining the community within which justice should apply, and of justice within and among animal species. If we enhance a fox's speed so that she can catch more rabbits, is that fair on other foxes, or on the rabbits? Without that first step of acknowledging interspecies justice, however, these issues will not even make it to the table. If we think that animals deserve equal consideration as moral subjects, we ought to recognize that the most important questions of justice raised by animal enhancement are not simply those of justice for and amongst humans, but of interspecies justice: justice for actual, as well as metaphorical, hedgehogs; for foxes and rabbits, chickens, mice and dogs, and any other creatures who matter morally.

Conclusions

This chapter has given a brief account of animal enhancement and some of the conceptual and ethical issues it raises, with reference to similar problems that arise in human enhancement.

This analysis suggests, firstly, that many of the modifications we perform upon animals perhaps should not be termed animal enhancement per se. Humans have a long history of altering the environment around them to suit their needs; animals are, in one sense, a part of that environment, but we must not forget that they are also creatures with a welfare of their own. To call it enhancement when it is in our interests and against theirs is problematic because it ignores that aspect.

Animal enhancement can also give us new insights into human enhancement, and reveal some of the faultlines in the debate, particularly around identity, harm and interests, and species-based accounts of function. In evaluating the moral effects of enhancement, both human and animal, the proper unit of consideration is the individual, not the species, and with reference to that individual's interests, not the idea of species-typicality or *telos*.

Finally, I suggest that an analysis of the ethics of animal enhancement also requires a fuller account of interspecies justice. Given that the majority of technological interventions on animals are performed for the benefit of humans, even if the animals themselves also benefit to some extent, we should ask whether the results are fair overall, to animals as well as humans.

Notes

[1] It should be noted here that I am treating interests and welfare as linked to capacities. On this account, plants do not have a welfare. Some animals probably also lack a welfare. I would not say, for example, that a plant has an interest in growing because it is in the plant's *telos* to do so. While there are other possible accounts of the interests of living beings, this approach is at least philosophically defensible, and broadly accords with both common intuition and practical approaches to animal welfare in agriculture and research.

[2] This problem is analysed by Sune Holm (2014).

References

Agar, N. (2010) Humanity's End: Why We Should Reject Radical Enhancement. MIT Press, Cambridge, Massachusetts.

Bennett, R. (2009) The fallacy of the Principle of Procreative Beneficence. Bioethics 23, 265–273.

Boorse, C. (1975) On the distinction between disease and illness. Philosophy and Public Affairs 5, 49–68.

Bosselman, K. (2006) Ecological justice and law. In: Richardson, B. and Wood, S. (eds) Environmental Law for Sustainability. Hart Publishing, Oxford, UK.

Buchanan, A., Brock, D.W., Daniels, N. and Wikler, D. (2000) From Chance to Choice: Genetics and Justice. Cambridge University Press, Cambridge, UK.

Chan, S. (2008) Humanity 2.0? Enhancement, evolution and the possible futures of humanity. EMBO Report 9(Suppl 1), S70–74.

Chan, S. and Harris, J. (2007) In support of enhancement. Studies in Ethics, Law and Technology 1, Article 10.

Daniels, N. (2000) Normal functioning and the treatment–enhancement distinction. Cambridge Quarterly Healthcare Ethics 9, 309–322.

Elliott, C. (2004) Better than Well: American Medicine Meets the American Dream. W.W. Norton, New York.

Glannon, W. (2002) Extending the human life span. Journal of Medical Philosophy 27, 339–354.

Harris, J. (1992) Wonderwoman and Superman: The Ethics of Human Biotechnology. Oxford University Press, Oxford, UK.

Harris, J. (2000) Is there a coherent social conception of disability? Journal of Medical Ethics 26, 95–100.
Harris, J. (2001) One principle and three fallacies of disability studies. Journal of Medical Ethics 27, 383–387.
Harris, J. (2007) Enhancing Evolution. Princeton University Press, Princeton, New Jersey.
Holm, S. (2014) Disease, dysfunction, and synthetic biology. Journal of Medical Philosophy 39, 329–345.
Juengst, E. (1998) What does enhancement mean? In: Parens, E. (ed.) Enhancing Human Traits: Ethical and Social Implications. Georgetown University Press, Washington, DC.
McLeod-Kilmurray, H. (2012) Commoditizing nonhuman animals and their consumers: industrial livestock production, animal welfare, and ecological justice. Bulletin of Science Technology & Society 32, 71–85.
Mehlman, M.J. (2003) Wondergenes: Genetic Enhancement and the Future of Society. Indiana University Press, Bloomington, Indiana.
Parens, E. (1998) Is better always good? The enhancement project. Hastings Center Report 28, S1–S17.
Parfit, D. (1984) Reasons and Persons. Oxford University Press, New York.
Persson, I. (1993) A basis for (interspecies) equality. In: Cavalieri, P. and Singer, P. (eds) The Great Ape Project. St Martin's Griffin, New York.
Roco, M.C. and Bainbridge, W. (2003) Converging Technologies for Improving Human Performance: Nanotechnology, Biotechnology, Information Technology and Cognitive Science. Kluwer Academic, Dordrecht.
Rollin, B.E (1995) The Frankenstein Syndrome: Ethical and Social Issues in the Genetic Engineering of Animals. Cambridge University Press, Cambridge, UK.
Rollin, B.E. (2015) Telos, conservation of welfare, and ethical issues in genetic engineering of animals. Current Topics in Behavioural Neurosciences 19, 99–116.
Savulescu, J. (2001) Procreative beneficence: why we should select the best children. Bioethics 15, 413–426.
Savulescu, J. (2005) New breeds of humans: the moral obligation to enhance. Reproductive Biomedicine Online 10(Suppl 1), 36–39.
Savulescu, J. (2006) Justice, fairness, and enhancement. Annals of the New York Academy of Science 1093, 321–338.

4 Working Equids: The Welfare of Those Worked to Their Limit

Melissa Upjohn* and Kimberly Wells

Brooke, Action for Working Horses and Donkeys, London

Introduction – Working Equids' Context

There are 113 million horses, donkeys and mules, collectively referred to as equids, worldwide (FAO, 2014). Of these, an estimated 85%, approximately 100 million, are working equids as distinct from the sports or leisure animals such as racehorses, professional and pleasure equine sports horses. Working equids are horses, donkeys and mules used by their owners or the people who hire them to perform draught, pack and transporter functions.

In a commercial setting, their task directly results in income generation for their owner or user. Examples include transporting raw and baked bricks (Fig. 4.1) within brick kilns where their owner's family works in countries such as Egypt, India, Nepal and Pakistan (Kandpal *et al.*, 2014), and pulling a taxi vehicle, such as a tonga, in India (Fig. 4.2) or a ghari in Ethiopia. As part of other value chains they may contribute indirectly to household income generation. Examples include transporting home produce such as milk to a processing centre or grain or vegetables to market, or transporting fodder (Fig. 4.3) to the homestead for consumption by livestock whose outputs are subsequently sold. Cash generated via either direct or indirect income activities can be used to buy food, other essential products or services such as healthcare and education.

Working equids may also assist with domestic tasks. These include reducing the physical burden on women and children involved in transporting water from its source to the homestead for consumption by humans or livestock; carrying home bulky or heavy food purchased at a market for family consumption; facilitating access to education by transporting children to school; enabling families to participate in social events such as a wedding or a funeral; or transporting sick people or animals, or women in labour to medical care centres (Valette, 2014). In these situations, equids do not generate income; rather they save paying another person to use their animal for the task, and they enable completion of day-to-day activities that would otherwise involve extra human effort and time, or would not happen at all.

The number of people directly supported by each equid might range from 1 to 21, depending on the country and the context (Brooke, unpublished data). Whilst not all equine owners meet the criteria for the world's poorest, according to United Nations scales (UNDP, 2015), their lives are financially vulnerable and they often barely survive from one day to the next.

Working equids are found across Asia, the Middle East, Africa, eastern Europe and Latin America, but peer-reviewed literature quantifying their contribution to their

*Corresponding author e-mail: Melissa.upjohn@dogstrust.org.uk

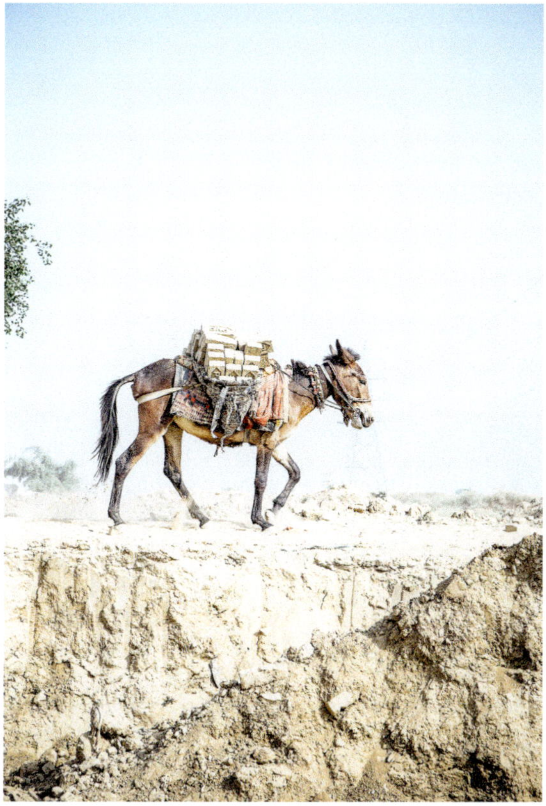

Fig 4.1. Mule working in a brick kiln in India (photo: Brooke, Action for Working Horses and Donkeys).

owner's, community's or the wider economy is limited (Valette, 2015). Since these animals, typically, facilitate food production or food purchase rather than being the source of a product with an objective market price, assigning monetary value to their contribution can be challenging. Financial contributions have generally been reported at household or community level (Arriaga-Jordán *et al.*, 2005; Martin Curran and Smith, 2005; Chang *et al.*, 2010; Nigatu and Abdelaw, 2010; Admassu and Shiferaw, 2011; Velazquez-Beltran *et al.*, 2011; Hassan *et al.*, 2013; Doumbia, 2014). This contrasts with developed countries' sport and pleasure horse industries, which have quantified their economic contribution at regional, national or international levels, thereby enabling government policy makers to contextualize their importance relative to other market sectors (American Horse Council Foundation, 2005). Governments in countries where working equids are found therefore often overlook their vital role in local and national economic activities and omit them from livestock and agricultural programmes and planning. This means that their physical and emotional welfare needs are also generally overlooked.

Welfare Consequences of Working Equids Being Pushed to Their Biological Limits

Working equids' context often results in them suffering physically and emotionally. The root causes of these problems may stem from a lack of understanding of their needs

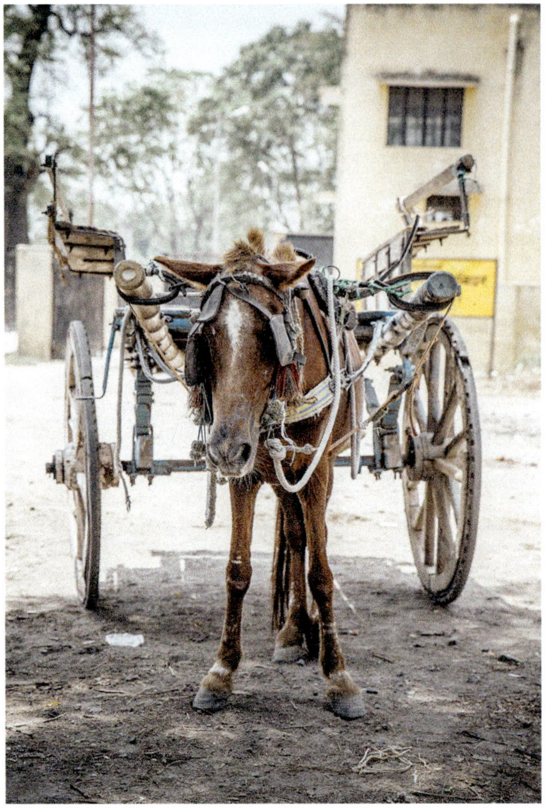

Fig 4.2. A horse drawn tonga carriage in India (photo: Brooke, Action for Working Horses and Donkeys).

and inadequate local infrastructure to meet them, or owners' inability to influence local environment due to power imbalances and resource limitations. Welfare issues are described under the headings used by the OIE's working equine welfare standards (OIE, 2016) and cover nutrition, environment, health, behaviour and mental domains described by Mellor (2016).

Access to food

Poor information access may mean that working equine owners lack understanding of a suitable diet for a working equid's maintenance and work-associated needs. Even if informed, they may struggle, logistically and financially, to source and store appropriate products and to determine the absolute and proportional quantities of different foodstuffs required for an individual animal. Consequently, working equids often suffer from inadequate nutrition, which contributes to them experiencing hunger and having below-optimum body condition score (BCS) using recognized rubrics (Carroll and Huntington, 1988). According to data collected by Brooke (Sommerville *et al.*, 2018) 72% of equids transporting goods by pack and cart in Kenya, 76% of equids transporting bricks or goods by cart and pack in Nepal, and 88% of equids transporting bricks by cart and pack in Pakistan have a suboptimal body condition score of below 2.5 on a five-point scale (Fig. 4.4).

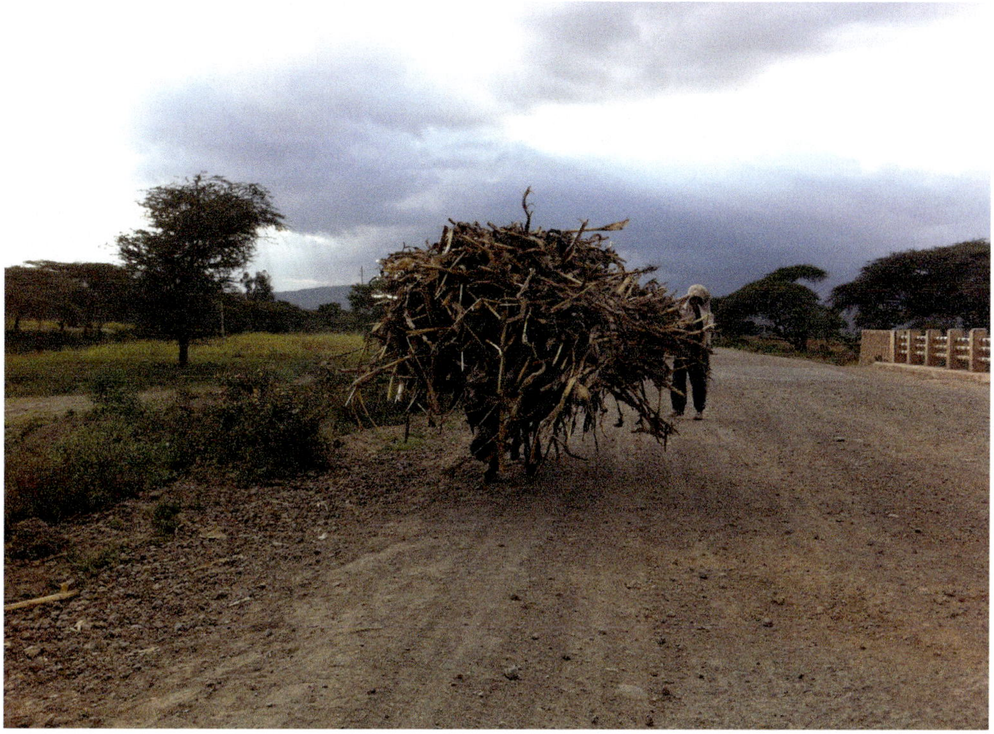

Fig 4.3. A donkey carrying fodder in Ethiopia (photo: Brooke, Action for Working Horses and Donkeys).

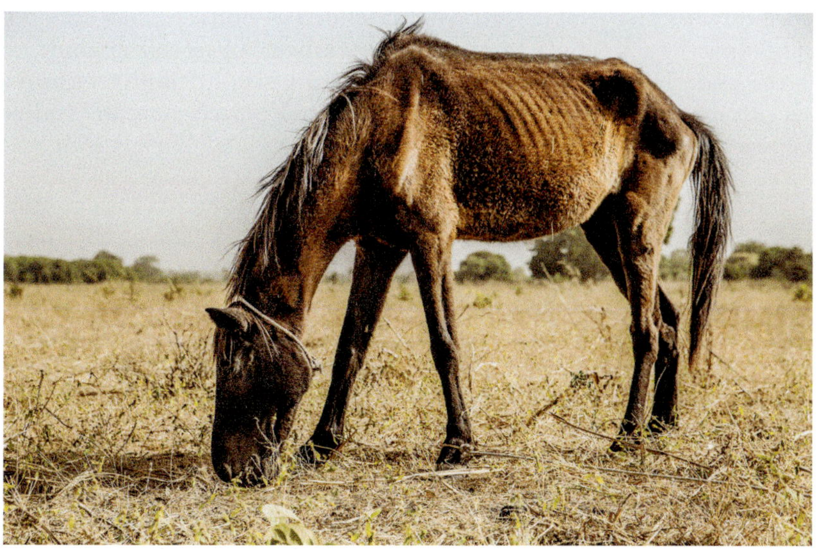

Fig 4.4. A horse with a suboptimal body condition score in Senegal (photo: Brooke, Action for Working Horses and Donkeys).

Poor nutrition may lead to impaired capacity to perform work expected of them, which may result in additional welfare issues since owners' economic situations often mean it is hard to make allowances for this impaired capacity. Suboptimal nutrition may also contribute to an impaired immune system, increasing susceptibility to disease.

In urban and industrial contexts there may be few or no grazing opportunities during or outside working hours. In rural situations, access to grazing may be limited, even outside working hours, due to owners' landless status, lack of access to suitable common land or concerns regarding theft. Where grazing opportunities do exist, owners may hobble or tether their equid to reduce risk of straying, which limits natural grazing activity and may also result in hobble-related injuries and pain. Whereas in developed countries the impact of lack of grazing on healthy gastrointestinal tract function may be able to be investigated, in low-resource environments this is generally not possible.

Long working hours and demanding performance targets for equids and their owners may be imposed by an institution such as a brick kiln, or arise from economic necessity due to the low piece rates earned for each task, over which owners have little influence due to market forces and power imbalances (Shah *et al.*, 2006). These working arrangements can result in equids' access to food being available only at limited time points, and those available during working hours being of relatively short duration. During short feeding slots, animals' working equipment and tack may not be removed, thereby limiting freedom to move, to adjust their feeding position and to masticate food if they are wearing a bit. If food is fed at ground level, whilst this mimics natural feeding behaviour, local environmental conditions may result in contamination with dirt or foreign bodies. If food is offered via a nosebag to avoid wastage or contamination, this may impair respiratory function and secretory drainage during feeding.

Structural and timing limitations on feeding may adversely affect gut health as equine species naturally trickle feed over extended periods. Equids eating inappropriate items (pica) such as waste products have been observed in some countries, although the underlying cause of these observations is not definitively proven. Consequences of pica include potentially fatal intestinal obstruction, depending on the product concerned, which often includes plastic materials (Curran *et al.*, 2014).

Access to water

Authorities managing infrastructure, particularly in industrial sites and urban centres, may not take account of working equids' welfare needs. This often results in limited or inappropriate water access facilities. Where water is available, it may be dirty or provided with insufficient time or space allowance within working schedules for equine drinking preferences (Pritchard *et al.*, 2008). Selected owners' traditional beliefs regarding adverse consequences of animals drinking (Lewa *et al.*, 2006) may also mean that they fail to offer their equids water even when it is accessible and suitable for their needs.

Although, traditionally, dehydration has been assessed using a skin pinch test, research has shown that this is an unreliable indicator of clinical dehydration (Pritchard *et al.*, 2008). The recommended approach to assess and resolve dehydration is to offer the animal access to clean water and allow time and space to drink if desired.

Owners' traditional beliefs regarding recognition and management of dehydration and heat stress may mean that appropriate action is not undertaken when early signs appear. These beliefs include that giving water to a sweating horse causes colic and that heat stress should be managed via feeding products such as jaggery (crystallized sugar). Consequently, working equids may be acutely or chronically dehydrated, even in moderate climatic conditions. When working in high temperatures such as those encountered in brick kilns (sometimes over 50° C) or in high humidity during a tropical summer, thermo-regulatory mechanisms may result in loss of large volumes of fluids and electrolytes on top of existing dehydration problems.

Weakness resulting from dehydration or heat stress reduces an equid's capacity to work and increases risk of collapse. Owners who are unable to recognize the root cause of this reduced work capacity may push their equid to continue working and unwittingly precipitate the animal's collapse, or, in extreme cases, death. Even if they recognize the need to seek veterinary services, the lack of suitably skilled providers may preclude timely and effective treatment of acute cases, so the animal remains pushed to its limits. Building owners' capacity to prevent dehydration is vital, via ensuring regular watering practices – for example by using their own buckets – and identifying and managing heat stress and dehydration as early as possible via additional watering and use of showering facilities.

Shelter

Authorities overseeing industrial or urban environments often also fail to recognize working equids' need during working hours for well ventilated shelter from adverse weather conditions such as direct sun, extreme heat and cold, wind, rain or snow. Combined with a lack of recognition by owners and service providers, in summer this may result in equids spending extended hours in direct sun in extreme temperatures or poorly ventilated environments, thereby increasing the risk of suffering heat stress, dehydration and impaired function, including respiratory disease (Shah *et al.*, 2006). In winter it may result in equids suffering from cold and using up some of their limited energy intake to maintain core body temperature rather than maintaining body condition. Blankets can mitigate this risk, but, if poorly designed, may bring associated risks of friction lesions.

Key stakeholders' improved understanding and engagement with the importance of these animals' need for shelter is required (Shah, 2016), alongside facilitation of construction of suitable structures and maintenance arrangements. For owners, interventions are needed to build owners' engagement with and understanding of their animals' needs and how these can be achieved in a cost-effective way.

Whilst owners may have greater influence over shelter outside work, lack of understanding of equine needs, and financial or other resource limitations may limit appropriate provision. This may result in them being housed in poorly ventilated or dirty conditions (Bradbury, 2002), where they are insufficiently segregated from other livestock species and lack sufficient dry bedding areas to enable them to move freely and lie down if and when they choose. The consequence for the equid is that they are vulnerable to disease and predation (Tesfaye *et al.*, 2006) and are unable to rest adequately.

Management of disease and injuries

Many diseases endemic in countries where working equids are found may negatively impact their welfare. Key infectious diseases include African horse sickness (AHS), epizootic lymphangitis (EZL), equine infectious anaemia (EIA), gastrointestinal nematodes, glanders, piroplasmosis, tetanus and trypanosomiasis (surra) (Stringer, 2014). Poorly resourced and low-skilled equine health service provision (Saville *et al.*, 2014), poor in-country availability of appropriate vaccines, lack of affordable diagnostic facilities and local non-availability of proprietary products to treat these diseases exacerbate the morbidity and mortality impacts on working equids. There may be complex comorbidity patterns of disease that are difficult to distinguish and manage effectively due to lack of accessible field diagnostics (Laing *et al.*, 2016; Mohite *et al.*, 2016). Owners' access to resources to inform their capacity to recognize these diseases may be limited. If their knowledge is sufficient to recognize the need to seek help, financial constraints and poor local accessibility of equine-appropriate health services may constrain treatment options.

Lack of data means that it is often difficult or impossible to quantify the occurrence, prevalence and distribution of many infectious diseases affecting these animals. Many countries known to have large populations of working equids do not have an OIE official status for certain diseases, and many countries have no reporting history regarding many infectious diseases (Stringer, 2014). Lack of data results in lack of policy maker recognition of the need to include equids in their animal health programmes. This often results in few preventive services such as vaccination for equids being provided, other than by non-government organizations (NGOs), whose operational areas may not be nationwide (Walker-Okello, 2010). Overcrowding and mixing of large numbers of non-familiar animals in environments such as equine fairs in India, or through involvement in transport services in and around commercial markets, risk transmission of infectious disease across wide geographical areas. The morbidity and mortality risks associated with potential outbreaks of infectious disease and their consequences for equine welfare are therefore substantial.

Similarly, population level morbidity data are lacking for symptoms of many non-disease-related equine welfare problems. Data are generated by individual organizations using bespoke tools for monitoring purposes (Brooke, 2012), but governments do not collect population level data on working equine welfare issues. A limited number of larger-scale studies indicate the most prevalent problems relate to lameness, body lesions and suboptimal BCS (Pritchard *et al.*, 2005; Ali *et al.*, 2016).

Adverse working environments for working equids often result in high risk of accidental injury and chronic overwork. These include poor underfoot conditions; encouraging the animal to move fast, stop or turn quickly on an unsuitable surface; and overloading; all compounded by poor communication to the animal by the driver. The economic imperative to earn a daily income limits owners' ability to allow an unsound animal time to recover from an injury and contributes to lameness being of high prevalence, often a multi-limb and high-severity problem for working equids (Pritchard *et al.*, 2005; Broster *et al.*, 2008; Broster *et al.*, 2009; Burn *et al.*, 2010a; Reix *et al.*, 2014; Regan *et al.*, 2015; Ali *et al.*, 2016).

Mixing of unfamiliar animals at environments such as equine fairs or other large gatherings may also increase the risk of fighting, particularly amongst males, and consequential traumatic injuries.

Handling and management practices

Lack of understanding of equids' physical and emotional needs by owners and others who interact with these animals may result in inappropriate handling. This in turn leads to fear responses and pain. Owners and service providers often lack basic skills in equine handling and behavioural understanding (McGreevy, 2004). Their misunderstanding of equine fight-or-flight response to environmental stressors may be misinterpreted as aggression or 'untrainability'. Examples seen during working hours include poor driving practices of cart-pulling equids, and owners beating working animals in the mistaken belief that this will make them go faster (Iqbal *et al.*, 2006; McLean *et al.*, 2010; Kawe, 2016). Poor practices result in physical lesions and adverse emotional states, which may in turn result in behavioural responses that elicit further poor handling practices (Scantlebury *et al.*, 2013; Starkey *et al.*, 2014).

Some animals are subject to extended confinement related to the nature of their work type. Ceremonial horses in India are used on very limited numbers of occasions per year according to schedules over which owners have limited influence (Reix *et al.*, 2015). When not being used for ceremonial work they are kept in a very restricted stall in darkness and/or tightly hobbled. This risks a negative feedback loop whereby adverse environmental conditions and lack of physical activity lead to increased risk of avoidance or aggressive behaviour, which elicits negative reactions by the owner such as hobbling. This in turn worsens the environment with which the animal has to cope.

Traditional handling and health management practices for animals have been passed down through generations of family and community members. Examples of these include nostril slitting in south Asia, believed to improve respiratory function (Fig. 4.5) (Nawaz *et al.*, 2010); burning of gums and soft palate to 'treat' perceived

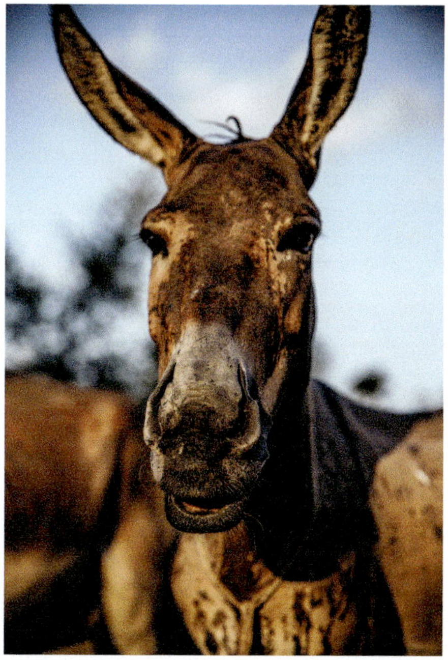

Fig. 4.5. A donkey with slit nostrils in Pakistan (photo: Brooke, Action for Working Horses and Donkeys).

swollen mucosae, sometimes referred to as lampas (Upjohn *et al.*, 2012); firing of wounds (Gogoi and Dennison, 2010), based on the same rationale as that historically proposed in Europe for treatment of tendon injuries (Hayward and Adams, 2001); traditional castration practices performed without local anaesthesia; use of inappropriate products on wounds (Getnet *et al.*, 2014); branding for cultural and identification purposes in Kenya (Fig. 4.6) and false perceptions of the necessity for, and effect of, essential husbandry (Lewa *et al.*, 2006). All of these practices result in pain, physical and emotional suffering and risk of systemic infection.

Behaviour

In urban environments, working equids are surrounded by loud and often unpredictable noise, which may induce fear, particularly in contexts where owners equip them with blinkers that reduce their field of vision. They are subject to conflicting commands to move forward at speed and then stop suddenly to avoid collisions with other vehicles or obstacles in overcrowded, poorly regulated street and industrial environments, or due to work-related pressures on their owners (Brown, 2014). These lead to confusion for the animals as to what is expected of them. Both noise and confusion may trigger stress-related behavioural responses from the animal, which, in turn, may be misinterpreted by their owner/user as resistance or aggression, and elicits further negative human–animal interaction.

In seasonal work situations, such as brick kilns in India and Nepal, which only operate during winter and spring, the animal is often expected to undertake a different work type during the primary work closed season. There may be limited or no time for the animal to adapt to a different physical and sensory environment, and poor

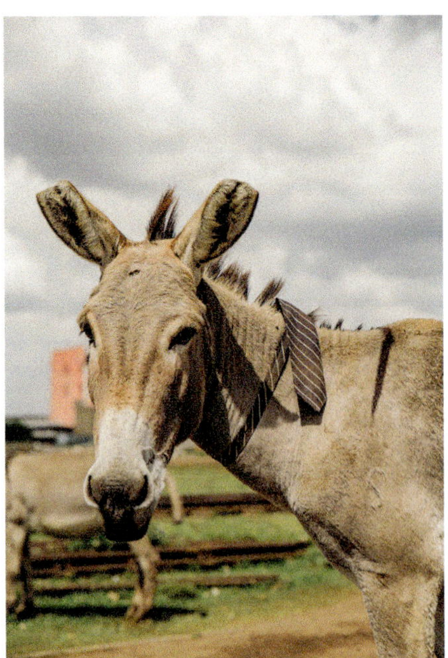

Fig. 4.6. A branded donkey in Kenya (photo: Brooke, Action for Working Horses and Donkeys).

understanding of the animal's training needs on the part of the owner or user. This regular presentation of stressors can result in induced fearfulness. Data are lacking on the training practices for different work types. These may involve different or conflicting demands on the animal, creating potential for confusion for the animal as to what is being expected of them. Pearson (2015) noted that horses have excellent long-term, but poor short-term, memory (Wolff and Hausberger, 1996; McLean and McLean, 2008), meaning that everything is learned through trial and error rather than problem solving. These characteristics may not be taken into consideration in working equine training activities, due to lack of owner/user awareness of them and their implications.

Evidence is lacking of stereotypies in working equids, but it is unclear whether this is due to it not being recognized, or whether it indicates that animals don't feel the need to exhibit these patterns, or that they don't have the opportunity to express them, for example due to the lack of 'cribs' or other suitable items to bite, or lack of space to weave or circle. In working equids, an alternative to stereotypies is seen in the form of apathy and learned helplessness, which may be a coping mechanism (Hall *et al.*, 2008). Multi-country research has shown that apathetic behaviour in working equids is associated with other indicators of poor physical welfare, such as low body condition and number and severity of skin lesions, as well as with old age (Burn *et al.*, 2010b). Apathy may contribute to working equids being pushed to their limits via a negative feedback loop, since they do not refuse to undertake tasks that other animals may be expected to resist, and therefore the tasks they are pushed to perform increase until they become physically impossible.

Donkeys' acknowledged different behavioural responses to pain or poor welfare, as compared with horses, mean that the subtle indicators of problems affecting them may be missed and result in additional misinterpretation of donkeys' welfare needs (Regan *et al.*, 2014).

Within a single country, there appear to be differences in patterns of behaviour categories between different species and different work types (Bhardwaj *et al.*, 2016), although the explanation for these is unclear. The multiple possible explanations for differences in behaviour between cart and pack equids, including variations in the burden of equipment between cart and pack animals, differences in training methods and differences in work-related handling and stimuli need further investigation. The high prevalence of head-shy equids in various contexts also needs further investigation to understand whether the underlying cause(s) relate to pain, medical or neurological issues or avoidance behaviour relating to previous adverse experiences.

Understanding of cumulative experience on an animal's welfare is well recognized in laboratory and experimental animals. It is not well investigated in the equine (Pearson, 2015) and needs further study in the working equine context to understand how best to manage an equid's reaction to its environment.

Many working equids are deprived of opportunities to display natural behaviour. Lack of choice access to grazing, non-availability of a rolling pit to relieve work- or heat-related discomfort, and limited or no opportunities to socialize with familiar conspecifics when desired or to develop natural social relationships, such as pair bonding in donkeys, are a few examples. Their impact on an equid's emotional well-being, on top of other physical and emotional welfare issues, may contribute to the prevalence of apathy seen in some populations.

Appropriate workloads and fitness to work

Owners' drive to generate sufficient income to feed their family means that they need to earn as many piece rates as possible in a given working day. This encourages a tendency to overload. Owners often lack understanding of weights, proportions and balances of loads that are physiologically reasonable for an equid to carry or pull in their specific context. Robust, locally relevant evidence on loading limits is scarce (Bouayad *et al.*, 2006) and absence of regulation or effective enforcement of any guidance mean that equids are often overloaded (Iqbal *et al.*, 2006). Consequently they suffer musculoskeletal injuries, wounds (Ali *et al.*, 2016), emotional stress, collapse and, in extreme cases, death due to acute trauma.

In order to generate income, owners may deliberately breed mares that are still working and are then required to continue to work late into pregnancy, with little or no reduction in workload. Evidence is lacking on the effect this has on maternal or neonatal health and welfare in this context. Mares with a foal at foot may start work again soon after foaling. Evidence is also lacking on the consequences for maternal attachment, opportunities for the foal to feed when desired, and weaning practices. The impact on mare and foal, foal growth rate and appropriate musculoskeletal development, if exposed to the working environment, is also unclear. Young equids may start work before they are skeletally mature, resulting in adverse musculoskeletal consequences. In low-resource environments, generating objective data on these issues is difficult.

Equipment and service provision – farriery and equipment

Farriery may be seen as a low-status profession, and it often comprises traditional practices passed down from one generation to another rather than formalized training being completed. Access to materials suitable for making shoes, availability of high-quality farriery tools and appropriate nails are often difficult or impossible. The consequence is that, even with training, farriers are unable to deliver a high-quality service. Equine owners' poor understanding of the importance of good foot care for their equids and how to recognize good farriery means that they are unwilling to pay for superior services, resulting in little incentive for farriers to improve the care they provide. Equids suffer poor foot trimming, balancing and shoeing, leading to poor foot conformation, resulting in musculoskeletal imbalances and lameness, which is associated with suffering through both acute and chronic pain. Poor shoeing may also increase the risk of injury due to poor traction on underfoot condition.

Working equids require pack saddles for loading, harnessing to attach a taxi or cart, effective bridles and bits with reins for steering, saddles for riders, carts and taxi vehicles that are fit for purpose. The absence of skilled equipment makers capable of supplying equipment that uses suitable materials to apply the principles of good designs and owners' resource limitations all have adverse welfare consequences (McLean *et al.*, 2010; Tesfaye *et al.*, 2010; Zaman *et al.*, 2010). Friction and imbalances arising from poor equipment result in acute and chronic skin lesions of varying severity, which cause pain and risk infection (Heleski *et al.*, 2009; Shafi *et al.*, 2014). Owners not appreciating the importance of maintaining and cleaning of equipment worsen these problems (Burn *et al.*, 2008; Zaman *et al.*, 2010). Load imbalances result in anatomical strain leading to joint, soft tissue and skeletal damage that manifest as acute or chronic musculoskeletal pathology.

End of working life

Ensuring optimal welfare in situations where working equids have reached the end of their working life is challenging. Owners' acknowledgement that an equid suffering chronic medical or lameness problems has reached the end of its working life is difficult to achieve when they rely on the animal to generate income that only covers the purchase of daily necessities. National livestock insurance schemes rarely include equids, and savings arrangements to put aside money for a replacement animal are rare (Kalita *et al.*, 2014). The non-working 'retirement' seen in developed countries is generally unworkable for economic, cultural and logistical reasons.

In many countries, discussing animal euthanasia is culturally sensitive, regardless of any acute or chronic pain or distress being suffered. In an emergency, such as limb fracture or a medically unresolvable colic, achieving owners' consent to euthanase the animal on welfare grounds can still be difficult. Chronically sick, work-unsuitable animals, such as horses suffering from epizootic lymphangitis in Ethiopia (Fig. 4.7) may be abandoned to be killed by wild carnivores. For abandoned animals, the legal framework for evidencing consent may be unclear. Capacity of local service providers to perform euthanasia may be limited since it is often not taught within the veterinary curriculum nor authorized for para-veterinary service providers. Non-availability of suitable drugs or firearms may limit delivery of a welfare-friendly end of life. Health and safety arrangements for carcass disposal must be reliable, and prevention of scavenging for drug-euthanased animals is essential. Any combination of these constraints

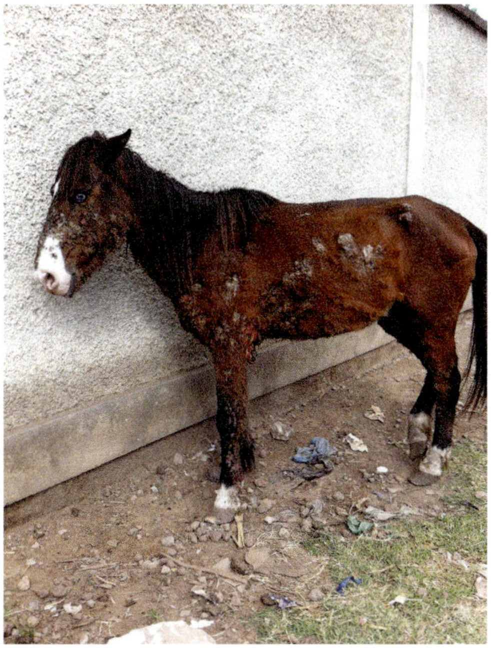

Fig. 4.7. A horse suffering from epizootic lymphangitis in Ethiopia (photo: Brooke, Action for Working Horses and Donkeys).

means that working equids often continue to work despite suffering severe and chronic welfare issues, and may suffer a slow or painful death rather than humane euthanasia.

Asian market demand for donkey hides and other carcass products in recent years has resulted in increased donkey slaughter in countries where they are used as working animals. Conditions of transport to slaughter, facilities for housing donkeys at the slaughterhouse, and slaughter techniques may all cause donkeys to experience physical and emotional welfare problems if they are not designed to meet their specific needs (Donkey Sanctuary, 2017).

Improving Life for Working Equids

When an acceptance of the nutritional, health, behavioural, environmental and mental welfare needs of equids is paired with an acceptance that solutions in low-resource settings require creativity, the daily and cumulative life experience of a working equid can be improved in the short and long term.

Practical suggestions for rectification at local level

Field experience has shown equids to access water through existing materials including: tyres (Fig. 4.8a), hollowed logs (Fig. 4.8b), buckets, collapsible troughs and permanent structures at strategic working and resting points.

Prevention or a reduction in harness sores could be achieved by organizing equipment-fitting sessions where minor adjustments can be made to improve cleanliness,

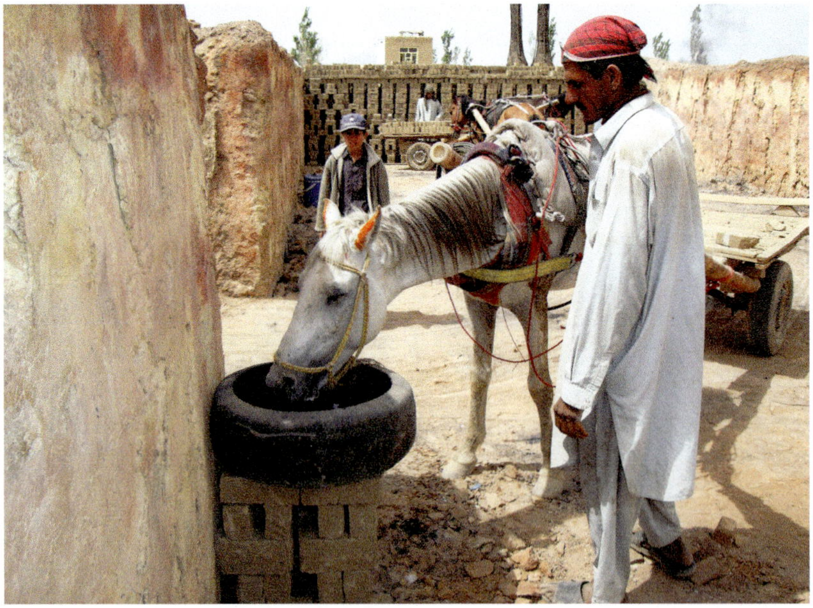

Fig. 4.8a. A water trough made from a tyre in Afghanistan (photo: Brooke, Action for Working Horses and Donkeys).

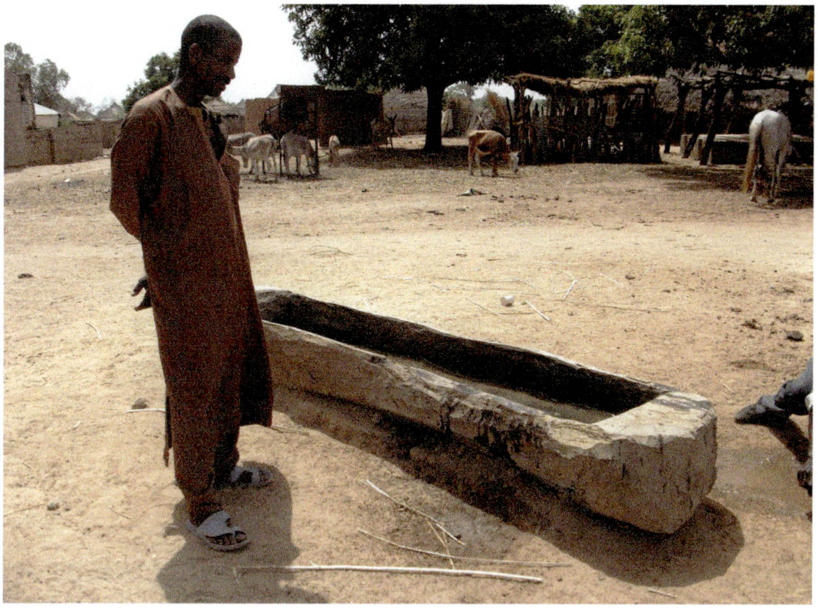

Fig. 4.8b. A water trough made from a log in Senegal (photo: Brooke, Action for Working Horses and Donkeys).

size, fit, material and balance of working equipment (Fig. 4.9). Daily grooming can be a positive experience for the animal and a bonding experience for its owner and will remove sweat and dirt that can cause harnesses to rub (Figs 4.10 and 4.11a).

Risk associated with trimming and balancing hooves is reduced by linking owners with quality, trained farriery professionals; daily cleaning of hooves using a locally made hoof pick (Fig. 4.11b) and ensuring a clean, dry place to stand and move, can ensure good foot health and prevent and avoid recurring bacterial infection (Fig. 4.12).

Further information on practical suggestions for relieving animals of welfare issues can be found within Brooke's *Welfare Interpretation Manual* and *Veterinary Manual* (Brooke, 2013; Brooke, 2016).

A Global Framework to Address Issues Associated with Working Equids Being Pushed to Their Limits

In 2016 the World Organisation for Animal Health (OIE) adopted a new chapter in its Terrestrial Animal Health Code covering standards for welfare of working equids (OIE, 2016). This means that member countries are expected to implement systems to address their needs. In many member countries, however, relatively low levels of equine specialist capacity exist in policy making and delivery departments and there is wide variation in supporting technical infrastructure. The standards' implementation will require the support of, and collaboration between, multiple stakeholders and via multi-party welfare platforms. Government policy makers and programme planners can engage with NGOs to support recognition of the issues that need addressing. The NGOs can offer generic and tailor-made resources in technical capacity building,

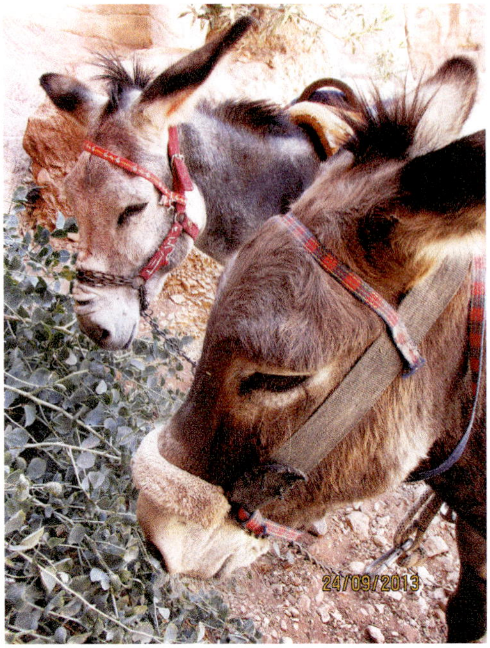

Fig. 4.9. A cover over a chain noseband on a donkey transporting tourists in Jordan (photo: Brooke, Action for Working Horses and Donkeys).

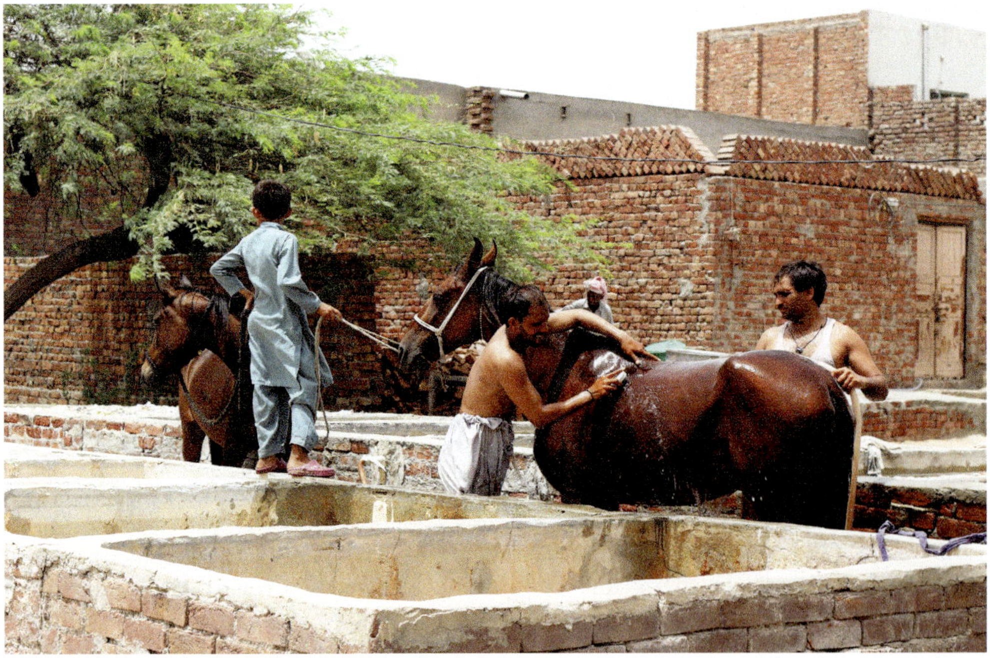

Fig. 4.10. A shower for a horse in Pakistan (photo: Brooke, Action for Working Horses and Donkeys).

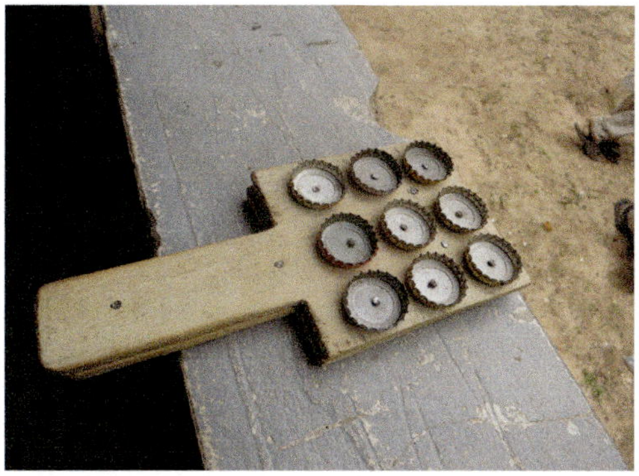

Fig. 4.11a. A locally made curry comb in Ethiopia (photo: Brooke, Action for Working Horses and Donkeys).

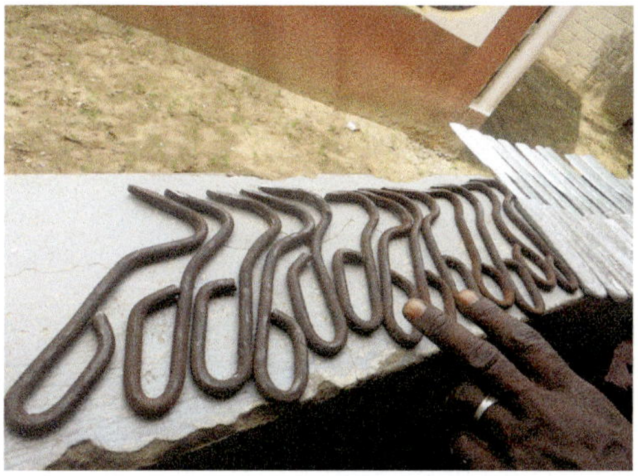

Fig. 4.11b. Locally made hoofpicks in Senegal (photo: Brooke, Action for Working Horses and Donkeys).

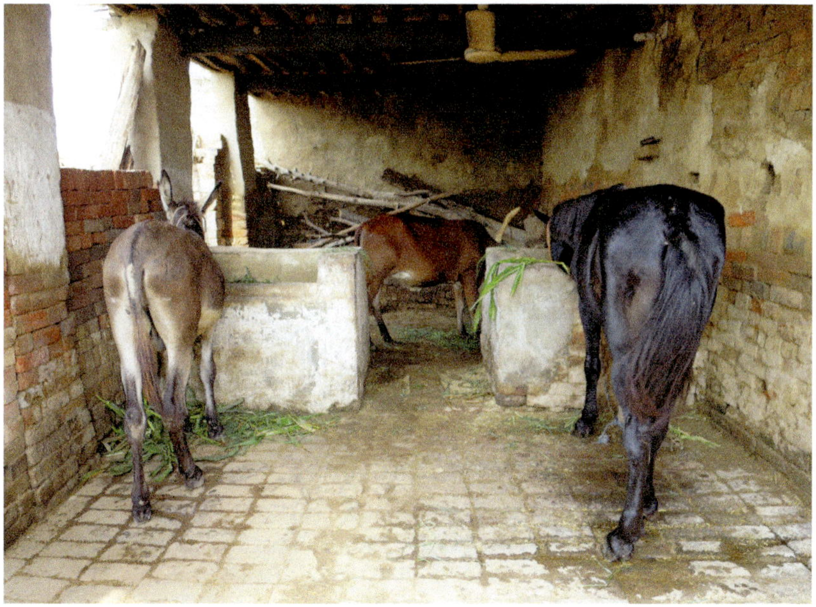

Fig. 4.12. An example of clean stables in Pakistan (photo: Brooke, Action for Working Horses and Donkeys).

which will be key to ensuring that sustainable progress is made on building context-specific local infrastructure to meet these animals' and owners' needs.

Conclusion

Working equids are pushed to their physical and emotional limits in the course of working with people who rely on them to support livelihoods but exist in low-resource settings. Investment in generation and dissemination of robust evidence regarding the welfare problems and potential solutions is required to inform understanding of priority issues and how local stakeholders can address them effectively. Interventions to address the often severe and high-prevalence welfare issues affecting these animals involve: recognition of infrastructure needs; facilitation of relevant capacity building for owners, users, service providers and policy makers; and the encouragement of social change to improve recognition of the importance of these animals' needs and how meeting them can be best effected.

References

Admassu, B. and Shiferaw, Y. (2011) Donkeys, Horses and Mules – Their Contribution to People's Livelihoods in Ethiopia. The Brooke, Addis Ababa.

Ali, A.B.A., El Sayed, M.A., Matoock, M.Y., Fouad, M.A. and Heleski, C.R. (2016a) A welfare assessment scoring system for working equids: a method for identifying at risk populations and for monitoring progress of welfare enhancement strategies (trialled in Egypt). Applied Animal Behaviour Science 176, 52–62.

Ali, A., Orion, S., Tesfaye, T. and Zambriski, J.A. (2016b) The prevalence of lameness and associated risk factors in cart mules in Bahir Dar, Ethiopia. Tropical Animal Health & Production 48(7), 1483–1489.

American Horse Council Foundation (2005) The economic impact of the horse industry on the United States. National Report, Deloitte. Available at: http://www.horsecouncil.org/product/2005-the-economic-impact-of-the-horse-industry-on-the-united-states-national-report/ (accessed 22 January 2018).

Arriaga-Jordán, C.M., Pedraza-Fuentes, A.M., Velázquez-Beltrán, L.G., Nava-Bernal, E.G. and Chávez-Mejía, M.C. (2005) Economic contribution of draught animals to Mazahua smallholder Campesino farming systems in the highlands of Central Mexico. Tropical Animal Health & Production 37(7), 589–597.

Bhardwaj, N., Negi, B. and Mohite, D. (2016) Behaviour of working equids engaged in different types of work. Proceedings of the 50th Congress of the International Society for Applied Ethology 12–15 July, Edinburgh, UK.

Bouayad, H., Ouragh, L. and Tah, M. (2006) Evaluation of the physical effort used by working animals in Marrakech. Proceedings of the 5th International Colloquium on Working Equids: The Future for Working Equines. 30 October–2 November, Addis Ababa, pp. 24–27.

Bradbury, H. (2002) Case study: the gharry horses of Gonder, Ethiopia – workable solutions for working horses. Proceedings of the 4th International Colloquium on Working Equines. 20–26 April 2002, Hama, Syria, pp. 232–236.

Brooke (2012) Standardised Equine Based Welfare Assessment Tool. Available at: https://www.thebrooke.org/sites/default/files/Professionals/SEBWAT.pdf (accessed 22 January 2018).

Brooke (2013) Veterinary Manual. Available at: https://www.thebrooke.org/for-professionals/working-equid-veterinary-manual (accessed 22 January 2018).

Brooke (2016) Welfare Interpretation Manual. Available at: https://www.thebrooke.org/for-professionals/welfare-interpretation-manual (accessed 22 January 2016).

Broster, C.E., Burn, C.C., Barr, A.R.S. and Whay, H.R. (2008) Lameness in the working equid: How lame can they get? Proceedings of the British Equine Veterinary Congress. 10–13 September, Liverpool, UK, pp. 322–323.

Broster, C.E., Burn, C.C., Barr, A.R.S. and Whay, H.R. (2009) The range and prevalence of pathological abnormalities associated with lameness in working horses from developing countries. Equine Veterinary Journal 41, 474–481.

Brown, A. (2014) Development of measures of human animal interaction for working equids. Proceedings of the 6th International Conference on the Assessment of Animal Welfare at Farm and Group Level. 3–5 September, Clermont-Ferrand, France.

Burn, C.C. Pritchard, J.C., Farajat, M., Twaissi, A.A. and Whay, H.R. (2008) Risk factors for strap-related lesions in working donkeys at the World Heritage Site of Petra in Jordan. The Veterinary Journal 178(2), 263–271.

Burn, C.C., Dennison, T.L. and Whay, H.R. (2010a) Environmental and demographic risk factors for poor welfare in working horses, donkeys and mules in developing countries. The Veterinary Journal 2010, 186, 385–392.

Burn, C.C., Dennison, T. and Whay, H.R. (2010b) Relationships between behaviour and health in working horses, donkeys, and mules in developing countries. Applied Animal Behaviour Science 126, 109–118.

Carroll, C.L. and Huntington, P.J. (1988) Body condition scoring and weight estimation of horses. Equine Veterinary Journal 20(1), 41–45.

Chang, C.R., Sapon, M. and Rodriguez, D. (2010) Economic valuation of the impact of the working equine in the Peten and Chimaltenango communities in Guatemala. Proceedings of the 6th International Colloquium on Working Equids. 30 November–2 December, pp. 106–110.

Curran, M.L., Stringer, A.P., Harry, J., Freeman, S.L. and Burford, J.H. (2014) Establishing clinical guidelines for the treatment of equine colic in developing countries. Abstract Programme, The Eleventh International Equine Colic Research Symposium. 7–10 July, Dublin.

Donkey Sanctuary (2017) Under the Skin: The Emerging Trade in Donkey Skins and Its Implications for Donkey Welfare and Livelihoods. The Donkey Sanctuary, Sidmouth, UK. Available at: https://www.thedonkeysanctuary.org.uk/sites/sanctuary/files/under_the_skin_report.pdf (accessed 11 December 2017).

Doumbia, A. (2014) The contribution of working donkeys to the livelihoods of the population in Mali. Proceedings of the 7th International Colloquium on Working Equids. Society for the Protection of Animals Abroad, 1–3 July, London, p. 35.

FAO (2014) Food and Agriculture Organization of the UN. Available at: http://faostat3.fao.org/browse/Q/QA/E (accessed 22 January 2018).

Getnet, F., Feyera, T., Alemu, F., Niguse, A. and Abera, T. (2014) Injuries in donkeys and mules: causes, welfare problems and management practices in Amhara region, northern Ethiopia. American-Eurasian Journal of Scientific Research 9(4), 98–104.

Gogoi, P. and Dennison, T. (2010) Firing (a mutilation) of working equines in India: a comparative ethnic practice in Delhi, Lucknow and Hyderabad cities. Proceedings of the 6th International Colloquium on Working Equids. 29 November–2 December, New Delhi, pp. 191–194.

Hall, C., Goodwin, D., Heleski, C., Randle, H. and Waran, N. (2008) Is there evidence of learned helplessness in horses? Journal of Applied Animal Welfare Science 11, 249–266.

Hassan, M.R., Steenstra, F.A. and Udo, H.M.J. (2013) Benefits of donkeys in rural and urban areas in northwest Nigeria. African Journal of Agricultural Research 8(48), 6202–6212.

Hayward, M. and Adams, D. (2001) The Firing of Horses: A Review for the Animal Welfare Advisory Committee of the Australian Veterinary Association. Available at: https://www.gungahlinvet.com.au/petcare-info/publications/the-firing-of-horses.pdf (accessed 22 January 2018).

Heleski, C.R., Amy, K.M. and Swanson, J.C. (2009) Practical methods for improving the welfare of horses, donkeys, and other working draught animals in developing areas. In: Temple, G. (ed.) Improving Animal Welfare: A Practical Approach. CAB International, Wallingford, UK.

Iqbal, A., Hassan, S., Ahsan-Ullah, R. and Riaz, M. (2006) Developments and research in equine husbandry and welfare: some issues in Pakistan. Proceedings of the 5th International Colloquium on Working Equids: The Future for Working Equines. 30 October–2 November, Addis Ababa, pp. 11–14.

Kalita, J., Singh, A., Kumar, N. and Pandey, G. (2014) Community-led insurance system among equine welfare associations. Proceedings of the 7th International Colloquium on Working Equids. 1–3 July, London, p. 113.

Kandpal, D.K., Zaman, S.F. and Kumar, A. (2014) Study on the contribution of equids to the livelihoods of landless people in Indian brick kilns. Proceedings of the 7th International Colloquium on Working Equids. 1–3 July, London, p. 37.

Kawe, N. (2016) Integrated approach to behavior change on donkey handling in Mwea, Kenya. The First International Conference on Human Behaviour Change for Animal Welfare, Dorking, UK. Available at: https://www.youtube.com/watch?v=RICu2kEtHjg (accessed 15 November 2017).

Laing, G., Christley, R., Stringer, A., Radford, A., Aklilu, N., Newton, R. and Pinchbeck, G. (2016) Unraveling the causes of respiratory disease in the working equids of Ethiopia: a cross sectional survey. Journal of Equine Veterinary Science 39, S98–S107.

Lewa, A.K., Mangero, J., Kajume, J.K.L. and Akumonyo, J. (2006) The unspoken enslavery. Proceedings of the 5th International Colloquium on Working Equids: The Future for Working Equines. 30 October–2 November, Addis Ababa, pp. 204–206.

Martin Curran, M. and Smith, D.G. (2005) The impact of donkey ownership on the livelihoods of female peri-urban dwellers in Ethiopia. Tropical Animal Health & Production 37(Suppl 1), 67–86.

McGreevy, P. (2004) Equine Behaviour: A Guide for Veterinarians and Equine Scientists. Saunders, UK.

McLean, A.K. and McLean, M. (2008) Academic Horse Training. Australian Equine Behaviour Centre, Clonbinane, Australia.

McLean, A.K., Heleski, C.R., Yokoyama, M.T., Wang, W., Doumbia, A. and Dembele, B. (2010) Improving working donkey (Equus Asinus) welfare in Mali, West Africa: measuring behaviour, heart rate variability associated with driving methods and pressure associated with harness and cart quality. Proceedings of the 6th International Colloquium on Working Equids. 29 November–2 December, New Delhi, pp. 20–26.

Mellor, D.J. (2016) Updating animal welfare thinking: moving beyond the 'five freedoms' towards 'a life worth living'. Animals 6, 21.

Mohite, D.S., Sheikh, C.S., Compston, P.C., Zaman, S.F. and Singh, S. (2016) Protozoal, EHV-1 and Japanese Encephalitis infection in Qalander community, northern India – seroprevalence in 113 equids. Journal of Equine Veterinary Science 39(2016), S98eS107.

Nawaz, S., Shah, Z., Soomro, N., Laghari, H., Kashif, M. and Brohi, S.A. (2010) Slitting nostrils in donkeys – a mythical but painful quack practice in the southern region of Brooke (Pakistan): coping through awareness. Proceedings of the 6th International Colloquium on Working Equids. 29 November–2 December, New Delhi, pp. 164–167.

Nigatu, A. and Abdelaw, Z. (2010) Socioeconomic impact of epizootic lymphangitis on horse drawn taxi business in central Ethiopia. Proceedings of the 6th International Colloquium on Working Equids. 29 November–2 December, New Delhi, pp. 83–86.

OIE (2016) Available at: http://www.oie.int/index.php?id=169&L=0&htmfile=chapitre_aw_working_equids.htm (accessed 22 January 2018).

Pearson, G. (2015) Practical application of equine learning theory, part 1. In Practice 37(5), 251–254.

Pritchard, J.C., Lindberg, A.C., Main, D.C.J. and Whay, H.R. (2005) Assessment of the welfare of working horses, mules and donkeys, using health and behaviour parameters. Preventive Veterinary Medicine 69, 265–283.

Pritchard, J.C., Burn, C.C., Barr, A.R.S. and Whay, H.R. (2008) Validity of indicators of dehydration in working horses: a longitudinal study of changes in skin tent duration, mucous membrane dryness and drinking behaviour. Equine Veterinary Journal 40(6), 558–564.

Regan, F.H., Hockenhull, J., Pritchard, J., Waterman-Pearson, A.E. and Whay, H.R. (2014) Behavioural repertoire of working donkeys and consistency of behaviour over time as a preliminary step towards identifying pain-related behaviours. PLOS ONE. Available at: http://dx.doi.org/10.1371/journal.pone.0101877 (accessed 22 January 2018).

Regan, F.H., Hockenhull, J., Pritchard, J.C., Waterman-Pearson, A.E. and Whay, H.R. (2015) Clinical abnormalities in working donkeys and their associations with behaviour. Veterinary Record Open 2, e000105. DOI: 0.1136/vetreco-2014-000105.

Reix, C.E., Burn, C.C., Pritchard, J.C., Barr, A.R.S. and Whay, H.R. (2014) The range and prevalence of clinical signs and conformation associated with lameness in working draught donkeys in Pakistan. Equine Veterinary Journal 46, 771–777.

Reix, C.E., Dikshit, A.K., Hockenhull, J., Parker, R.M.A., Banerjee, A., Burn, C.C., Pritchard, J.C. and Whay, H.R. (2015) A two-year participatory intervention project with owners to reduce lameness and limb abnormalities in working horses in Jaipur, India. PLOS ONE. DOI: 10.1371/journal.pone.0124342.

Saville, K., Skippen, L., Compston, P. and Hirson, T. (2014) Disseminating knowledge further: a model for cascade training following continuing professional development workshops. Available at: https://www.thebrooke.org/sites/default/files/Animal%20Welfare/Cascade-training_0.pdf (accessed 20 October 2016).

Scantlebury, C.E., Aklilu, N., Reed, K., Knottenbelt, D.C., Gebreab, F. and Pinchbeck, G.L. (2013) Ocular disease in working horses in Ethiopia: a cross-sectional study. Veterinary Record 172(4), 99.

Shafi, M., Shah, S.Z.A., Nawaz, S., Laghari, H., Shah, S.N.A. and Brohi, S. (2014) Minimising prevalence and severity of croup lesions in cart pulling donkeys through community awareness in Jacobabad, Pakistan. Proceedings of the 7th International Colloquium on Working Equids. 1–3 July, London, p. 146.

Shah, Z. (2016) Brick kilns in Peshawar – improving comfort for working equids. The First International Conference for Human Behaviour Change for Animal Welfare, Dorking, UK. Available at: http://www.hbcforanimals.com/hbcaw1--2016.html (accessed 1 November 2017).

Shah, Z., Khan, S., Nawaz, S. and Suhail, S.M. (2006) Effect of working hours, housing and water provision on body condition and saddle sores in working equines in brick kilns in Peshawar, Pakistan. Proceedings of the 5th International Colloquium on Working Equines: The Future for Working Equines. 30 October–2 November, Addis Ababa.

Sommerville, R., Brown, A.F. and Upjohn, M. (2018) A standardised equine-based welfare assessment tool used for six years in low and middle income countries. *PLOS ONE* 13 (2), e0192354. https://doi.org/10.1371/journal.pone.0192354.

Starkey, E., Matas, M. and Verheyen, K.L.P. (2014) Ocular disease in the working horses of Cholutecca, Honduras. Proceedings of the 7th International Colloquium on Working Equids. 1–3 July, London, pp. 176–178.

Stringer, A.P. (2014) Infectious diseases of working equids. Veterinary Clinics of North America Equine Practice 30(3), 695–718.

Tesfaye, M., Feseha, G., Bojia, E., Alemayehu, F., Ayele, G. et al. (2006) Hyena bite: a potential threat to the lives of working donkeys in central Ethiopia. Proceedings of the 5th International Colloquium on Working Equines: The Future for Working Equines. 30 October–2 November, Addis Ababa.

Tesfaye, M., Bojia, E., Feseha, G., Ayele, G., Alemayehu, F. (2010) Community-based harness development initiative for pack donkeys: a progress report: Ethiopia. Proceedings of the 6th International Colloquium on Working Equids. 29 November–1 December, Delhi, pp. 284–291.

United Nations Development Programme (UNDP) (2015) Available at: http://hdr.undp.org/en/content/multidimensional-poverty-index-mpi (accessed 22 January 2018).

Upjohn, M.M., Shipton, K., Pfeiffer, D.U., Lerotholi, T., Attwood, G. and Verheyen, K.L.P. (2012) Cross-sectional survey of owner knowledge and husbandry practices, tack and health issues affecting working horses in Lesotho. Equine Veterinary Journal 44(3), 310–318.

Valette, D. (2014) Invisible Helpers: Voices from Women. The Brooke London. Available at: https://www.thebrooke.org/sites/default/files/Advocacy-and-policy/Invisible-helpers-voices-from-women.pdf (accessed 1 November 2016).

Valette, D. (2015) Invisible Workers. The Brooke London. Available at: https://www.thebrooke.org/sites/default/files/Advocacy-and-policy/Invisible-workers-report.pdf (accessed 30 October 2016).

Velazquez-Beltran, L.G., Sanchez-Vera, E. and Nava-Bernal, E.G. (2011) The role of working equines to livelihoods in current day campesino hill-slope communities in central Mexico. Tropical Animal Health & Production 43, 1623–1632.

Walker-Okello, A. (2010) Opportunities for NGOs involved with the draught sector to contribute to national livestock policy frameworks in developing countries. Proceedings of the 6th International Colloquium on Working Equids. 29 November–2 December, New Delhi, pp. 80–82.

Wolff, A. and Hausberger, M. (1996) Learning and memorisation of two different tasks in horses: the effects of age, sex and sire. Applied Animal Behaviour Science 46, 137–143.

Zaman, S.F., Aravindan, M., Thanammal, S.R., Roy, C., Childs, A.C. and Eager, R.A. (2010) Risk factors for wither lesions in tourist-riding mules of Uttarakhand, India. Proceedings of the 6th International Colloquium on Working Equids, 29 November–2 December, New Delhi, pp. 272–275.

5 Genetics and Other Technologies for Increasing the Productivity of Cattle, Sheep and Pigs: Welfare Implications

Temple Grandin*

Department of Animal Sciences, Colorado State University, USA

Introduction

Through the use of selective breeding, the productivity of farm animals has greatly increased. Milk production has tripled and carcass weights in US beef cattle have risen. Most of the increases in milk and meat production are due to genetic selection. Scientists are becoming increasingly concerned that the functionality of farm animals has declined (Otenocu and Broom, 2010; Rodenbury and Turner, 2012). Rauw and Gomez-Raya (2015) also state that animals bred for high productivity might have more behavioural, physiological or metabolic problems. Most of the great increases in production described in this chapter were achieved with conventional breeding. None of the animals covered in this chapter is a product of a genetically modified organism (GMO), where DNA from another species was inserted into the genome.

This chapter will cover six main areas: (i) problems with lameness and poor leg conformation; (ii) difficulty maintaining body condition in breeding females; (iii) behaviour problems associated with genetic selection that may be detrimental to animal welfare; (iv) loss of disease resistance; (v) heart and circulatory problems; and (vi) reproductive problems. Other areas that will be discussed are the effects of production-enhancing feed additives and hormones, and issues with providing adequate nutrition for high-producing animals. All of these concerns can be classified as possible biological overload where the animal's biological systems stop functioning normally (Grandin, 2014).

One example of a loss of functionality is the huge increase in milk production in dairy cows, associated with a steep decline in fertility (Spencer, 2013). The decline in fertility may be due to negative energy balance (Walsh *et al.*, 2011). Negative energy balance occurs when an animal is not able to eat sufficient nutrients to prevent loss of body condition. Many dairy managers have reported that getting Holsteins to re-breed quickly is a problem. Years ago, I wrote that if you over-select for any single production, appearance or behaviour trait, you will wreck your animal (Grandin and Deesing, 1998). At the time of writing this chapter, some sectors of the livestock industry are approaching a tipping point where the biological system is

*E-mail: cheryl.miller@colostate.edu

becoming overloaded. Single-minded genetic selection for a few narrow production traits may cause welfare problems.

There are always trade-offs. For example, in wild sheep, ewes with lower immune function have more lambs, and ewes with greater immune function have fewer lambs (Graham *et al.*, 2010). There is a trade-off between immune function to fight gastrointestinal parasites and body weight (Greer, 2008). Instead of attempting to achieve maximum production, we need to select animals for optimum production and still have sufficient immune function to fight parasites and disease.. Doing this will help prevent the serious problems that may occur when the animal's biology is so overloaded that it starts to fail. Some breeders are now using a more balanced approach. This is already underway in poultry and dairy cow breeding. Poultry breeders started making changes when both leg problems and death losses had greatly increased (Gonzáles-Cerón *et al.*, 2014). Leg growth had become so abnormal that the broilers had twisted legs. This is called tibial dychondroplasia. A shorter generational interval in poultry also made it easier to start correcting the leg problems.

The poultry, dairy and pork industries are correcting some of their breeding mistakes. Unfortunately, there are some people in the beef cattle industry who are repeating these same mistakes. In the dairy industry, some progressive breeders are taking a more balanced approach to dairy cow selection. Unfortunately, there are others who single-mindedly select for milk production. This can result in problems with maintaining adequate body condition and increased lameness (Randall *et al.*, 2015). Animal breeders need to get out of their breed-specific silos and see what breeders of other species are doing. Each species has its own journals and cattle breeders usually do not read many poultry journals.

Lameness, Leg Problems and Body Condition

Dairy cows

Lameness in dairy cows is still a huge issue and it has not improved. Roughly a quarter of all lactating dairy cows are lame (Bennett *et al.*, 2014; Cook *et al.*, 2015). Lameness (difficulty in walking) is highly detrimental to welfare because it causes pain. Both lameness and poor body condition are related. High-producing cows have less fat cushion tissue in their feet and less body condition (Green *et al.*, 2014; Oikonomou *et al.*, 2014). Cows with low body condition also have more leg lesions (Fulwider *et al.*, 2007). Both studies show that high-producing cows have lower fat reserves. A study done by Randall *et al.* (2015) indicated that dairy cows with a body condition score of less than 2 on a five-point scale were at greater risk of lameness. Pritchard *et al.* (2013) examined the records of over 75,000 dairy cows in over 2000 herds. There may be an antagonistic relationship between selecting for both reduced mastitis and lameness with milk production. Excellent management of cows bred and fed for high production reduced the average percentage of lame cows in Wisconsin to 13% (Cook *et al.*, 2015). There was a big difference between the best and worst dairies. Out of 66 high-producing dairies in Wisconsin, the best one had 2.8% lame cows and the worst one had 36% (Cook *et al.*, 2015).

Progressive dairy managers have learned that they need to reduce milk production slightly and select for smaller cows with better longevity. This will result in a cow that will last three to four years of milking instead of only two years. This optimal cow will be more profitable because heifer development costs will be less. Another benefit is that when it is time to remove the cow from the milking line, she will be a better source of beef with greater body condition. The trade-offs are clear. Cows with a longer production lifespan have significantly lower estimated breeding values for milk production (Abfalter *et al.*, 2016). Another study showed that selecting dairy cows for feed efficiency increases the potential for the negative consequence of reducing energy balance (Spurlock *et al.*, 2012). Put simply, the cow will get skinnier because she will not be eating enough to maintain body condition. In high-producing dairy herds, management factors such as housing, feed availability and hoof trimming greatly reduced death losses. A cluster analysis of 557 Wisconsin dairies had many interesting findings. In dairies managed for the highest production, the death losses were 6.8% in the best cluster and 12.5% in the worst cluster (Brotzman *et al.*, 2015). These figures clearly show the benefits of best management practices such as deep loose bedding and easy access to feed (Brotzman *et al.*, 2015). To maintain an adequate level of welfare in high-producing cows requires excellent management. It is likely that lower-producing cows may be more tolerant of sloppy management.

Pigs

In the late 1980s, lean, rapidly growing lines of hybrid pigs were introduced. A breeder with one of the major breeding companies told me that they only selected for three economically important traits. These were: rapid weight gain, large loin eye size and thin lean back fat. Within ten years, producers realized that there were now severe problems with lameness in both market-weight pigs and sows. When the author watched pigs being unloaded from trucks at a slaughter plant, up to 50% of the fed market weight animals were lame. There was no disease or injury in their feet; the problem was due to leg conformation. They were either post legged (too straight) or the pastern had collapsed. This resulted in the pig walking on the dew claws. Unfortunately, exclusive selection for meat traits was linked to poor leg conformation. Today the best pig breeders and producers are selecting breeding stock that is free of leg conformation problems.

A Swedish study has shown that selecting gilts for good mobility and proper leg conformation will help sows produce more live piglets (Le *et al.*, 2015a). Selection for good leg conformation improves sow longevity (Le *et al.*, 2015b). Sows will also last longer and have more piglets when gilts are selected for leg conformation (Le *et al.*, 2015b). Highly productive sows that have heavier litters at weaning have thinner back fat and more shoulder lesions (Lundeheim, *et al.*, 2014).

Selection for more efficient feed conversion

To improve sustainability, breeders are now selecting pigs for improved feed conversion. This reduces the amount of feed required by 12–15% to produce a kilogram of pork (Azarpajouh *et al.*, 2016). Selecting for feed conversion has trade-offs that are both positive and negative for pig welfare. On the positive side, the young growing market pigs may have some welfare advantages such as less reactive, calmer behaviour

(Colpays *et al.*, 2014, 2015), better disease resistance (Dunkelberger *et al.*, 2015; Merlot *et al.*, 2015) and lower cortisol (Colpays *et al.*, 2014). On the negative side the feed-efficient sows selected for residual feed intake lost more body condition during lactation (Young *et al.*, 2012) and sow lameness and leg conformation problems may increase (Mumm *et al.*, 2016). The bottom line was that more efficient conversion of feed into meat benefited the young growing offspring but was detrimental to their mothers.

The researchers at Iowa State University who did these studies on feed conversion were surprised that there were positive benefits (Azarpajouh *et al.*, 2016). The author hypothesizes that there is a possible evolutionary reason for this effect. The wild ancestors of pigs may have made an adaptation for times when food was scarce. In this situation there may be a better chance of survival if all resources are put into the offspring and the older mother is sacrificed. Sows selected for efficient feed conversion had more pigs, but lost significantly more body condition (Young, 2012; Azarparjouh *et al.*, 2016).

Beef cattle

Until recently, lameness due to leg conformation was never an issue. Unfortunately, some breeders of beef cattle may be repeating mistakes that pig breeders made in the 1980s and 1990s. The author has started to see some genetic lines of Angus beef cattle with similar leg conformation problems as the pigs. This problem started when the industry started selecting for carcass traits such as marbling and lean back fat. Many top show bulls are post legged and a few animals are showing up at the slaughter plant with the same collapsed pasterns that I have observed in many pigs. Kacee Vollmar at Colorado State University did a survey of over 2000 cattle in Colorado and Texas feed lots. Newly arrived cattle were evaluated for leg conformation and for crooked claw. This condition is also called corkscrew claw or crossed toes. Crooked claw may not be genetically related to other leg structure traits. Claw health and hoof abnormalities in dairy cows was not related to leg conformation (Odegard *et al.*, 2014). Fortunately, selective breeding can probably be used to reduce claw abnormalities (Van der Spek *et al.*, 2015). One must remember that dairy cows and beef cows are selected for different traits of milk and meat. The author has observed that obvious foot abnormalities or leg conformation problems appear to be more related by selecting for meat traits.

In her survey, Vollmar (2016) found that crooked claw was significantly more likely to occur in calves originating from northern ranches. Texas calves had more normal hooves. The most likely explanation for this is that Texas cattle originate from small farms with less intense genetic selection. Northern cattle originate from large ranches that would have more intensive breeding selection programmes. In many breeding programmes there is an emphasis on selection for carcass traits.

Many breeders use EPD (Expected Progeny Difference) numbers to select bulls. A particular sire may have EPDs for calving ease or weight gain. EPDs for calving ease have greatly improved welfare by reducing dystocia difficult calving. EPDs have also been added for carcass traits such as beef marbling. Unfortunately, some breeders only go by the numbers and do not visually appraise bulls and cows kept for breeding stock. The author has observed beef cattle from a large breeder who breeds only by the numbers. He tells everybody that visual appraisal is obsolete. During handling of his cattle, the author observed some of the worst post legged bulls. They were lame and walked stiffly. Visual appraisal is still needed to keep breeders out of trouble and to insure that animals can walk and function normally.

Lameness can also occur in grain fed cattle that have acidosis. When cattle are fed high grain rations to achieve maximum weight gain, it must be done carefully to avoid acidosis. Shifting the ration too quickly from forage to grain can be a problem. Acidosis in grain fed cattle can also occur if they suddenly go off feed. A severe weather event or other problem that interrupts feed delivery can also cause acidosis. Feeding cattle for maximum gain is a balancing act. When it is done correctly, the welfare of the cattle is acceptable. Another issue is liver abscesses. They can vary from a few small spots to hundreds of spots. Research is needed to determine at which level liver abscesses affect welfare. There appear to be genetic factors. Holstein dairy steers get twice as many liver abscesses as beef breed steers (Amachawadi and Nagaraja, 2015).

Genetics: Effects on Behaviour Problems

Pigs

In the late 1980s, when new lean-line pigs were introduced in the USA, the author observed a threefold increase in tail bite wounds and fighting in market pigs arriving at the slaughter plant. These pigs were also extremely excitable. When the author walked through the lairage and rattled the pen gates, these new pigs would explode into a frenzy of squealing and jumping. Shaking the gate in the next pen of pigs bred from older genetic lines had no effect. When I asked the breeder about my observations he replied, 'You are not a geneticist.' I told him that I had one important qualification: during my work in many large slaughter plants I had observed many different pigs with lots of different genetics. When you see different genetic lines of pigs in adjacent pens, it becomes obvious that some of the new pigs had problems. Nobody would deliberately breed aggressive pigs, but these breeders never had the opportunity to see their pigs beside pigs with different breeding. Research shows very clearly that behaviour traits are heritable in pigs (Rohrer, *et al.*, 2013; Rydhmer and Canario, 2014).

The pigs that were so aggressive and excitable in the late 1980s were bred for three traits: (i) rapid weight gain; (ii) thin back fat; and (iii) large loin eye size. The breeders accidentally selected for aggression, because the pigs that gained a lot of weight pushed other pigs away from the feeders.

In Europe, young market weight pigs are kept intact and fed as boars. This eliminates painful castration. In other countries pigs are castrated due to concerns about boar smell (boar taint) in the meat. In 2014, the author had the opportunity to observe multiple truckloads of intact boar pigs from both Dutch and German genetic lines arriving at a slaughter plant. When the young boars from many German producers arrived at the plant, they quietly unloaded from the truck and lay down in the pens. The Dutch white boars were totally different. After unloading they engaged in both fighting and mounting of each other. The behaviour of the two genetic lines was totally different. From a welfare standpoint, the Dutch pigs would have had poorer welfare.

Beef cattle

Temperament is definitely heritable in cattle. Many studies have shown that beef cattle that remain calm during handling gain more weight and have better-quality meat. Beef cattle that struggle during restraint or run quickly when exiting a race have lower weight gain (Voisinet *et al.*, 1997; Hoppe *et al.*, 2008). They also have poorer meat quality, are more likely to have dark cutting beef and have higher physiological measures of stress (King *et al.*, 2006; Café *et al.*, 2010; Hall *et al.*, 2011). Many beef breed associations now have EPDs for cattle temperament. Selecting calm cattle has improved animal welfare. This has been especially important for cattle raised on extensive range land. Calmer more docile animals are safer for people to handle and they are less likely to get injured during handling. Breeders must be careful not to over-select for a docile temperament. Too much of the docility trait may result in a loss of mothering ability or motivation to forage on rough ground. Flöercke *et al.* (2012) found that there were definite differences in the mothering behaviour of Red Angus beef cows. Some mothers are more vigilant to threats, and a few poor mothers walked off and left their young calves.

Cardiac Weakness, Acidosis and Liver Abscesses

Poultry breeders have known for years that fast-growing broilers would often die from 'flip over' disease. Birds bred for meat have a higher susceptibility to cardiac arrhythmias (Olkowski and Classen, 2010). Muscle can grow so rapidly that the circulatory system cannot keep up. In extreme cases, an area of necrosis will form in the middle of a turkey muscle (Velleman, 2015).

In beef cattle, some animals living at very high altitudes have cardiac problems. Some are more resistant to the hypoxic effects of high altitudes than others (Will *et al.*, 1975; Newman *et al.*, 2011, 2015). Beef cattle bred to have superior carcass traits may have more difficulty living at high altitudes.

Unfortunately, ranchers are starting to observe cardiac problems in cattle that were originally only seen at high altitudes. Heart issues are occurring at much lower elevations (Neary *et al.*, 2015). It is likely that breeding selection for larger cattle and improved carcass traits has contributed to this problem. Heavy Angus steers with increased levels of adiposity (fat) were at increased risk of heart failure during finishing (fattening) (Neary *et al.*, 2015). Researchers at Kansas State University have described a new condition in beef cattle called fatigued cattle syndrome (Thomson *et al.*, 2015). It is most likely to occur in very large grain fed cattle when they are subjected to physical exertion. Cattle that become non-ambulatory have high lactic acid levels (Thomson *et al.*, 2015). This is similar to fatigued pigs.

Amachawadi and Nagaraja (2015) reported that 10–20% of fed beef cattle get liver abscesses. The problem is worse in grain fed Holstein cattle (Amachawadi and Nagaraja, 2015). Researchers in New Zealand found similar problems with an increased incidence of liver abscesses in pastured bulls. Meat inspection reports from 137,675 bulls indicated that dairy breed bulls had 10.3% abscessed livers and the beef breed had only 4.7% (Trotter, 2016). Both studies illustrate that there is a genetic effect on the likelihood that an animal will get liver abscesses.

Not Enough Feed to Support It

Animals that are hardy and live in a rugged environment are often smaller. There is a simple reason for this: small animals and slow-growing animals need less food. On sparse range land such as the American west or the Australian outback, the forage cannot support big cows. In the 1970s, when the first European Continental cattle arrived in the USA, AL Lane, the University of Arizona county agent, said: 'There is not enough groceries on the Arizona desert to feed those big cows' (AL Lane, personal communication, early 1970s). The small local Hereford cattle survived and almost always produced a calf. There are trade-offs; animals that are well adapted to rugged sparse range will be smaller and less productive. A larger cow would starve on the Arizona desert.

Breeders often fail to see that there is a limit to continuous genetic selection for a few narrow production traits. Even when new genomic selection methods are used for choosing breeding stock, physics will still set limits. Enhanced production requires more inputs. A major discussion in US organic agriculture is the use of synthetic methionine in broiler diets (Burley *et al.*, 2016). Modern birds are growing so fast that they need this supplement (Burley *et al.*, 2016). The solution to this problem is to either feed methionine or use slower-growing poultry. Highly productive animals require more nutritional inputs.

It now appears that pig genetics is hitting a feed barrier. A high-producing pork producer who is doing all his management practices right may be more likely to have pigs with Mulberry heart disease. This causes sudden death in weanling pigs. Steve Ensley, a veterinarian at Iowa State University, stated that, normally, Mulberry heart can be prevented by supplementing with Vitamin E and selenium (Neutkens, 2010). The latest information shows that MHD may be related to rapid growth. Ensley concludes, 'Genetics is so high, disease control and nutrition are so good and then boom, the animal can't compensate for rapid growth and we've got a pig that has outgrown our ability to provide nutrition.'

Issues with Growth Promoters and Hormones

An animal's biology can either be overloaded by over zealous genetic selection for production traits or by administering too many growth or milk production promoters. Unless it is used very carefully, the hormone rBST, which is used for increasing milk production, has caused problems in dairy cows. The cow may have increased difficulty maintaining her body condition and suffer more illness from mastitis (Willeberg, 1993; Kronfeld, 1994, 2000; Collier *et al.*, 2001).

Beta-agonists (zilpateral and ractopomine) both increase muscle mass (Scamlin *et al.*, 2009). These products are not hormones or antibiotics. They also make meat tougher (Shook *et al.*, 2009; Jean *et al.*, 2014). Both the author and other people who work in slaughter plants have observed that cattle fed high doses of beta-agonists are sometimes lame and stiff when they arrive (Grandin, 2010). The problem is more likely to occur in hot weather. Hagenmaier *et al.* (2017) also reported increased lameness in feedlot cattle during unloading at the abattoir during hot weather. Physical exertion and muscle fatigue during handling and transport may make it worse. Observations in the field indicate that problems are more likely to occur during hot weather over 90° F on the day of slaughter (Grandin, 2010). Higher doses tend to worsen the detrimental effects. When pigs are fed a high dose of ractopamine they were more difficult to handle (Marchant-Forde *et al.*, 2003; Ritter, 2017). Aggression between pigs also increased in pigs fed high doses (>10 mg) of ractopomine (Poletto *et al.*, 2008). During hot weather, death losses in cattle may be increased (Montgomery *et al.*, 2008; Longeragan *et al.*, 2014). Pigs fed ractopomine were more likely to become stressed if they were handled roughly (James *et al.*, 2013). An increase in downed non-ambulatory pigs was related to the dose. A dose of 5 mg/kg had no effect and a dose of 7.5 mg/kg, fed for 28 days, increased downed fatigued pigs (Peterson, *et al.*, 2015). Another study showed that ractopomine fed at a dose of 10 mg for 28 days increased epinephrine levels and had only minor effects on handling (Puls *et al.*, 2015). One study shows that heat stress may be increased in sheep fed beta-agonists (Marcias-Cruz *et al.*, 2010). Another study done with zilpaterol showed minor heat effects (Boyd *et al.*, 2015). The cattle were 78% with red hides and the temperature during the beta-agonist feeding period was high but dropped into the 80s on the day of slaughter. In the USA, zilpaterol has a three-day withdrawal period prior to slaughter. The cattle in this study had an extra day of withdrawal. There is a possibility this may have reduced detrimental effects during handling and transport. There is also evidence that high doses may be associated with hoof cracking in pigs (Poletto *et al.*, 2009) and abnormal lateral lying posture in 31% of the cattle (Tucker *et al.*, 2015). In the worse case, sloughing of the outer hoof shells was possibly associated with beta-agonists combined with large amounts of potato starch in the feed (Thomson *et al.*, 2015). These cattle were also fed a high starch diet of potato waste. Most problems are related to a combination of either high doses or hot temperatures greater than 90° F, either shortly before or on the day of slaughter.

Use of Growth Promoters to Reduce the Effects of Detrimental Genetic Selection

Like most people, the author had a knee jerk reaction thinking that all growth promoters such as beta-agonists should be banned. If a whole-systems approach is used, a low dose of beta-agonists late in the feeding period could be used to produce fed market animals with more muscle. This would reduce the motivation of breeders to select parent animals for high muscle growth. Slower growing, hardier parents may be more suitable for use in range land environments where feed is scarce. There are large land areas in both the USA and the Australian outback where there is insufficient water for crops.

Future Genetic Issues

Pushing an animal's biology to the biological overload point can be done by either genetic selection or feed additives. In the future, some of the greatest problems may occur when genomic selection tools become readily available for selection of breeding stock. Powerful genetic tests will make it easier to change animal genetics very quickly. Genomics are genetic 'power tools'. A visual analogy can be used: power tools are good things, but if you make a mistake, a power saw will cut your hand off quicker than a handsaw. Power tools must be used carefully because mistakes that are made in animal selection will be magnified.

Animals Suitable for the Environment

Some American Holsteins are so highly bred for milk production that they have a difficult time living in a hot climate. The OIE in its General Principles of Animal Welfare states that genetic selection should always take into account the health and welfare of the animals (OIE, 2014). A Black Angus bull that performs really well in a temperate zone may have heat stress problems in a hot desert location. Black-hided cattle get hotter. In the hot Mexican tropics, Holsteins are crossed with local cattle to provide resistance to heat stress (Galukande *et al.*, 2013).

Loss of Disease Resistance

In both crops and cattle, monoculture is fabulous in the short term because both crop yields and animal protein yields are increased. In the long term there may be problems due to disease. A narrow minded focus on selecting for production may result in lower disease resistance. It is likely that the price that will have to be paid for increased disease resistance is slightly lowered productivity. Pigs bred for high productivity may have lowered disease resistance (Jiang *et al.*, 2013). In the USA, a big epidemic of porcine epidemic diarrhoea and avian influenza killed 9% of the piglet supply and 11% of laying hens. The PED virus is extremely difficult to remove from feed handling equipment (Schumacher *et al.*, 2017).

The Bright Side of Genetic Technologies

People are too quick to condemn genetic technology. The genomic tests that have been described previously are not a GMO. They are either blood, hair or saliva tests, which measure different parts of the genetic code. Breeding stock chosen with these tests are bred with either natural breeding or artificial insemination. They are tests for choosing breeding animals, not modifying them.

Gene editing can be used to remove horns from cattle. No new DNA is added from another species. When gene editing is used, pieces of genetic code are either removed or rearranged. There is some exciting new research on disease resistance. Whitworth *et al.* (2016) describe a gene editing procedure where a piece of genetic code was removed. This resulted in a pig that had no response to the PRRS virus. When challenged with the virus, nothing happened; there was no sickness and no immune response. The pig's system did not have to use energy to fight the virus. Dosing the pig with the PRRS virus had absolutely no effect. Traits are often linked in unexpected ways. Could an undesirable trait be linked to the PRRS resistance trait? Research with gene editing with CRISPR makes it easy to change the spot pattern on a butterfly's wing (Zhang and Reed, 2016). One must be careful, because the same gene edit may have an effect on the length of the insect's legs. When CRISPR is used to edit genes, it will sometimes edit other genetic code that was not specifically targeted (Chapman *et al.*, 2017; Tykco *et al.*, 2017). To prevent unintended consequences from off-target editing, the entire new genome should be sequenced (Schaefer *et al.*, 2017). Genomic sequencing should be used to 'proofread' the genome for off-target edits.

Conclusions

When farm animals are made more productive with genetic selection, hormones or drugs, people often have a hard time determining what is the optimum level of production. After reading many studies there appear to be basic trade-offs. An animal or bird can be genetically selected to either live a long time and be able to survive on little food, or it is selected to produce lots of milk, meat or eggs and have shorter longevity and higher feed requirements. A common principle in studies with cattle, pigs and poultry shows that excessive selection for production sacrifices traits that would be required for longevity, such as strong bones and maintaining body condition of breeding females. The consumer is going to become increasingly interested in both animal welfare and sustainability. A dairy cow selected to optimize production would require less concentrate such as grain or other feeds high in energy. The cow would be able to eat a diet higher in forages, which would reduce competition with humans for grain (Otenacu and Broom, 2010).

References

Abfalter, K., Brade, W. and Distl, O. (2016) Comparison of breeding values among cows with exceptional longevity and contemporary herdmates in German Holsteins. *Archiv fuer Tierzucht* 59(1), 71–77.

Amachawadi, R.G. and Nagaraja, T.G. (2015) Liver abscesses in cattle: a review of incidence in Holsteins and of bacteriology and vaccine approaches to control in feedlot cattle. *Journal of Animal Science* 94, 1620–1632.

Azarpajouh, S., Colpoys, J., Dekkers, J., Gabler, N., Patience, J. and Johnson, A. (2016) Selection for feed efficiency helps pigs adapt to stressors. *National Hog Farmer* April, 20–25.

Bennett, R., Barker, Z.E., Main, D.C.J., Whay, H.R. and Leach, K.A. (2014) Investigating the value dairy farmers place on a reduction of lameness in their herds using a willingness to pay approach. *The Veterinary Journal* 199, 72–75.

Boyd, B.M., Shackelford, S.D., Hales, K.E., Brown-Brandt, T.M. *et al.* (2015) Effect of shade and feeding zilpaterol hydrochloride to finishing steers on performance, carcass quality, heat stress, mobility and body temperature. *Journal of Animal Science* 93, 5801–5811.

Brotzman, R.L., Dofner, D., Foy, M.R., Hess, J.P., Nordlund, K.V., Bennett, T.B. and Cook, N.B. (2015) Survey of facility and management characteristics of large upper Midwest dairy herds clustered by dairy herd improvement records. *Journal of Dairy Science* 98, 8245–8261.

Burley, H.K., Anderson, K.E., Patterson, P.H. and Tillman, P.B. (2016) Formulation challenges of organic poultry diets with readily available ingredients and limited synthetic methionine. *Journal of Applied Poultry Research* 25(3), 443–454.

Café, L.M., Robinson, D.L., Ferguson, D.M., McIntyre, B.L., Geesink, G.H. and Greenwood, P.L. (2010) Cattle temperament: persistence of assessments and associations with productivity, efficiency, carcass, and meat quality traits. *Journal of Animal Science* 89, 1452–1465.

Collier, R.J., Byatt, J.C., Denham, S.C., Eppard, P.J., Fabellar, A.C. *et al.* (2001) Effects of sustained release bovine somatotropin (sometribove) on animal health in commercial dairy herds. *Journal of Dairy Science* 84, 1098–1108.

Colpays, J.D., Abell, C.E., Young, J.M., Keating, A.F., Gabler, N.K., Millman, S.T., Siegford, J.M. and Johnson, A.K. (2014) Effects of genetic selection for residual feed intake on behavioral reactivity of castrated male pigs to novel stimuli tests. *Applied Animal Behaviour Science* 159, 34–40.

Colpays, J.D., Abell, C.E., Gabler, N.K., Keating, A.F., Millman, S.T., Siegford, J.M., Young, J.M. and Johnson, A.K. (2015) Feed efficiency effects on barrow and gilt behavioral reactivity to novel stimuli. *Journal of Animal Science* 93, 1267–1275.

Cook, N.B., Hess, J.P., Foy, M.R., Bennett, T.B. and Brotzman, R.L. (2015) Management characteristics, lameness, and body injuries of dairy cattle housed in high performance dairy herds in Wisconsin. *Journal of Dairy Science* 99, 1–13.

Dunkelberger, J.R., Boddicker, N.J., Serao, N.V.L., Young, J.M., Rowland, R.R.R. and Dekkers, J.C.M. (2015) Response of pigs divergently selected for residual feed intake to experimental infection with the PRRS virus. *Livestock Science* 177, 132–141.

Floercke, C., Engle, T.E., Grandin, T. and Deesing, M.J. (2012) Individual differences in calf defense patterns in Red Angus beef cows. *Applied Animal Behaviour Science* 139, 203–208.

Fulwider, W.K., Grandin, T., Garrick, D.J., Engle, T.E., Lamm, W.D. *et al.* (2007) Influence of freestall base or tarsal joint lesions and hygiene in dairy cows. *Journal of Dairy Science* 90, 3559–3566.

Galukande, E., Mulindwa, H., Wurzinger, M., Roshinsky, R., Mwai, A.O. *et al.* (2013) Crossbreeding cattle for milk production in the tropics: achievements, challenges, and opportunities. *Animal Genetic Resources* 52, 111–125.

Gonzáles-Cerón, F., Rekaya, R., Anthony, N.B. and Aggrey, S.E. (2014) Genetic analysis of leg problems and growth in random mating broiler population. *Poultry Science* 94(2), 162–168.

Graham, A.L., Hayward, A.D., Watt, K.A., Pilkington, J.G., Pemberton, J.M. and Nussy, D.H. (2010) Fitness correlates to heritable variation in antibody responsiveness in a wild mammal. *Science* 330, 662–665.

Grandin, T. (2010) *Improving Animal Welfare: A Practical Approach*. CAB International, Wallingford, UK.

Grandin, T. (2014) Animal welfare and society concerns: finding the missing link. *Meat Science* 98(3), 461–469.

Grandin, T. and Deesing, M.J. (1998) Behavioral genetics and animal science. In: Grandin, T. (ed.) *Genetics and the Behaviour of Domestic Animals*. Academic Press (Elsevier), San Diego, California, pp. 1–30.

Green, L.E., Huxley, J.N., Barks, C. and Green, M.J. (2014) Temporal associations between low body condition lameness and milk yield in a UK dairy herd. *Preventative Veterinary Medicine* 113, 63–71.

Greer, A.W. (2008) Trade-offs and benefits: implications of promoting a strong immunity to gastrointestinal parasites in sheep. *Parasite Immunology* 30, 123–132.

Hagenmaier, J.A, Reinhardt, C.D., Ritter, M.J., Calvo-Lorenzo, M.S. *et al.* (2017) Effects of ractopomine hydrochloride on growth performance, carcass characteristics and physiological response to different handling techniques. *Journal of Animal Science* 35, 1977–1998.

Hall, N.L., Buchanan, D.S., Anderson, V.L., Ilse, B.R., Carlin, K.R. and Berg, E.P. (2011) Working chute behavior of feedlot cattle can be an indicator of cattle temperament and beef carcass composition and quality. *Meat Science* 89, 52–57.

Hoppe, S., Brandt, H.R., Konig, S.E. and Gauly, M. (2008) Temperament traits of beef calves measured under field conditions and their relationships to performance. *Journal of Animal Science* 88, 1982–1989.

James, B.W., Tokoch, M.D., Goodband, R.D., Nelssen, J.L., Dritz, S.S. *et al.* (2013) Effects of dietary L-Camitine and ractopomine HCl on the metabolic response to handling in finishing pigs. *Journal of Animal Science* 91, 4426–4439.

Jean, I.J., Thompson, J.M. and Dunshea, F.R. (2014) A meta-analysis of Zilpaterol and ractopomine effects on feedlot performance, carcass traits, and shear force strength of meat in cattle. *PLOS ONE* 9(12): el 15904. Available at: http://journals.plos.org/plosone/article?id=10.1371/journal.pone.0115904 (accessed 6 February 2018).

Jiang, C., Xing, F., Xing, J., Jiang, Y. and Zhou, E. (2013) Different expression patterns of PRRSV indicator genes in the lung tissues of PRRSV resistant and susceptible pigs. *Developmental and Comparative Immunology* 39, 127–131.

King, D.A., Schuehle-Pfeiffer, C.E., Randel, R.D., Welsh Jr, T.H., Oliphint, R.A. *et al.* (2006) Influence of animal temperament and stress responsiveness on the carcass quality and beef tenderness of feedlot cattle. *Meat Science* 74, 546–556.

Kronfield, D.S. (1994) Health management of dairy herds treated with bovine somatotropin. *Journal of American Veterinary Medical Association* 204, 116–130.

Kronfield, D.S. (2000) Recombinant somatogropin and animal welfare. *Journal of the American Veterinary Medical Association* 216, 1719–1722.

Le, T.H., Madsen, P., Lundeheim, N., Nilsson, K. and Norberg, E. (2015a) Genetic association between leg conformation in young pigs and sow longevity. *Journal of Animal Breeding and Genetics* 133(4), 283–290.

Le, T.H., Nisson, K., Norberg, E. and Lundeheim, N. (2015b) Genetic association between leg conformation in young pigs and sow longevity. *Livestock Science* 176, 9–17.

Longeragen, G.H., Thomson, D.U. and Scott, H.M. (2014) Increased mortality in groups and cattle administered the ß-adrenergic agonists ractopamine hydrochloride and zilpaterol hydrochloride. *PLOS ONE.* DOI:10.1371/journal.pone.0091177.

Lundeheim, N., Lundgren, H. and Rydhmer, L. (2014) Shoulder ulcers in sows are genetically correlated to leanness of young pigs and to litter weight. *Acta Agriculturae Scandinavica, Section A – Animal Science*, 64, 67–72.

Marchant-Forde, J.N., Lay, D.C. Jr, Pajor, J.A., Richert, B.T. and Schinckel, A.P. (2003) The effects of ractopomine on the behavior and physiology of finishing pigs. *Journal of Animal Science* 81, 416–422.

Marcias-Cruz, U., Alvarez-Valenzuela, F.D., Torrentera, N., Velaquez- Morales, J.V., Correa-Calderon, A. *et al.* (2010) Effect of zilpaterol hydrochloride on feedlot and carcass characteristics of ewe lambs under heat stress condition. *Animal Production Science* 50, 983–989.

Merlot, E., Gilbert, H. and LeFloch, N. (2015) Metabolic responses to inflammatory challenge in pigs divergently selected for feed intake. *Journal of Animal Science* 94, 563–573.

Montgomery, J.L., Krehiet, C.R., Cranston, J.J., Yates, D.A., Hutcheson, J.P., Nichols, T., Streete, M.N., Swingle, R.S. and Montgomery, T.H. (2008) Effects of dietary zilpaterol hydrochloride on feedlot performance and carcass characteristics of beef steers fed without monensin and tylosin. *Journal of Animal Science* 87, 1013–1023.

Mumm, J.M., Stalder, K.J., Stock, J.D., Dekkers, J.C.M. and Calderon Diaz, J.A. (2016) Identification of the range of hock angles in replacement gilts. *Journal of Animal Science* 94 (Suppl. 2), 37.

Neary, J.M., Garry, F.B., Holt, T.N., Thomas, M.G. and Enne, R.M. (2015) Mean pulmonary arterial pressures in Angus steers increase from cow-calf to feedlot finishing phases. *Journal of Animal Science* 93, 3854–3861.

Neutkens, D. (2010) When good pigs die young. *National Hog Farmers*, 16 November.

Newman, J.H., Holt, T.N., Hedges, L.K., Womack, B., Memon, S.S. *et al.* (2011) High-altitude pulmonary hypertension in cattle (brisket disease): candidate genes and gene expression profiling of peripheral blood mononuclear cells. *Pulmonary Circulation* 1, 462–469.

Newman, J.H., Holt, T.N., Cogan, J.D., Wormack, J.A. *et al.* (2015) Increased prevalence of EPASI variant in cattle with high altitude pulmonary hypertension. *Nature Communications* 6, article 6833. DOI: 10-1038/ncomms7863.

Odegard, C., Svendsen, M. and Herringstad, B. (2014) Genetic correlation between claw health and feet and leg conformation in Norwegian red cows. *Journal of Dairy Science* 97, 4622–4629.

OIE (World Organization for Animal Health) (2014) Article 7.1.4. General principles for the welfare of animals in livestock production systems. In: Chapter 7.1 Introduction to the Recommendations for Animal Welfare, Terrestrial Animal Health Code, OIE, Paris.

Olkonomou G., Trojacenec, P., Ganda, E.K., Bicalho, M.L.S. and Bicalho, R.C. (2014) Association of digital cushion thickness with sole temperature measured with use of infrared thermography. *Journal of Dairy Science* 97, 4208–4216.

Olkowski, A.A. and Classen, H.L. (2010) High incidence of cardiac arrhythmias in broiler chickens. *Journal of Veterinary Medicine* 45, 83–91.

Otenocu, P.A. and Broom, D.M. (2010) The impact of genetic selection for increased milk yield on the welfare of dairy cows. *Animal Welfare* 19, 39–49.

Peterson, C.M., Pilcher, C.M., Rothe, H.M., Marchant-Forde, J.N., Ritter, M.J., Carr, N., Puls, C.L. and Ellis, M. (2015) Effect of feeding ractopomine hydrochloride on the growth performance and responses to handling and transport in heavy-weight pigs. *Journal of Animal Science* 93, 1239–1249.

Poletto, R., Garner, J., Cheng, H.W. and Marchant-Forde, J. (2008) The effects of ractopomine, gender and social rank on aggression and peripheral monoamine levels in finishing pigs. *Journal of Animal Science* 86(E.Suppl2) (Abstract 352).

Poletto, R., Rostagno, M.H., Richert, B.T. and Marchant-Forde, J.N. (2009) Effects of a 'step up' ractopomine feeding program, sex, and social rank on growth performance, hoof lesions, and Enterobacteriaceae shedding in finishing pigs. *Journal of Animal Science* 87, 304–313.

Pritchard, T., Coffey, M., Mrode, R. and Wolf, E. (2013) Genetic parameters for production, health, fertility, and longevity traits in dairy cows. *Animal* 7634–7646.

Puls, G.L., Trout, W.E., Ritter, M.J., McKeith, F.K., Carr, S.N. and Ellis, W. (2014) Impact of ractopomine hydrochloride on growth performance, carcass and pork quality characteristics, and responses to handling and transport in finishing pigs. *Journal of Animal Science* 93, 1229–1238.

Randall, L.V., Green, M.J., Chagunda, M.G.G., Mason, C., Archer, S.C., Green, L.E. and Huxley, J.N. (2015) Low body condition predisposes cattle to lameness: an 8-year study of one dairy herd. *Journal of Dairy Science* 98, 3766–3777.

Rauw, W.M. and Gomez-Raya, L. (2015) Genotype by environmental interaction and breeding for robustness in livestock. *Frontiers in Genetics* 6, 310.

Ritter, M.J., Johnson, A.K., Benjamin, M.E., Carr, S.N., Ellis, M., Faucitano, L., Grandin, T. and Goldhawk, C. (2017) Review: effects of ractopomine hydrochloride (Paylean) on welfare indicators for market weight pigs. *Translational Animal Science* 1, 533–558.

Rodenbury, T.B. and Turner, S.P. (2012) The role of breeding and genetics in the welfare of farm animals. *Animal Frontiers* 2, 16–21.

Rohrer, G.A., Brown-Brandt, T., Rempel, L.A. and Hall, J. (2013) Genetic analysis of behavior traits in swine production. *Livestock Science* 157, 28–37.

Rydhmer, L. and Canario, L. (2014) Behavioral genetics in pigs and relations to welfare. In: Grandin, T. and Deesing, M.J. (eds) *Genetics and the Behavior of Domestic Animals* (2nd edn). Academic Press (Elsevier), London.

Scamlin, S.M., Platter, W.J., Gomez, R.A., McKeith, F.K. and Killefer, J. (2009) Comparative effects of ractopomine hydrochloride and zilpateral hydrochloride on growth performance, carcass traits, and longissimus tenderness of finishing steers. *Journal of Animal Science* 88, 1823–1829.

Schaefer, K.A., Wu, W.H., Golgan, D.F., Tsang, S.H. *et al.* (2017) Unexpected modifications after CRISPR Cas9 editing in vivo. *Nature Methods* 14, 547–548.
Schumacher, L.L., Huss, A.R., Cochrane, R.A., Stark, C.R. *et al.* (2017) Characterizing the rapid spread of porcine epidemic diarrhea virus (PED) through an animal food manufacturing facility. *PLOS ONE* 12(11). Available at: http://journals.plos.org/plosone/article?id=10.1371/journal.pone.0187309 (accessed 6 February 2018).
Shook, J.N., Van Overbeke, D.L., Kinman, L.A., Krehbiel, C.R., Holland, B.P. and Streeter, M.N. (2009) Effects of zilpaterol hydrochloride and zilpaterol hydrochloride withdrawal on beef carcass cutability, composition, and tenderness. *Journal of Animal Science* 87, 3677–3685.
Serenius, T., Sevon-Aimonen, M.L. and Mantysaan, E.A. (2001) The genetics of leg weakness in Finnish large white and landrace populations. *Livestock Production Science* 69, 101–111.
Spencer, T.E. (2013) Early pregnancy: concepts, challenges, and potential solutions. *Animal Frontiers* 3, 48–55.
Spurlock, D.W., Dekers, J.C.W., Fernando, R., Koltes, D.A. and Woic, A. (2012) Genetic parameters for energy balance, feed efficiency and related traits in Holstein cattle. *Journal of Dairy Science* 95, 5393–5402.
Thomson, D.L., Longeragan, G.H., Hennington, J.N., Ensley, S. and Bawa, B. (2015) Description of novel fatigue syndrome of finished feedlot cattle following transportation. *Journal of the American Veterinary Medical Association* 247, 66–72.
Trotter, C. (2016) Liver abscesses in pasture based beef bulls in the South Island of New Zealand: the incidence and effect on carcass weight. *Animal Production*. Australian Society of Animal Production, *Proceedings* 109, Abstract NZSp-9.
Tucker, C.B., Calvo-Lorenzo, M.S. and Mitlochner, F.M. (2015) Effect of growth promoting technology on feedlot cattle behavior in the 21 days before slaughter. *Applied Animal Behavior Science* 182, 1–8.
Tycko, J., Myer, V.E. and Hsu, P.D. (2016) Methods of optimizing CRISPR-Cas9 genome editing specificitiy. *Molecular Cell* 63, 355–370.
Van der Spek, D., Van Arendonk, J.A. and Bovenhuis, H. (2015) Genome wide association study for claw disorders and trimming status in dairy cattle. *Journal of Dairy Science* 2, 1286–1295.
Velleman, S.G. (2015) Relationship of skeletal muscle development and growth to breast muscle myopathies: a review. *Avian Diseases* 59, 525–531.
Voisinet, B.D., Grandin, T., Tatum, J.D., O'Connor, S.F. and Struthers, J.J. (1997) Feedlot cattle with calm temperaments have higher average daily gains than cattle with excitable temperaments. *Journal of Animal Science* 75, 892–896.
Vollmar, K. (2016) Survey of prevalence of conformational leg defects in feedlot receiving cattle in the United States. Master's thesis, Colorado State University.
Walsh, S.W., Williams, E.J. and Evans, A.C. (2011) A review of the causes of poor fertility in high milk producing dairy cows. *Animal Reproduction Science* 123, 127–138.
Whitworth, K.M., Rowland, R.R.R., Ewen, C.L., Trible, B.R., Kerrigan, M.A. *et al.* (2016) Gene-edited pigs are protected from porcine reproductive and respiratory syndrome virus. *Nature Biotechnology* 34, 20–22.
Will, D.H., Hicks, J.L., Card, C.S. and Alexander, A.F. (1975) Inherited susceptibility of cattle to high altitude pulmonary hypertension. *Journal of Applied Physiology* 38, 491–494.
Willeberg, P. (1993) Bovine somatotropin and clinical mastitis: epidemiological assessment of the wellbeing risks. *Livestock Science* 36, 55–66.
Young, J.M., Bergsma, R., Knol, E.F., Patience, J.F. and Dekkers, J.C. (2010) Effect of selection for residual feed intake during the grow/finish phase of production on sow reproductive performance and lactation efficiency. *Journal of Animal Science* 94, 4120–4132.
Zhang, L. and Reed, R.D. (2016) Genome editing in butterflies reveals that spalt promotes and distal-less represses eye spot color patterns. *Nature Communications* 7, 11769.

6 Technologies for Increasing the Productivity of Poultry: Welfare Implications

STEFAN GUNNARSSON*

Swedish University of Agricultural Sciences (SLU); Department of Animal Environment and Health, Skara, Sweden

Introduction

Poultry production has been successful in supplying consumers with high-quality protein food, such as chicken meat and hen eggs at a moderate price. Previously, those were expensive in relation to the general cost of living. This development can be illustrated by the price history of frozen whole chicken (recalculated in relative value for comparison), which in Sweden, in 1961, cost around €10/kg, and in 2012 the price had decreased to around €3/kg (Swedish Board of Agriculture and Statistics Sweden, 2013). During the same period, the bird health, in general, improved with regard to infectious diseases. However, the breeding and management procedures that made this dramatic increase in productivity possible have had side effects in terms of the emerging manmade diseases and challenges to animal welfare. In order to make the poultry production sustainable and ethically acceptable to the public, further development in breeding, housing and management of the broiler chickens and the laying hens needs to focus on improvements in bird welfare.

The Common Background of Broiler and Layer Chickens

The red jungle fowl (*Gallus gallus*), originating from southeast Asia, is the main ancestor of the domestic fowl (Gallus *Gallus domesticus*), i.e. the broiler chicken, as well as the laying hen (Hughes *et al.*, 2004). Genetic studies have demonstrated that the domestication occurred about 8000 years ago (Rubin *et al.*, 2010) and recent studies of the chicken genome have revealed that the grey jungle fowl (*Gallus sonneratii*) was involved in the development of the domestic fowl (Eriksson *et al.*, 2008).The primary reason for the domestication was for religious cock fighting, whereas meat, eggs and feathers were probably then by-products of the rearing of fighting cockerels (Hughes *et al.*, 2004). Later, the main purpose for keeping the birds was to get eggs, with the by-product of chicken meat, although in ancient Rome, several breeds were used for various purposes (Wood-Gush, 1959). The management of the domestic fowl in small farmyard flocks appears to have stayed more or less unchanged in Asian and European agriculture

*E-mail: Stefan.Gunnarsson@slu.se

from the start of the domestication until the beginning of the 20th century (Hughes *et al.*, 2004). Eggs and meat were a seasonally restricted but appreciated food source, and the bird flocks were kept extensively outdoors and occasionally offered shelter indoors. The birds were expected to find food by themselves with supplementation of some additional food, mainly domestic waste products. This extensive farming allowed the birds to perform all natural behaviours and establish groups on their own (Hughes *et al.*, 2004). The breeding until industrialization was concerned with various body features including colouring. However, liveability, health and productive performance can be assumed to have influenced their domestication over the centuries. The large genetic variation and adaptability of the domestic fowl made it suitable for almost all climates, from the tropics to the temperate zones (Hughes *et al.*, 2004).

The Conflicting Breeding Goals for Meat and Egg Production

Industrialization brought substantial restructuring of animal production. Thus, poultry production also became specialized and more efficient, and people could no longer have their own backyard chickens in the growing cities. The division in a meat-producing strain versus an egg-producing one occurred around 1900 (Rubin *et al.*, 2010). During the 20th century, intense housing indoors (seasonally or completely) made it possible to control the day length and light intensities with artificial lighting systems, and supported a series of improvements in management and housing in order to reduce risk of disease and increase profit. A higher yield could be obtained from each individual bird, as birds were better fed in relation to their genetic potential.

The breeding of birds specifically for meat production or egg production resolved the conflict of having dual breeding goals, i.e. that demand that the bird should have substantial muscle growth and still lay many eggs. Production was enhanced in both laying hens and broiler chickens, and in general, poultry productivity has increased almost threefold over the last 100 years (Hafez and Hauck, 2005). However, this was not achieved without negative side effects for health and welfare.

Intense breeding, which aimed at increased meat production, made the breeders of broiler chickens consciously select for a large body size, relatively larger pectoral muscles, and rapidity, whereas the layer strains were selected for high egg production (Zuidhof *et al.*, 2014). The breeding process made both broiler and layer chicks larger than the jungle fowl chicks at hatching, but the growth rate is slower in layer chicks than in broilers, and the layer hens have relatively smaller pectoral muscles than broilers, similar to the jungle fowl. The difference in development can be illustrated by the fact that broiler chickens at 42 days old weigh five times more than layer chickens at the same age (Zhao *et al.*, 2004; Druyan, 2010).The body organs of the laying hen have similar proportions to the organs of the jungle fowl, but the laying hen has relatively lighter and shorter intestines than the broiler chicken. Still, both layers and broilers have been intentionally selected for high feed efficiency (Jackson and Diamond, 1996). In studies of molecular genetics, it has been found that the genetic development of the hormonal mechanisms of appetite control in broilers and layers seems to play a main part in the breeding for increased production (Buzala and Janicki, 2016) and that this has been a common breeding path for both broilers and layer chickens. However, it has been found that layer chicks are better in utilizing feed when fed a suboptimal diet (Zhao *et al.*, 2004). There are also indications that the immune capacity of the broiler chickens is inferior or at least different to that of laying hen strains (Koenen *et al.*, 2002; Buzała *et al.*, 2015).

Intentional breeding has side effects on other body morphology and physiology (Jackson and Diamond, 1996). Domestication has general effects on animals, such as increased reproduction and relaxation of behaviours such as fear of humans (Mignon-Grasteau *et al.*, 2005). Nevertheless, it has been found that domestication of the chicken has not led to a regression of the brain mass in the birds, which might be expected judging by what has been found in other species (Henriksen *et al.*, 2016).

Genetic Improvements and Side Effects in Broiler Chickens

Genetics, combined with nutrition and other management changes, has, since the 1950s, resulted in broiler chickens that require less than one third of the time to reach target weight (1815 g) and more than a threefold decrease in the amount of feed consumed (using 2001 as a reference year) (Havenstein *et al.*, 2003a, b). More recent studies have found the same pattern, and Zuidhof *et al.* reported in 2014 that since the 1960s, broiler chickens have seen an increase of 400% growth rate, while the feed conversion ratios have decreased by 50% (Zuidhof *et al.*, 2014).

The increased body growth has changed the body constitution of the broiler chicken considerably, i.e. the breast muscle is double the size in modern broiler chickens compared to birds from strains that have not altered since the 1950s (Schmidt *et al.*, 2009). However, the relative size of the heart is smaller in modern lines compared to heritage line birds, whereas the liver matures earlier and the intestines are 20% longer, possibly due to an adaptation to a more carbohydrate-rich diet (Schmidt *et al.*, 2009).

The rapid changes associated with growth have brought welfare challenges for the broiler chickens. The genetic aims have been to achieve a broiler chicken from fast-growing strains intended for use in production systems with a short rearing period of 4–6 weeks. Thus, this aim has had several side effects, e.g. the increased weight gain and large breast muscles have changed the centre of gravity of the bird, and thereby altered its walking pattern (Corr *et al.*, 2003). The physiological and anatomical changes, together with a high live weight, have been found to be associated with leg weakness and thus decreased activity (Bokkers and Koene, 2004). The limited mobility observed in birds of heavy broiler strains is thought to be an indication of high pressure on a relatively undeveloped skeleton and joints (Corr *et al.*, 2003), which can cause pain (Naas *et al.*, 2009).

In addition, the increasing knowledge of poultry feeding has been crucial for achieving high productivity in modern poultry production (Elwinger *et al.*, 2016). However, when analysing the background to the high productivity in broilers, it has been found that genetic selection has contributed about 85–90% of the change and nutritional development has provided 10–15% (Havenstein *et al.*, 2003a, b). Therefore, it can be assumed that the negative side effects of the increase in productivity can be attributed to genetic transformation, rather than to nutritional aspects. Nevertheless, the negative side effects can be modulated by optimizing feeding, housing and management, e.g. diminishing leg problems in broiler chickens can be observed in flocks where identified risk factors have been eliminated (Knowles *et al.*, 2008).

Health and behavioural problems are related to the fast growth of the broilers, as well as skeletal-biomechanical and other imbalances, and may result in lameness, foot pad dermatitis and circulatory collapse disorders (Havenstein *et al.*, 2003a, 2003b; Bessei, 2006). In particular, heavy birds, including adult birds of broiler strains, i.e. broiler breeders, are increasingly predisposed to pulmonary arterial hypertension, due to increased energy demands on muscle tissue that exceed the capacity of the cardiovascular system to supply oxygen to the body, and thus the circulatory system is more exposed to heart failure and ascites (Buzała *et al.*, 2015).

The Welfare of Broiler Breeders

The breeding of a strain involves several generations including grandparents (GP) and parents (P) and involves housing and managing of birds in order to enhance not only defined breeding goals, but also the health and welfare of all generations.

As mentioned earlier, broiler chickens are increasingly predisposed to pulmonary arterial hypertension, due to increased energy demands of muscle tissue exceeding the capacity of the cardiovascular system to supply oxygen to the body (Buzała *et al.*, 2015). These problems are aggravated with age. Thus, growth effects that are highly productive in broiler chickens reared for early slaughter may have detrimental effects in adult birds. In addition to the previous challenges to broiler health and welfare, the selection in broiler breeder flocks has led to compromised reproductive function due to reduced egg production and decreased fertility and hatchability, and these health problems have been associated with abnormalities in the skeletal system and increased carcass fatness that adult birds may develop (Buzała *et al.*, 2015).

Other welfare problems in broiler breeders are related to the necessary mating between cockerels and hens. The males are quite commonly causing damage to the hens at the moment of mating, e.g. aggressive behaviour and injuries when the cockerels are courting and mounting the hens (De Jong and Guémené, 2011). Paradoxically, it has been found that broiler males show low libido, but, at the same time, more aggressive and rough behaviour during mating, partially due to over-mating (De Jong and Guémené, 2011). In some countries, mutilations, like beak trimming of both males and females, and despurring and toe clipping of males, are performed as a standard procedure to prevent excessive damage, although EU legislation is banning all mutilation (De Jong and Guémené, 2011).

The genetic capacity of the birds is difficult to mitigate with suboptimal food and management factors. However, in order to slow down the growth process to avoid skeletal and circulatory problems, the birds have to be restricted in feeding. A food restriction that would substantially reduce the growth speed is considerable, i.e. the chicks would need to eat only about 50% or less of the ad libitum ration, as applied previously in broiler breed flocks. This means that birds would be hungry throughout the production period, with severe consequences for their welfare (De Jong and Guémené, 2011). The reduction of feed intensity has sometimes been performed using a diet that consists of more bulk, e.g. increased content of non-digestible fibres. Feed restriction in itself has been found to decrease flock uniformity, and the rushed eating and increased competition for feed that go along with it may increase the injurious pecking and other problems. However, the identifying characteristics of individual birds and the habituation to restricted feeding may improve stress coping mechanisms and bird welfare (Lindholm *et al.*, 2015), although the welfare problem of semi-starved birds is not solved, merely moderated.

Genetic Improvements and Side Effects in Laying Hens

In the early 20th century, laying hens were kept in free-range systems; the flock size was a few hundred birds, maximum, and the egg production averaged about 200 eggs/hen/year. Mortalities of 20–30% per year were not uncommon (Leenstra *et al.*, 2016). Thereafter, egg production as well as mortality improved; so in 2015, an average hen is laying 340 eggs/year and the mortality is approximately 6% during a production cycle of 75 weeks (Leenstra *et al.*, 2016). In the selection of laying hens, production, egg weight, body weight, egg quality traits, feed efficiency, disease resistance and single gene traits are important selection criteria. The latter traits are required to sex chicks immediately after hatching (Leenstra *et al.*, 2016). A comprehensive review of the breeding of laying hens has been published by Leenstra *et al.* (2016).

In contrast to the broiler chickens, laying hens are primarily bred for high egg production, but the breeding traits have been associated with development of metabolic diseases such as fatty liver, haemorrhagic syndrome, necrotic haemorrhagic hepatitis and osteoporosis (pathological calcium metabolism). In addition, genetic selection had a less detrimental effect on the immune system of layer hens compared to broiler breeders, which makes the layers more likely to be robust (Buzała *et al.*, 2015).

Since the middle of the 20th century until the beginning of the 21st century, the compact battery cages with small groups of hens in a barren environment have been the dominating housing system. However, increased knowledge of animal welfare and increased public concern about the welfare of the laying hens has required the development of alternative housing systems (Leenstra *et al.*, 2016). Systems replacing battery cages pose different requirements on the birds and genetic selection has to meet these demands. Thus, breeding programmes, recently, have become more diversified in order to supply different systems with more robust birds. Furthermore, in order that the laying hens function well in alternative systems, e.g. decreasing risk of injurious pecking and avoidance of eggs on the floor, rearing involves the pullets in complex housing systems (Gunnarsson *et al.*, 1999; Janczak and Riber, 2015).

In some cases the genetic development has been considered to cause an increase in health and welfare problems, such as injurious pecking, and its behavioural background has been investigated in several studies. It has been found that there is a genetic background to the phenomenon (Jensen *et al.*, 2005). The red jungle fowl is performing feather pecking when housed in indoor pens, so it is not something that has solely come with domestication (Vestergaard *et al.*, 1993). The common way to prevent injurious pecking has been to beak trim the chicks, but the measure is not always effective, and the welfare of the chicks undergoing the mutilation is threatened, even if treatment at younger age is associated with less pain (Gentle, 2011). Several environmental risk factors have been identified for injurious pecking, and minimizing or eliminating these factors, e.g. inadequate feed or litter, improves the situation substantially (Lambton *et al.*, 2013). Genetic advances will probably decrease the risk of developing injurious pecking in laying hens (Leenstra *et al.*, 2016) but it seems unlikely at the moment that it will completely eliminate the behavioural disorder in commercial egg production.

Development and Improvement of Management Methods

Applying the principle of 'all in, all out', i.e. all old birds should be removed from a compartment before new birds are put in, careful cleaning effectively reduced the transmission of disease between bird groups of different ages. To be completely efficient, the 'all in, all out' principle means that all birds in a group should have been hatched and reared together.

Another important part in disease fighting was the development of confined housing systems. They aim to restrict the birds' ability to access manure, and thereby prevent extended spread of intestinal infections such as helminths and coccidia. Cage housing has advantages in limiting not only parasitism but also injurious pecking as the group size of the birds can be limited. However, the restriction of bird behaviour and the barren environment associated with the cage environment affect the behaviour and welfare of laying hens (Elson, 2015). The challenges for the future are to capitalize on the advantages of caged systems and still enhance the natural behaviour and physical exercise of the birds.

Contemporary advances in microbiology made it possible to recognize infectious agents and to systematically test for disease. Suspected disease carriers could be identified and eliminated. This, in combination with the development of antibiotics that could be used against bacterial infections and coccidiosis, made it possible to create the industrial poultry production as we know it today (Hughes *et al.*, 2004). The advances of efficient vaccines for detrimental viral diseases, such as bronchitis and avian encephalomyelitis, cannot be underestimated. These medical advances made it possible to maintain good health in large groups of birds during whole production cycles.

Since the 1940s, antibiotics have been widely used in animal production in order to cure diseases, but shortly after the introduction of therapeutic treatment antibiotics it was found that antibiotic agents (bactericides as well as bacteriostatic drugs) had a growth-stimulating effect in laboratory animals as well as in farm animals (Black *et al.*, 1941; Weber *et al.*, 1952). Quite early on, it was also found that usage of antibiotics could increase production performance by promoting weight gain and increased feed conversion, and already in 1952 Weber *et al.* report that tetracycline, aureomycin or combinations of antibiotic substances were, at that time, widely used in commercial poultry production (Weber *et al.*, 1952). The effect on growth rate was reported to be substantial, e.g. broiler chickens and turkeys may increase their growth rate up to an average of 30% with feed additive of various antibiotics (Weber *et al.*, 1952). The growth promotion effect was thought to depend on reduction of clinical and subclinical disease caused by bacteria and fungi, including the suppression of bacterial toxin production. However, additional physiological effects, e.g. protein metabolism were also postulated (Weber *et al.*, 1952). Since the discovery of antibiotics as a tool for improving animal production in an inexpensive way, the development has been that more antibiotics were used in sub-therapeutic doses in order to achieve growth-promoting effects and preventing subclinical diseases (Silbergeld *et al.*, 2008).

In poultry production, anthelmintics as well as antibiotics are commonly used, although large variations between countries are found; for example, broiler producers in Sweden used a minimum of antibiotics since antibiotics as a feed additive without veterinary prescription were banned in 1988 (Cogliani *et al.*, 2011; Grave *et al.*, 2012). Dutch studies of the epidemiology of extended-spectrum beta-lactamase

(ESBL)-producing bacteria in food-producing animals, and contamination of retail meat, may contribute to increased incidences of infections with ESBL-producing bacteria in humans. These findings are suggestive of transmission of ESBL genes, plasmids and E. coli isolates from poultry to humans, most likely through the food chain (Leverstein-Van Hall *et al.*, 2011). There are indications from the USA that an improvement in the prevalence of antibiotic resistant Salmonella can be achieved due to on-farm changes that make it possible to reduce antibiotics voluntarily in large scale poultry facilities that perform a transition from conventional to organic practices (Sapkota *et al.*, 2014).

In intense broiler chicken production, the usage of drugs, in particular antibiotics, is substantial, and in many countries efficient antibiotics can still be considered a necessity for the development of intense broiler production. Thus, the risk factors associated with intense production need to be tackled in order to enable animal production with minimal antibiotics usage (Gleeson and Collins, 2015). For example, in order to avoid disease outbreaks, the biosecurity needs to be rigorous, but still anti-parasitic drugs are used widely in order to prevent disease outbreaks.

Coccidiosis is a costly parasitic disease in poultry production and mainly affects young and growing birds. Vaccination today is predominately carried out with laying hens, whereas broiler production mainly relies on coccidiostats (Elwinger *et al.*, 2016). In most countries prophylactic antibiotics are used for specific targeting of bacterial diseases, e.g. clostridia (Skinner *et al.*, 2010), but some coccidiostats also have an effect on bacteria, e.g. prophylaxis of clostridia infection (necrotic enteritis caused by *Clostridium perfringens*) (Brennan *et al.*, 2001; Williams, 2002). Therefore withdrawal of coccidiostats would potentially increase the risk of intestinal clostridia infections occurring, if no other measures are taken.

Within the EU, anticoccidial drugs are considered as feed additives and may be put in feed to prevent coccidiosis without veterinary prescription, even if prescription is required in, e.g., Sweden (Elwinger *et al.*, 2016). There are reports of a development of microbial resistance to coccidiostats, but previously these drugs have been considered to have no negative effect on public health (Elwinger *et al.*, 2016). The effects of coccidiostats in poultry is well documented but little is known concerning the consequences of human exposure to coccidiostats-resistant bacteria or to coccidiostats. An extended scientific report has been published in Norway (VKM, 2015). Partly as a consequence of the report, the broiler producers of Norway have decided to phase out the usage of coccidiostats in conventional broiler production. Furthermore, there have been discussions about phasing out coccidiostats within the EU; but although the future status of coccidiostats is uncertain at the current time, the surveillance and control will probably increase in Europe (Elwinger *et al.*, 2016).

In order to fight the common parasitic and bacterial infections in broiler production, the interest in the use of other types of additive that might promote growth or provide other health benefits has increased. For example, probiotic and prebiotic preparations containing non-pathogenic bacteria and different molecules have been marketed as replacements (Elwinger *et al.*, 2016). However, it has been found that antibiotic resistance can be spread by products marketed as probiotics (Sharma *et al.*, 2014), and therefore the introduction of substances replacing antibiotic or antiparasitic drugs should be made with care, and non-chemical prevention should always be considered, i.e. genetic development and improvement of housing and management.

In conventional broiler production, the chickens are reared in large houses with controlled climate at a stocking density of approx. 20 birds/m^2 (i.e. >42 kg live weight). The birds are slaughtered at ~5 weeks of age at target weight of ~2 kg, with a feed conversion rate of ~1.6 kg feed/kg body weight. The housing systems are litter-based; therefore a crucial factor for achieving a low prevalence of contact dermatitis (including foot pad dermatitis, hook burns and breast blisters) is to maintain the litter dry and viable, with adequate ventilation and controlled air humidity (Bessei, 2006). Furthermore, if birds are sitting more on the litter due to locomotor problems, the problems may be more severe (Bessei, 2006).

The housing of laying hens has been transformed substantially since the 1980s, when the battery cage system was common in the entire industrial world. Public concerns for animal welfare, as well as the increased incidence of production diseases, e.g. osteoporosis and feet injuries, initiated intense work on developing alternative housing systems, such as loose housing systems and furnished cages. These systems aim to allow hens to perform essential behaviours such as pecking/scratching, dust-bathing and nesting, and still maintain a good animal environment and high production (Leenstra *et al.*, 2016).

Cage systems provide the birds with a less variable environment and restrict the group size, which decreases the risk of injurious pecking. The hygiene of the few facilities available in the caged system is easier to maintain and less dependent on the quality of the management. Therefore, the risk of exposing the birds to severe welfare threats (including intestinal parasites) is less in caged systems than in more complex systems such as free-range outdoor systems. Furthermore, the production performance and mortality is usually worse in free-range systems than in caged systems, but over the years there are signs of improvement, e.g. the productivity gap between furnished cages and organic production is decreasing, but still there is a difference (Leenstra *et al.*, 2014). However, it has been argued that the modern laying hen strains have poor welfare, irrespective of production systems, and that the high prevalence of emaciation, loss of plumage, fractures and stress are of concern across all housing systems. It suggests that the welfare of modern genotypes is poor in general (Sherwin *et al.*, 2010).

Welfare Concerns in Production of *Foie gras*

The highly specialized production of *foie gras* has been the target of extended animal welfare debate. Although some countries are producing water fowl liver in order to obtain the assumed delicatessen liver with an increased content of fat, French legislation defines the specific product *foie gras* as the liver of a duck or goose fattened by force feeding. The procedure is performed with a feeding tube used in force feeding a corn based diet.

The production of *foie gras* has historically involved geese (*Anseranser*), but in contemporary production it is the mule ducks that constitute the majority of the production (approx. 80%). These are a hybrid between the female common duck (*Anasplatyrhynchos*) and the male muscovy duck (*Cairinamoschata*). In the production of *foie gras*, only livers from force-fed, male mule ducks are accepted, although both sexes are accepted in *foie gras* from geese and muscovy ducks. The production birds are fed ad libitum from hatching until 6–9 weeks of age, then they are fed restrictively for 3–5 weeks. Prior to the force feeding period the birds are fed ad libitum again for 3–10 days in order to increase the digestion capacity of the birds, i.e. increasing crop size and digestive secretion. During this phase the liver steatosis is promoted, although it is considered to be a (pre-)pathological condition in other species. The birds are then prepared for the force feeding, which is typically performed twice daily for 9–12 days and for geese, three times a day for approx. 17 days. Then the ducks are slaughtered at 10–14 weeks and the geese at 16 weeks.

The areas of concerns have been the housing conditions, and the management procedure of the force feeding, which includes catching the bird, introducing a tube into its oesophagus and forcing a large amount (500–600 g per meal) twice daily for almost two weeks (Guémené and Guy, 2004). Although the negative effects of the force feeding procedure – inflammation in the upper digestive tract walls where the tube and forced bolus are introduced – have been considered to be moderate (Serviere *et al.*, 2011), there is controversy about the welfare of the birds in production.

Some aspects of *foie gras* production have been scientifically studied, e.g. the pathology of the accumulation of fat in the liver, but there is still a lack of scientific evidence that force feeding is detrimental to birds, causing pathology, stress and pain. The negative effect of the rearing in individual cages in which ducks are prevented from expressing important behaviours have been cited, even if the scientists performing the studies conclude that it cannot be considered detrimental, as stereotyped behaviour was found to be rare (Guemene *et al.*, 2006). However, it was found that signs of acute and possibly chronic stress were observed in the force feeding and handling procedure (Guemene *et al.*, 2006). Therefore, it may be suggested that the welfare of the *foie gras*-producing birds should be considered througout their whole life as the capture and handling is intermingled with the force feeding procedure. Furthermore, it has been suggested that improvements in housing and management can partly decrease negative impacts on bird welfare (Guemene *et al.*, 2006). Although the different production steps of *foie gras* may not solely be considered detrimental to bird welfare, there are scientific indications that some production steps are associated with negative welfare compared to other possible housing and management of the birds.

Animal Welfare, Animal Ethics, Conflicts and the Possible Future Improvements

As described previously, the development of productivity in poultry production has been most rapid within animal production, possibly competing with fish farming. This process can mainly be attributed to extraordinary genetic development for egg laying hens, but particularly for broiler chickens. Yet methods associated with traditional poultry breeding have been used, i.e. no GMO technique, which has been widely used for increasing productivity.

Enhanced production achievements have been very lucrative as high-quality protein products are produced in large amounts in an inexpensive way; life cycle assessments have found that the resources and energy needed for producing 1 kg of chicken meat is only a fraction of that required for producing pork or beef. Subsequently, the negative environmental impacts of poultry products are diminished in comparison (Cederberg and Flysjö, 2004; Bengtsson and Seddon, 2013; Sonesson *et al.*, 2015). On the other hand, genetic transformations have substantially changed the body and the physiology of the birds, and yet most aspects of the birds' basic behavioural needs have stayed the same. The domestic fowl has the same behavioural needs as the old jungle fowl, although the body of the domestic fowl has been substantially modified.

Thus, features of poultry production really put ethical considerations at the centre. But are these conflicts inevitable? Even if there is an association between speedy growth and impaired welfare (e.g. disproportional body development) in broiler chickens, and this association has been considered to be very strong, this view has been challenged by Dawkins and Layton (2012). This view is partly confirmed by recent genetic analyses of the relationship between body weight, breast meat yield, conformation score and leg soundness traits, which found, in general, a negative but low correlation. Thus, selecting for improved leg health would be possible and still will have little adverse effect on production efficiency (Rekaya *et al.*, 2013). As the productivity improvement of the broiler chick, i.e. its genetic potential, has made the production inexpensive, it is questionable whether a further increase in growth capacity will substantially improve general profitability. The flattening out of the productivity increase due to improved growth speed may make room for improvements in broiler welfare (including health), in terms of breeding a more robust bird. That would probably increase the net productivity and gain wider consumer acceptance.

The spectrum of welfare problems in laying hens varies between production systems. Depending on how much emphasis is put on mortality, morbidity, behavioural needs and natural behaviour, caged and non-caged systems, indoors or outdoors, will score slightly differently in an animal welfare scheme. Animal welfare science and consumer attitudes will, during the foreseeable future, maintain a dynamic market for egg production in various types of housing systems. Thus, there will be a need for breeding and rearing layer chicks in various ways in order for them to function well in the system designated for them. In short, there is a need for bird strains that are adapted to each production system. A way forward here has been proposed by Leenstra *et al.* (2016), which is to widen the breeding into broader objectives in order to produce crossbred birds that are suitable for egg production in various housing systems, including organic systems.

In a distant but not unimaginable future, the techniques of genetic modification may be able to redesign strains of the domestic fowl and alter a single gene of larger parts of the genome. So far, the genetic modification of the chicken has made strains resistant to single infectious diseases, which can produce pharmaceutical substances for treating chronic diseases in humans (Van Eenennaam, 2017). Even though the difficulties of genetic modification of complex features in the chicken should not be underestimated, the history of the modern fowl teaches us that development can be very rapid, if resources are put into target areas like egg and meat production. Let us hope that in the future the public debate on science and ethics continues and that the future sustainability challenges can be mitigated in a responsible way.

References

Bengtsson, J. and Seddon, J. (2013) Cradle to retailer or quick service restaurant gate life cycle assessment of chicken products in Australia. *Journal of Cleaner Production* 41, 291–300. DOI: 10.1016/j.jclepro.2012.09.034.

Bessei, W. (2006) Welfare of broilers: a review. *World's Poultry Science Journal* 62, 455–466. DOI: 10.1079/wps2005108.

Black, S., Mckibbin, J.M. and Elvehjem, C.A. (1941) Use of sulfaguanidine in nutrition experiments. *Experimental Biology and Medicine* 47, 308–310. DOI: 10.3181/00379727-47-13121p.

Bokkers, E.A.M. and Koene, P. (2004) Motivation and ability to walk for a food reward in fast- and slow-growing broilers to 12 weeks of age. *Behavioural Processes* 67, 121–130.

Brennan, J., Bagg, R., Barnum, D., Wilson, J. and Dick, P. (2001) Efficacy of narasin in the prevention of necrotic enteritis in broiler chickens. *Avian Diseases* 45, 210–214. DOI: 10.2307/1593030.

Buzala, M. and Janicki, B. (2016) Review: effects of different growth rates in broiler breeder and layer hens on some productive traits. *Poultry Science* 95, 2151–2159. DOI: 10.3382/ps/pew173.

Buzała, M., Janicki, B. and Czarnecki, R. (2015) Consequences of different growth rates in broiler breeder and layer hens on embryogenesis, metabolism and metabolic rate: a review. *Poultry Science* 94, 728–733. DOI: 10.3382/ps/pev015.

Cederberg, C. and Flysjö, A. (2004) Life cycle inventory of 23 dairy farms in south-western Sweden. *SIK Rapport*, p. 59.

Cogliani, C., Goossens, H. and Greko, C. (2011) Restricting antimicrobial use in food animals: lessons from Europe. *Microbe Magazine* 6, 274–279. DOI: 10.1128/microbe.6.274.1.

Corr, S.A., Gentle, M.J., McCorquodale, C.C. and Bennett, D. (2003) The effect of morphology on walking ability in the modern broiler: a gait analysis study. *Animal Welfare* 12, 159–171.

Dawkins, M.S. and Layton, R. (2012) Breeding for better welfare: genetic goals for broiler chickens and their parents. *Animal Welfare* 21, 147–155. DOI: 10.7120/09627286.21.2.147.

De Jong, I.C. and Guémené, D. (2011) Major welfare issues in broiler breeders. *World's Poultry Science Journal* 67, 73–82. DOI: 10.1017/S0043933911000067.

Druyan, S. (2010) The effects of genetic line (broilers vs. layers) on embryo development. *Poultry Science* 89, 1457–1467. DOI: 10.3382/ps.2009-00304.

Elson, H.A. (2015) Poultry welfare in intensive and extensive production systems. *World's Poultry Science Journal* 71, 449–460. DOI: 10.1017/S0043933915002172.

Elwinger, K., Fisher, C., Jeroch, H., Sauveur, B., Tiller, H. and Whitehead, C.C. (2016) A brief history of poultry nutrition over the last hundred years. *World's Poultry Science Journal* 72, 701–720. DOI: 10.1017/S004393391600074X.

Eriksson, J., Larson, G., Gunnarsson, U., Bed'hom, B., Tixier-Boichard, M. *et al.* (2008) Identification of the yellow skin gene reveals a hybrid origin of the domestic chicken. *PLOS Genetics* 4, e1000010. DOI: 10.1371/journal.pgen.1000010.

Gentle, M.J. (2011) Pain issues in poultry. *Applied Animal Behaviour Science* 135, 252–258. DOI: 10.1016/j.applanim.2011.10.023.

Gleeson, B.L. and Collins, A.M. (2015) Under what conditions is it possible to produce pigs without using antimicrobials? *Animal Production Science* 55, 1424–1431. DOI: 10.1071/AN15271.

Grave, K., Greko, C., Kvaale, M.K., Torren-Edo, J., Mackay, D., Muller, A. and Moulin, G. (2012) Sales of veterinary antibacterial agents in nine European countries during 2005–09: trends and patterns. *Journal of Antimicrobial Chemotherapy* 67, 3001–3008. DOI: 10.1093/jac/dks298.

Guémené, D. and Guy, G. (2004) The past, present and future of force-feeding and 'foie gras' production. *World's Poultry Science Journal* 60, 210–222. DOI: 10.1079/WPS200314.

Guemene, D., Guy, G., Noirault, J., Destombes, N. and Faure, J.M. (2006) Rearing conditions during the force-feeding period in male mule ducks and their impact upon stress and welfare. *Animal Research* 55, 443–458. DOI: 10.1051/animres:2006028.

Gunnarsson, S., Keeling, L.J. and Svedberg, J. (1999) Effect of rearing factors on the prevalence of floor eggs, cloacal cannibalism and feather pecking in commercial flocks of loose housed laying hens. *British Poultry Science* 40, 12–18. DOI: 10.1080/00071669987773.

Hafez, H.M. and Hauck, R. (2005) Genetic selection in turkeys and broilers and their impact on health conditions. World Poultry Science Association, 4th European Poultry Genetics Symposium, Dubrownik, Croatia.

Havenstein, G.B., Ferket, P.R. and Qureshi, M.A. (2003a) Carcass composition and yield of 1957 versus 2001 broilers when fed representative 1957 and 2001 broiler diets. *Poultry Science* 82, 1509–1518.

Havenstein, G.B., Ferket, P.R. and Qureshi, M.A. (2003b) Growth, livability, and feed conversion of 1957 versus 2001 broilers when fed representative 1957 and 2001 broiler diets. *Poultry Science* 82, 1500–1508.

Henriksen, R., Johnsson, M., Andersson, L., Jensen, P. and Wright, D. (2016) The domesticated brain: genetics of brain mass and brain structure in an avian species. *Scientific Reports* 6, 34031. DOI: 10.1038/srep34031.

Hughes, B.O., Appleby, M.C. and Mench, J.A. (2004) *Poultry Behaviour and Welfare*. CAB International, Wallingford, UK.

Jackson, S. and Diamond, J. (1996) Metabolic and digestive responses to artificial selection in chickens. *Evolution* 50, 1638–1650. DOI: 10.2307/2410900.

Janczak, A.M. and Riber, A.B. (2015) Review of rearing-related factors affecting the welfare of laying hens. *Poultry Science* 94, 1454–1469. DOI: 10.3382/ps/pev123.

Jensen, P., Keeling, L., Schütz, K., Andersson, L., Mormède, P. *et al*. (2005) Feather pecking in chickens is genetically related to behavioural and developmental traits. *Physiology & Behavior* 86, 52–60.

Knowles, T.G., Kestin, S.C., Haslam, S.M., Brown, S.N., Green, L.E. *et al*. (2008) Leg disorders in broiler chickens: prevalence, risk factors and prevention. *PLOS ONE* 3, e1545. DOI: 10.1371/journal.pone.0001545.

Koenen, M.E., Boonstra-Blom, A.G. and Jeurissen, S.H.M. (2002) Immunological differences between layer- and broiler-type chickens. *Veterinary Immunology and Immunopathology* 89, 47–56. DOI: 10.1016/S0165-2427(02)00169-1.

Leenstra, F., Maurer, V., Galea, F., Bestman, M., Amsler-Kepalaite, Z., Visscher, J., Vermeij, I. and Van Krimpen, M. (2014) Laying hen performance in different production systems: Why do they differ and how to close the gap? Results of discussions with groups of farmers in The Netherlands, Switzerland and France: benchmarking and model calculations. *European Poultry Science* 78. DOI: 10.1399/eps.2014.53.

Leenstra, F., Ten Napel, J., Visscher, J. and Van Sambeek, F. (2016) Layer breeding programmes in changing production environments: a historic perspective. *World's Poultry Science Journal* 72, 21–35. DOI: 10.1017/S0043933915002743.

Leverstein-Van Hall, M.A., Dierikx, C.M., Stuart, J.C., Voets, G.M., Van Den Munckhof, M.P. *et al*. (2011) Dutch patients, retail chicken meat and poultry share the same ESBL genes, plasmids and strains. *Clinical Microbiology and Infection* 17, 873–880. DOI: 10.1111/j.1469-0691.2011.03497.x.

Lindholm, C., Calais, A., Jonsson, J., Yngwe, N., Berndtson, E., Hult, E. and Altimiras, J. (2015) Slow and steady wins the race? No signs of reduced welfare in smaller broiler breeder hens at four weeks of age. *Animal Welfare* 24, 447–454. DOI: 10.7120/09627286.24.4.447.

Mignon-Grasteau, S., Boissy, A., Bouix, J., Faure, J.M., Fisher, A.D. (2005) Genetics of adaptation and domestication in livestock. *Livestock Production Science* 93, 3–14. DOI: 10.1016/j.livprodsci.2004.11.001.

Naas, I.A., Paz, I.C.L.A., Baracho, M.S., Menezes, A.G., Bueno, L.G.F., Almeida, I.C.L. and J.M.D. (2009) Impact of lameness on broiler well-being. *Journal of Applied Poultry Research* 18, 432–439.

Rekaya, R., Sapp, R.L., Wing, T. and Aggrey, S.E. (2013) Genetic evaluation for growth, body composition, feed efficiency, and leg soundness. *Poultry Science* 92, 923–929. DOI: 10.3382/ps.2012-02649.

Rubin, C.-J., Zody, M.C., Eriksson, J., Meadows, J.R.S., Sherwood, E. *et al*. (2010) Whole-genome resequencing reveals loci under selection during chicken domestication. *Nature* 464, 587–591.

Sapkota, A.R., Kinney, E.L., George, A., Hulet, R.M., Cruz-Cano, R. *et al.* (2014) Lower prevalence of antibiotic-resistant Salmonella on large-scale US conventional poultry farms that transitioned to organic practices. *Science of the Total Environment* 476, 387–392. DOI: 10.1016/j.scitotenv.2013.12.005.

Schmidt, C.J., Persia, M.E., Feierstein, E., Kingham, B. and Saylor, W.W. (2009) Comparison of a modern broiler line and a heritage line unselected since the 1950s. *Poultry Science* 88, 2610–2619. DOI: 10.3382/ps.2009-00055.

Serviere, J., Carriere, M., Duvaux-Ponter, C., Guy, G. and Roussel, S. (2011) Neurogenic inflammation in the upper digestive tract of the mule duck: effect of a chemical algogen and force-feeding. *British Poultry Science* 52, 792–799. DOI: 10.1080/00071668.2011.640660.

Sharma, P., Tomar, S.K., Goswami, P., Sangwan, V. and Singh, R. (2014) Antibiotic resistance among commercially available probiotics. *Food Research International* 57, 176–195. DOI: 10.1016/j.foodres.2014.01.025.

Sherwin, C.M., Richards, G.J. and Nicol, C.J. (2010) Comparison of the welfare of layer hens in 4 housing systems in the UK. *British Poultry Science* 51, 488–499. DOI: 10.1080/00071668.2010.502518.

Silbergeld, E.K., Graham, J. and Price, L.B. (2008) Industrial food animal production, antimicrobial resistance, and human health. *Annual Review of Public Health* 29, 151–169. DOI: 10.1146/annurev.publhealth.29.020907.090904.

Skinner, J.T., Bauer, S., Young, V., Pauling, G. and Wilson, J. (2010) An economic analysis of the impact of subclinical (mild) necrotic enteritis in broiler chickens. *Avian Diseases* 54, 1237–1240. DOI: 10.1637/9399-052110-Reg.1.

Sonesson, U.G., Lorentzon, K., Andersson, A., Barr, U.-K., Bertilsson, J. *et al.* (2015) Paths to a sustainable food sector: integrated design and LCA of future food supply chains: the case of pork production in Sweden. *The International Journal of Life Cycle Assessment* 1–13. DOI: 10.1007/s11367-015-0969-5.

Swedish Board of Agriculture and Statistics Sweden, S. (2013) Jordbruksstatistisk årsbok 2014 (*Yearbook of Agricultural Statistics 2014*).

Van Eenennaam, A.L. (2017) Genetic modification of food animals. *Current Opinion in Biotechnology* 44, 27–34. DOI: 10.1016/j.copbio.2016.10.007.

Vestergaard, K.S., Kruijt, J.P. and Hogan, J.A. (1993) Feather pecking and chronic fear in groups of red junglefowl: their relations to dustbathing, rearing environment and social status. *Animal Behaviour* 45, 1127–1140.

Vkm (2015) *The Risk of Development of Antimicrobial Resistance with the Use of Coccidiostats in Poultry Diets (Opinion of the Panel on Animal Feed of the Norwegian Scientific Committee for Food Safety)*. Panel on Animal Feed of the Norwegian Scientific Committee for Food Safety, Oslo. Available at: https://brage.bibsys.no/xmlui/handle/11250/2463088 (accessed 24 January 2018).

Weber, E.M., Luther, H.G. and Reynolds, W.M. (1952) Antibiotics as animal-growth stimulants. *Bulletin of the World Health Organization* 6, 149–161.

Williams, R.B. (2002) Fifty years of anticoccidial vaccines for poultry (1952–2002). *Avian Diseases* 46, 775–802. DOI: 10.1637/0005-2086(2002)046[0775:fyoavf]2.0.co;2.

Wood-Gush, D.G.M. (1959) A history of the domestic chicken from antiquity to the 19th century. *Poultry Science* 38, 321–326.

Zhao, R., Muehlbauer, E., Decuypere, E. and Grossmann, R. (2004) Effect of genotype–nutrition interaction on growth and somatotropic gene expression in the chicken. *General and Comparative Endocrinology* 136, 2–11. DOI: 10.1016/j.ygcen.2003.11.009.

Zuidhof, M.J., Schneider, B.L., Carney, V.L., Korver, D.R. and Robinson, F.E. (2014) Growth, efficiency, and yield of commercial broilers from 1957, 1978, and 2005. *Poultry Science* 93, 2970–2982. DOI: 10.3382/ps.2014-04291.

7 Selective Breeding, Cloning and Gene Editing of Dogs and Cats for Appearance and Performance Traits

Rowena M.A. Packer*

Department of Clinical Science and Services, Royal Veterinary College, University of London

Introduction

Humans have manipulated and altered animals by domestication and selective breeding for thousands of years, breeding and rearing a multitude of species to meet their varied needs. Extremes of selection for specific traits have been documented to lead to unintended changes in other traits, which can be pathological, e.g. lameness in highly productive dairy cows and broiler chickens, and birthing complications in heavily muscled Belgian Blue cattle. Complications of selection are not limited to production animals, and indeed the species that often live in the closest proximity to human beings, companion animals, are increasingly affected by welfare problems associated with selective breeding. It is estimated that in the UK alone over 10.5 million dogs and 10.3 million cats are kept as companion animals (Murray *et al.*, 2010). These animals represent a vast array of breeds and crossbreeds, with a huge human appetite for variation and often extreme appearance in their pets. This chapter will focus on the process of domestication and selective breeding in the dog (*Canis familiaris*) and cat (*Felis silvestris*), how these processes have resulted in the modern-day cat and dog, and how pushing the limits of these species' biology has led to concerns about their welfare. Finally, it will explore the future of genetically manipulating companion animals, with advances in biotechnology opening new avenues to moulding man's best friends.

Domestication of the Dog and Cat

The dog (*Canis familiaris*) is believed to be the first animal to be domesticated by man (Robinson, 1999) and the only member of the Canidae family to be fully domesticated. Domestication has been defined as: 'The capture and taming by man of animals of species with particular behavioural characteristics, their removal from their natural living area and breeding community, and their maintenance under breeding conditions

*E-mail: rpacker@rvc.ac.uk

for mutual benefits' (Bökönyi, 1989). The wild gray wolf (*Canis lupus*) is widely accepted to be the ancestral species of the dog (Vila *et al.*, 1997). Archaeological evidence has indicated that domestication may have occurred as early as 14,000–15,000 years ago (Nobis, 1979); however, more recent genetic studies of mtDNA have estimated over 100,000 years ago (Vila *et al.*, 1997). The near eastern wildcat (*Felis silvestris lybica*) is considered the progenitor species of the modern cat, attracted to human food sources in early agricultural settlements, with evidence for close cat–human relationships from archaeological sources in Cypus *c.*9500 years ago (Vigne *et al.*, 2012) and depictions of domesticated cats in Egyptian art *c.*4000 years ago (Faure and Kitchener, 2009). In contrast to dogs, cats are only considered semi-domesticated, with many populations of cats not isolated from wildcats, with humans not controlling their food supply or breeding (Cameron-Beaumont *et al.*, 2002).

Impact of domestication

Many physical changes are commonly induced by domestication, including alterations in body and brain size, external appearance, gaining a fat layer beneath the skin and a reduction of the facial skull (Clutton-Brock, 1999). Alterations in the proportions of the skull and a reduction in cranial capacity is typical of many different species of mammal being domesticated (Hemmer, 1990). These physical changes are considered a by-product of selection for docility (Wayne, 2001). The concomitant morphological changes of domestication were observed in the seminal silver fox domestication experiments of Belyaev, in which selection for a purely behavioural trait (tameness) had surprising morphological consequences, including floppy ears, rolled/shortened tails and maloccluded teeth, along with coat colour mutations that are often seen in domesticated mammals (Trut, 1999). The signatures of selection in the domestic cat genome are primarily linked to behaviour, including genes associated with memory, fear-conditioning behaviour, and stimulus reward learning (Montague *et al.*, 2014). Morphological divergence between the domestic cat and the near eastern wildcat is unremarkable, with increased gracility and variation in pigmentation the only exceptions. In contrast to the cat, the morphology of the domestic dog is markedly different from the gray wolf. Dogs have undergone pedomorphosis, with traits previously only seen in juvenile wolves observed in adult dogs (Goodwin *et al.*, 1997). Along with a general decrease in body size, domestic dogs exhibit smaller teeth, a shortening of the skull, a change in hair colour and tail carriage, and a decrease in the brain-to-body size ratio (Clutton-Brock, 1995).

Artificial Selection of the Dog and Cat

Although passive morphological change associated with domestication had an influence upon morphology, the dogs and cats that we see today are not just the product of thousands of years of domestication; they also show the effects of selective breeding, a process that has the power to bring about rapid morphological changes (O'Regan and Kitchener, 2005). Indeed, the development of the Pekingese skull from that of the wolf has been described as 'one of the most extraordinary examples known of morphological variation within a single biological species' (Clutton-Brock, 1995). Selective breeding in the early stages of the domestic dog was likely to have been heavily based on behavioural characteristics, with only tractable, obedient dogs being bred from; however, in the later stages, morphological selection led to different 'types' of dog (groups with recognizable morphologies) being developed to fulfil varied human requirements (Clutton-Brock, 1995). The description of the functions and co-occurring morphologies of groups of dogs has been documented since the Romans, before AD 70. The Romans are considered the first to have developed primitive 'breeds' of dog including *Canes pastorales* (sheepdogs), *Canes villatici* (watch-dogs), and *Canes venatici* (hunting dogs) (Drury, 1903). The segregation of 'types' of dog has continued over the last 800 years, with the era for the great proliferation of dog 'types' in Europe primarily during the Middle Ages, from the 13th to the 15th centuries. In John Caius's book *De Canibus Britannicus*, four main groups of dog were defined: hunting dogs, spaniel gentle or comforter, farm dogs and mongrels (Caius, 1576). This classification was built upon by Linnaeus, first to name the domestic dog *familiaris* in his work *Systema naturae* (Linnaeus, 1792).

The domestic cat was first classified as *Felis catus* in 1758 by Linnaeus, and this nomenclature is still the most commonly used. Despite the wide and rapid initial spread of the cat across the world, cats have remained remarkably similar in form and function to their ancestors (Dobney and Larson, 2006), in part influenced by gene flow between feral and tame domestic cats and their wild subspecies (Beaumont *et al.*, 2001). Selection of cats has historically been based on appearance, with cats unsuited to the herding, hunting and guardianship roles fulfilled by domestic dogs. Consequently, the development of 'types' and formalized breeds was less prominent and occurred at a later date. Much of the initial variation in domestic cats was thought to represent regional variation, with 'natural breeds' that predate pedigree cat breeding still recognized today (Wastlhuber, 1991).

Companion Animal Breeds

Today, domestic cats and dogs are primarily kept as companion animals. The development of breeds is common to many domesticated species, with a breed defined as animals of 'uniform groups with similar physical characteristics, shaped by selection rooted in human preferences' (Bjornerfeldt *et al.*, 2008). At present, 220 individual breeds of dog are recognized by the Kennel Club (UK), with the level of morphological variation displayed in them exceeding that observed in wild species, and comparable to the disparity throughout the Order Carnivora (Drake and Klingenberg, 2010). The proliferation in cat breeds has been more limited, with 30–40 genetically distinct cat breeds identified (Kurushima *et al.*, 2013), 36 registered with the Governing Council of the Cat Fancy (GCCF). To create new breeds, discrete mutations (also termed 'sports') that resulted in novel phenotypic characteristics were captured and selected for by breeders (Darwin, 1859). To fix these traits, animals exhibiting these mutations were inbred to increase homozygosity and reduce genetic variation, so that desired physical and behavioural traits became increasingly heritable (Arman, 2007). The rapid genesis of breeds from small founding populations suggests that a small number of genes with large effects are responsible for many characteristics that define breeds (Pollinger *et al.*, 2005). The formalized reproductive isolation of breeds is considered a recent human invention, with the majority of cat and dog breeds created since the mid-19th century. Pedigree registration bodies worldwide have played a pivotal role in the development and maintenance of 'breed' rather than 'type', enforcing 'breed barrier' rules, whereby no animal may become a registered member of a breed unless both its dam and sire are registered members. Breed barriers ensures relatively closed gene pools and were first introduced by the Victorians in the 19th century in the UK, with the Kennel Club founded in 1873, and the Governing Council of the Cat Fancy founded in 1910. The first canine stud book was published by the Kennel Club in 1874 listing 40 breeds, and the first feline stud book published in 1910 with just five breeds listed.

Breed Standards

During this early period, breeding organizations developed the concept of the breed standard, the blueprint for the 'perfect' example of each breed, described by qualitative and quantitative descriptors. During cat and dog shows, animals entered are judged on the extent to which they conform to the breed standard. Once created, breeds are not necessarily phenotypically static due to within-breed variation allowing for refinement of desired traits over generations, with breed standards also revised over time. There are now major concerns that many modern breed standards no longer encourage healthy, functional morphologies, and encourage body shapes that no longer confer on dogs the capability to perform the tasks for which they were originally bred (Arman, 2007). Rather than a desire for utility, many breeders are now thought to select for 'showy' or 'stylish' looks that often become distorted, mimicked exaggerations of the original breed standards (Fox, 1972). This has led to 'extreme' breeds, exhibiting increasingly exaggerated characteristics in the pursuit of type, where the attitude of 'if something in a dog's appearance is good, then more of it must be better' prevails. This may be due to several reasons, including:

1. **Loss of physical function**. The original functions of some breeds are now no longer required, allowing for the selection of phenotypes which may have previously hindered performance. For example, when bull baiting was banned in the 1800s, bulldogs were no longer used for this sport, which allowed bulldog breeders to select for non-functional traits, such as larger heads and less athletic body shapes (Fig. 7.1). In 1998, the bulldog breed standard stated: 'The skull should be very large, the larger the better.'
2. **Lack of physical utility**. Some breeds were originally bred for a purely companion role, in which physical demands are low. This is true for the majority of cats and some dog breeds including those considered 'lap dogs' or 'sleeve dogs', e.g. the Pekingese, one of the oldest breeds of dog originally bred in ancient China to fit inside the sleeves of a man's robe (Parker *et al.*, 2004). In this role, physical expectations are minimal and selection pressures can divert from physical function to appearance and behaviour.
3. **The advent of 'show lines'**. Some dogs within breeds that maintain a working function are not all used for that purpose, instead being bred for competition in conformational shows. The primary selection pressure in this role is upon appearance and meeting the breed standard as closely as possible.

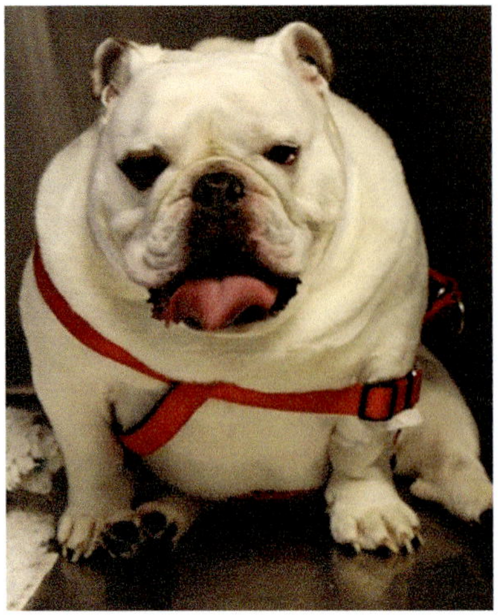

Fig. 7.1. A modern bulldog exhibiting a large, broad skull, flattened face, broad shoulders and obese body condition (photo: R.M.A. Packer).

Separating Form and Function and the Reversal of Natural Selection

Separation of form and function has potentially profound effects upon canine health. When form follows function and performance is the primary characteristic selected for, health and conformation are indirectly selected for, as to be able to perform well in a functional working role only healthy dogs with healthy conformations will perform well (Maki *et al.*, 2005). In contrast, when appearance is prioritized, traits that are directly implicated in health problems can be allowed to proliferate, and even be encouraged, and insufficient selection pressure may be exerted on traits that would improve animal welfare (McGreevy and Nicholas, 1999). In nature, animals predisposed to health problems would have correspondingly lower evolutionary fitness and would therefore be less likely to successfully compete with healthier counterparts, reproduce and survive. Under human care, animals predisposed to health problems may survive and intentionally be selected for, encouraging traits that are not in an animal's best interests. In some cases, pathological characteristics have been favoured, with animals 'protected' from the effects of natural selection by veterinary intervention, allowing such characteristics to be perpetuated. Human selection for pathological morphologies has literally reversed the effects of natural selection. A startling example of this is the selection of dogs with large heads and narrow pelvic girdles who are unable to give birth naturally due to fetopelvic disproportion (where the skull of the pups is too large to pass through the mother's pelvis naturally). Caesarean sections are required to allow these conformations to persist; indeed, the rate of caesareans in the Boston terrier, English bulldog and French bulldog exceeds 80% (Evans and Adams, 2010). The similar conformation of the Persian cat is also considered at increased risk of obstruction in the birth canal (Wilkinson, 1984). Without veterinary interventions, many mothers and offspring would not survive, and breeds exhibiting these characteristics could not exist.

Extreme Morphologies

The selection of extreme morphologies that run counter to dog welfare is a major concern in pedigree dog and cat breeding. Indeed, it has been thought that many companion animal breeds effectively have become 'handicapped' by selection for traits that appeal to our anthropomorphic perceptions (Serpell, 2002). In Germany, the word *qualzuchten* ('torture breeding') has been used to describe 'defective breeds' that have been bred for extreme morphological, physiological or behavioural characteristics (Steiger, 2005). Evidence for the link between exaggerated morphologies and inherited disease is often based on the high prevalence of specific conditions in breeds exhibiting shared extreme phenotypes. A recent systematic review of inherited disease in dogs identified 63 disorders directly associated with conformation in the top 50 Kennel Club breeds (Asher *et al.*, 2009). Table 7.1 outlines several exaggerated conformations that have been linked to inherited disorders in the veterinary literature.

Recent evidence in dogs has demonstrated that as conformations become more exaggerated, the risk of disease correspondingly increases (Packer *et al.*, 2013; Packer *et al.*, 2015a, b). For example, as relative back length increases, the risk of painful and debilitating intervertebral disc extrusions increases, in 'long and low' breeds such as dachshunds (Packer *et al.*, 2013) (Fig. 7.2).

Table 7.1. Exaggerated conformations linked to inherited disorders in the veterinary literature.

Conformational feature	Associated disorder(s)	Example breeds
Short muzzle	Brachycephalic obstructive airway syndrome (Packer *et al.*, 2015b) Dental disease (Hale, 2013) Epiphora (Schlueter *et al.*, 2009)	Pug, Bulldog, French Bulldog, Pekingese, Boston Terrier, Persian
Large head	Dystocia (Evans and Adams, 2010)	Bulldog
Large eyes	Corneal ulcers (Packer *et al.*, 2015a)	Pug, Cavalier King Charles Spaniel
Small eyes	Entropion (Barnett, 1988)	Chow Chow
Corkscrew tail	Fold dermatitis (Hodgman, 1963) Pyoderma (Toma *et al.*, 2008) Hemivertebrae (Done *et al.*, 1975)	Pug, Bulldog
Pendulous ears	Otitis externa/media (Hayes *et al.*, 1987)	Cocker Spaniel, Basset Hound
Heavy facial fold	Fold dermatitis (Hodgman, 1963) Pyoderma (Toma *et al.*, 2008) Corneal ulcers (Packer *et al.*, 2015a)	Pug, Bulldog
Drooping eyelid conformation – 'diamond eye'	Ectropion and entropion (Hodgman, 1963)	Basset Hound, Saint Bernard, Bloodhound
Deep chest	Splenic torsion (Neath *et al.*, 1997) Gastric torsion (Brockman *et al.*, 1995) Lung lobe torsion (Neath *et al.*, 2000)	Great Dane, German Shepherd Dog
Wrinkled skin	Cutaneous mucinosis (Muller, 1990)	Shar Pei
Long back	Intervertebral disc extrusion (Goggin *et al.*, 1970)	Dachshund, Basset Hound, Pekingese

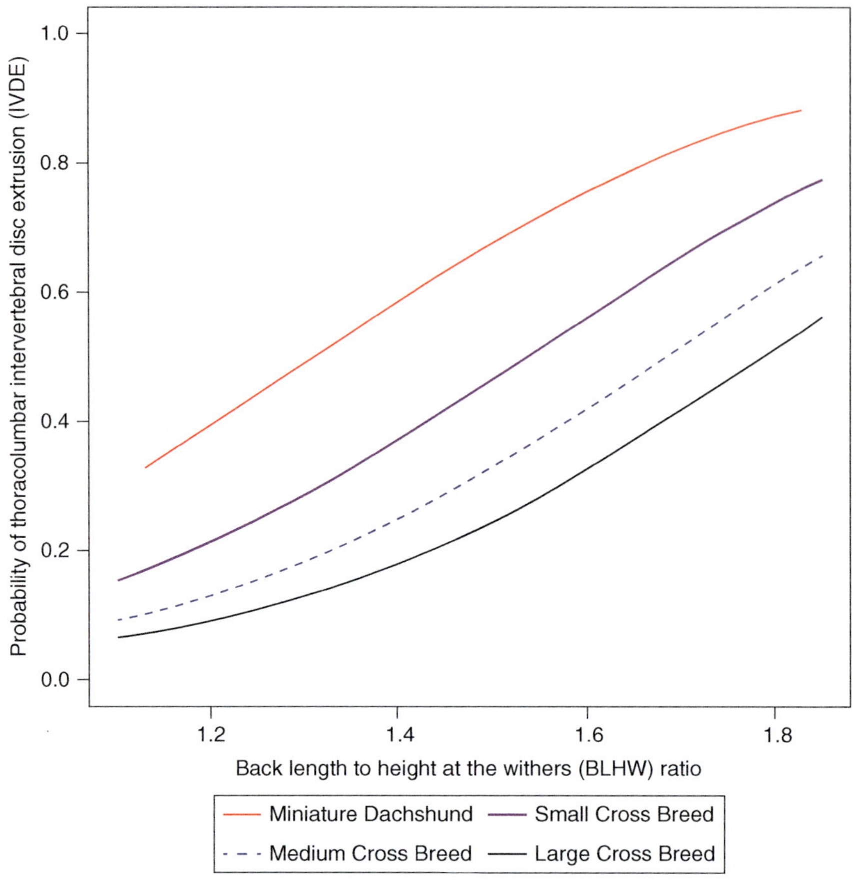

Fig. 7.2. The probability of being affected by a thoracolumbar intervertebral disc extrusion ('slipped disc') across the relative back length spectrum. As relative back lengths become longer, the risk increases. The miniature dachshund is the highest-risk breed for this disorder.

Case Study: Extreme Brachycephaly

A prominent example of the consequences of extreme conformation is that of brachycephaly, breeding for a short and wide skull shape with a markedly foreshortened muzzle. This conformation is encouraged in breed standards through phrases such as 'muzzle short' and has been selected to extremes in breeds such as the pug (Fig. 7.3). The dramatically shortened skeleton of muzzle of brachycephalic breeds results in a 'space problem', where the soft tissues of the head and neck, including the soft palate, tongue and tonsils, no longer fit, obstructing the larynx during respiration. This obstruction is often compounded by the nasal turbinates often being abnormally positioned in the nasopharynx (Ginn *et al.*, 2008), and congenitally narrowed nostrils ('stenotic nares') reducing nasal airflow and impeding thermoregulation. This disorder, brachycephalic obstructive airway syndrome, manifests as laboured and difficult breathing, abnormal respiratory noise, exercise intolerance and overheating. As muzzles get relatively shorter (as reflected by the 'craniofacial ratio'), the risk of BOAS increases dramatically, with the most extreme flat faces almost inevitably affected (Fig. 7.4) (Packer *et al.*, 2015b). In addition to the lack of space for soft tissues, teeth are often crammed within the mouth, predisposing brachycephalic dogs to periodontal disease (Hale, 2013).

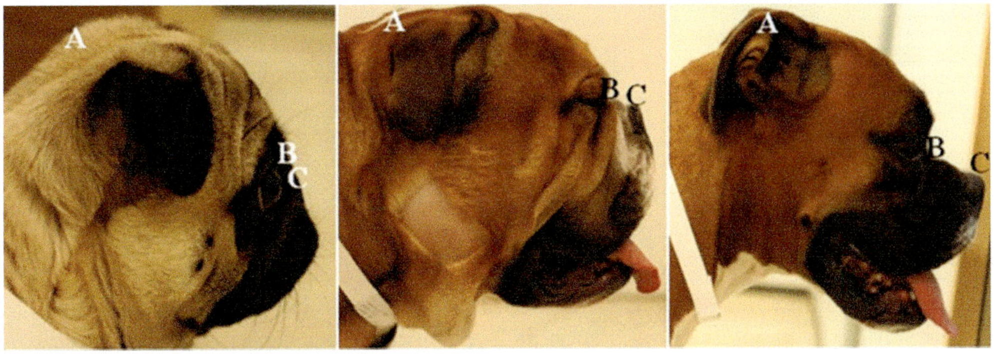

Fig. 7.3. Three brachycephalic dogs demonstrating differing degrees of brachycephaly. From left to right, the pug (extreme brachycephalic), a bulldog cross (moderately brachycephalic) and a boxer (mildly brachycephalic). Note the reduction in distance between (B) the stop and (C) the dorsal tip of the nasal planum in comparison to the distance between (A) the occipital protuberance and (B). (Photo: R.M.A. Packer).

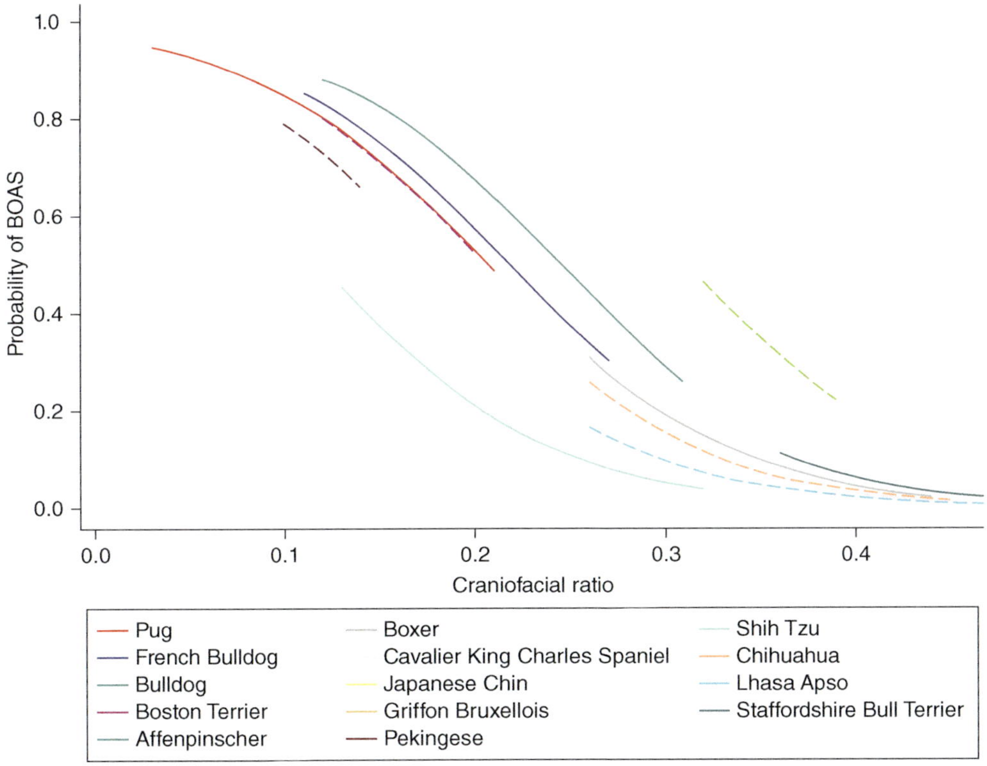

Fig. 7.4. Predicted probability of brachycephalic dog breeds being affected by brachycephalic obstructive airway syndrome (BOAS) across relevant craniofacial ratio (CFR) ranges. As craniofacial ratio decreases (muzzles become shorter), the risk of BOAS increases.

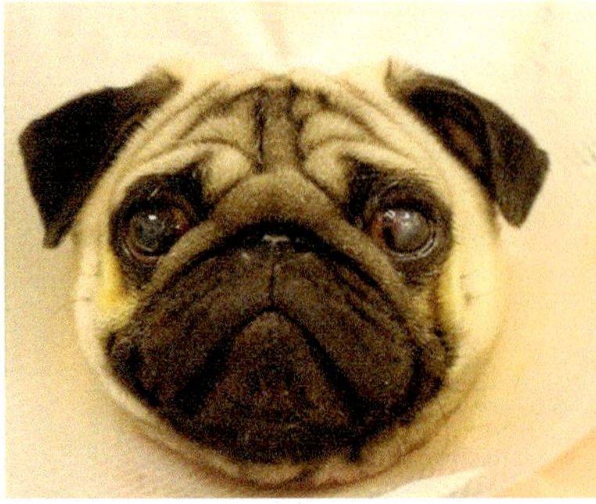

Fig. 7.5. A pug undergoing treatment for corneal ulceration as a result of chronic exposure to the cornea. This is a consequence of extreme brachycephaly and shallow orbits. This dog also exhibits a prominent nasal fold which can result in nasal fold trichiasis (photo: R.M.A. Packer).

Flat faces are often accompanied by prominent, protruding eyes, caused by a combination of shallow orbits and large palpebral fissure openings. Although encouraged in breed standards through phrases such as 'eyes large', this conformation can result in chronic exposure and drying of the eye due to an inability to blink fully, open to trauma, and can lead to painful corneal ulcers. Larger eyelid openings and flatter faces have been demonstrated to increase the risk of ulceration (Packer *et al.*, 2015a) (Fig. 7.5). In cats, shorter facial bones are associated with rotation of the canine teeth and deformation of the nasolacrimal drainage system, leading to persistent epiphora (Schlueter *et al.*, 2009).

Limiting the Extremes

Due to the mounting evidence that extremes of companion animal conformation lead to unacceptably high risks of disease, strategies to reduce the prevalence of conformation-related disorders are urgently required. As disease risk scales with conformation, strategies to reduce disease prevalence require a component of conformational change, to move away from high-risk extremes. To date, the Kennel Club (UK), in 2009, revised breed standards to include terminology to discourage exaggeration (e.g. addition of terms such as 'fairly', 'relatively' and 'moderately'); however, the subjective nature of this terminology allows room for interpretation by breeders. The Council of Europe suggested the implementation of 'conformational limits' to breed standards, setting maximum and minimum values for conformational features including muzzle length, the proportion between length and height of short-legged dogs, and height and weight of giant or miniature dogs (Council of Europe, 1995). These 'supply' based strategies must be complemented by demand based initiatives, to educate the public regarding the consequences of purchasing animals with extreme conformations. With almost 1 in 7 (14%, 31,654 dogs) of all Kennel Club registrations in 2016 being either a pug, French bulldog or bulldog, compared to 1 in 50 in 2005 (2%, 5437 dogs), the public appetite for extreme dogs is clearly increasing, and to protect animal welfare, this issue must be strongly addressed.

The Future of Companion Animal Breeding? Cloning and Gene Editing

Advances in biotechnology may facilitate a new age of companion animal breeding, with more rapid and precise manipulations of genetics than selective breeding alone.

Gene targeting CRISPR technology (clustered regularly interspaced short palindromic repeats), may allow for the creation of 'designer dogs' by genetic engineering, and has recently been used to create knockout beagles for the myostatin gene (a negative regulator of skeletal muscle mass). This resulted in dogs with doubled muscle mass (Zou *et al.*, 2015). The authors of this work speculated that this approach may facilitate the generation of novel dog models for biomedical research, but also the creation of new strains of dogs with favourable traits for other purposes. Double muscling has been naturally reported in whippets (the 'bully whippet') and genetically characterized (Mosher *et al.*, 2007). As little is known about the health issues and potential risks associated with the myostatin-mutation, and negative consequences observed in other species with this mutation (e.g. birthing difficulties and decreased organ size in Belgian Blue cattle (Webster, 2002)), using gene editing to select for this and other such traits is of welfare and ethical concern. As CRISPR technology is so new, the long-term effects are still unclear and should be treated with caution. Cloning technologies have been commercially available to pet owners for over a decade, with a Korean company, Sooam Biotech (http://en.sooam.com/dogcn/sub01.html), reported to have cloned 700 dogs between 2007 and 2015 (Taylor, 2015). Due to the high failure and mortality rates, and evidence of health problems in cloned animals, there are serious ethical and welfare concerns associated with this technology. In addition, cloning animals with extreme conformations may contribute to the perpetuation of disorders associated with these body shapes.

Conclusions

Mankind has successfully manipulated the phenotype of cats and dogs to satisfy their appetite for variation in appearance. This has led to exaggeration in both body size and shape, and due to increasing evidence that these extremes are associated with inherited disorders, they pose a major threat to animal welfare. Although relaxed functional demands may have facilitated diversification of companion animal's morphologies, health should be one of the primary considerations in all breeding decisions, and biological limits of body shape should be respected to protect animal welfare.

References

Arman, K. (2007) A new direction for Kennel Club regulations and breed standards. *Canadian Veterinary Journal-Revue Veterinaire Canadienne* 48, 953–964.

Asher, L., Diesel, G., Summers, J.F., McGreevy, P.D. and Collins, L.M. (2009) Inherited defects in pedigree dogs. Part 1: Disorders related to breed standards. *The Veterinary Journal* 182, 402–411.

Barnett, K. (1988) Inherited eye disease in the dog and cat. *Journal of Small Animal Practice* 29, 462–475.

Beaumont, M., Barratt, E., Gottelli, D., Kitchener, A., Daniels, M., Pritchard, J. and Bruford, M. (2001) Genetic diversity and introgression in the Scottish wildcat. *Molecular Ecology* 10, 319–336.

Bjornerfeldt, S., Hailer, F., Nord, M. and Vila, C. (2008) Assortative mating and fragmentation within dog breeds. *Bmc Evolutionary Biology* 8.

Bökönyi, S. (ed.) (1989) *Definitions of Animal Domestication*. Unwin, London.

Brockman, D.J., Washabau, R.J. and Drobatz, K.J. (1995) Canine gastric dilatation/volvulus syndrome in a veterinary critical care unit: 295 cases (1986–1992). *Journal of the American Veterinary Medical Association* 207, 460–464.

Caius, J. (1576) *De canibus Britannicis – 'Of Englishe dogges, the diversities, the names, the natures, and the properties: a short treatise written in latine' by Johannes Caius of late memorie, and newly drawn into Englishe by Abraham Fleming, 1880*. A. Bradley, London.

Cameron-Beaumont, C., Lowe, S. and Bradshaw, C. (2002) Evidence suggesting pre-adaptation to domestication throughout the small Felidae. *Biology Journal of the Linnean Society London* 75, 361–366.

Clutton-Brock, J. (ed.) (1995) *Origins of the Dog: Domestication and Early History*. Cambridge University Press, Cambridge, UK.

Clutton-Brock, J. (1999) *A Natural History of Domesticated Mammals*. Cambridge University Press, Cambridge, UK.

Council of Europe (1995) Resolution on the breeding of pet animals: multilateral consultation of parties to the European Convention for the Protection of Pet Animals (ETS 123). Document CONS 125(95)29, Council of Europe, F 67075, Strasbourg-Cedex, France.

Darwin, C. (1859) *On the Origin of Species by Means of Natural Selection*. Murray, London.

Dobney, K. and Larson, G. (2006) Genetics and animal domestication: new windows on an elusive process. *Journal of Zoology* 269, 261–271.

Done, S.H., Drew, R.A., Robins, G.M. and Lane, J.G. (1975) Hemivertebra in the dog: clinical and pathological observations. *The Veterinary Record* 96, 313–317.

Drake, A.G. and Klingenberg, C.P. (2010) Large-scale diversification of skull shape in domestic dogs: disparity and modularity. *American Naturalist* 175, 289–301.

Drury, W.D. (1903) *British Dogs, Their Points, Selection, and Show Preparation*. Gill, London.

Evans, K.M. and Adams, V.J. (2010) Proportion of litters of purebred dogs born by caesarean section. *Journal of Small Animal Practice* 51, 113–118.

Faure, E. and Kitchener, A.C. (2009) An archaeological and historical review of the relationships between felids and people. *Anthrozoös* 22, 221–238.

Fox, M.W. (1972) *Understanding Your Dog*. St Martin's Griffen, New York.

Ginn, J., Kumar, M., Mckiernan, B. and Powers, B. (2008) Nasopharyngeal turbinates in brachycephalic dogs and cats. *Journal of the American Animal Hospital Association* 44, 243–249.

Goggin, J.E., Li, A.S. and Franti, C.E. (1970) Canine intervertebral disk disease – characterization by age, sex, breed, and anatomic site of involvement. *American Journal of Veterinary Research* 31, 1687.

Goodwin, D., Bradshaw, J.W.S. and Wickens, S.M. (1997) Paedomorphosis affects agonistic visual signals of domestic dogs. *Animal Behaviour* 53, 297–304.

Hale, F. (2013) Stop brachycephalism, now! *Canadian Veterinary Journal* 54, 185–186.

Hayes, H.M., Pickle, L.W. and Wilson, G.P. (1987) Effects of ear type and weather on the hospital prevalence of canine otitis externa. *Research Veterinary Science* 42, 294–298.

Hemmer, H. (1990) *Domestication: The Decline of Environmental Appreciation*. Cambridge University Press, Cambridge, UK.

Hodgman, S.F.J. (1963) Abnormalities and defects in pedigree dogs. i. An investigation into the existence of abnormalities in pedigree dogs in the British Isles. *Journal of Small Animal Practice* 4, 447–456.

Kurushima, J.D., Lipinski, M.J., Gandolfi, B., Froenicke, L., Grahn, J.C., Grahn, R.A. and Lyons, L.A. (2013) Variation of cats under domestication: genetic assignment of domestic cats to breeds and worldwide random bred populations. *Animal Genetics* 44, 311–324.

Linnaeus, C.T. and R.B.R.K. (1792) *'Systema Naturae' – The Animal Kingdom; or, Zoological System of the Celebrated Sir Charles Linnaeus. Class I: Mammalia and Class II: Birds*. Murray, London.

Maki, K., Liinamo, A.E., Groen, A.F., Bijma, P. and Ojala, M. (2005) The effect of breeding schemes on the genetic response of canine hip dysplasia, elbow dysplasia, behaviour traits and appearance. *Animal Welfare* 14, 117–124.

McGreevy, P.D. and Nicholas, F.W. (1999) Some practical solutions to welfare problems in dog breeding. *Animal Welfare* 8, 329–341.
Montague, M.J., Li, G., Gandolfi, B., Khan, R., Aken, B.L. *et al.* (2014) Comparative analysis of the domestic cat genome reveals genetic signatures underlying feline biology and domestication. *Proceedings of the National Academy of Sciences* 111, 17230–17235.
Mosher, D.S., Quignon, P., Bustamante, C.D., Sutter, N.B., Mellersh, C.S., Parker, H.G. and Ostrander, E.A. (2007) A mutation in the myostatin gene increases muscle mass and enhances racing performance in heterozygote dogs. *PLOS Genetics* 3, e79.
Muller, G.H. (1990) Skin diseases of the Chinese shar-pei. *Veterinary Clinics of North America – Small Animal Practice* 20, 1655–1670.
Murray, J.K., Browne, W.J., Roberts, M.A., Whitmarsh, A. and Gruffydd-Jones, T.J. (2010) Number and ownership profiles of cats and dogs in the UK. *Veterinary Record* 166, 163–168.
Neath, P.J., Brockman, D.J. and Saunders, H.M. (1997) Retrospective analysis of 19 cases of isolated torsion of the splenic pedicle in dogs. *Journal of Small Animal Practice* 38, 387–392.
Neath, P.J., Brockman, D.J. and King, L.G. (2000) Lung lobe torsion in dogs: 22 cases (1981–1999). *Journal of the American Veterinary Medical Association* 217, 1041–1044.
Nobis, G. (1979) Der alteste Haushund lebte vor 14,000 Jahren. *UMSHAU* 19, 610.
O'Regan, H.J. and Kitchener, A.C. (2005) The effects of captivity on the morphology of captive, domesticated and feral mammals. *Mammal Review* 35, 215–230.
Packer, R.M.A., Hendricks, A., Volk, H.A., Shihab, N.K. and Burn, C.C. (2013) How long and low can you go? Effect of conformation on the risk of thoracolumbar intervertebral disc extrusion in domestic dogs. *PLOS ONE* 8, e69650.
Packer, R.M.A., Hendricks, A. and Burn, C.C. (2015a) Impact of facial conformation on canine health: corneal ulceration. *PLOS ONE* 10, e0123827.
Packer, R.M.A., Hendricks, A., Tivers, M.S. and Burn, C.C. (2015b) Impact of facial conformation on canine health: brachycephalic obstructive airway syndrome. *PLOS ONE* 10, e0137496.
Parker, H., Kim, L., Sutter, N., Carlson, S., Lorentzen, T. *et al.* (2004) Genetic structure of the purebred domestic dog. *Science* 304, 1160–1164.
Pollinger, J.P., Bustamante, C.D., Fledel-Alon, A., Schmutz, S., Gray, M.M. and Wayne, R.K. (2005) Selective sweep mapping of genes with large phenotypic effects. *Genome Research* 15, 1809–1819.
Robinson, R. (1999) *Genetics for Dog Breeders*. Elsevier Health Sciences.
Schlueter, C., Budras, K.D., Ludewig, E., Mayrhofer, E., Koenig, H.E., Walter, A. and Oechtering, G.U. (2009) Brachycephalic feline noses: CT and anatomical study of the relationship between head conformation and the nasolacrimal drainage system. *Journal of Feline Medicine and Surgery* 11, 891–900.
Serpell, J.A. (2002) Anthropomorphism and anthropomorphic selection – beyond the 'cute response'. *Society and Animals* 10, 437–454.
Steiger, A. (ed.) (2005) *Breeding and Welfare*. Springer, Dordrecht, The Netherlands.
Taylor, D. (2015) UK couple have dead dog cloned in South Korea. Available at: www.theguardian.com/science/2015/dec/23/uk-couple-await-birth-of-two-clones-of-dead-dog (accessed 17 November 2017).
Toma, S., Colombo, S., Cornegliani, L., Persico, P., Galzerano, M., Gianino, M.M. and Noli, C. (2008) Efficacy and tolerability of once-daily cephalexin in canine superficial pyoderma: an open controlled study. *Journal of Small Animal Practice* 49, 384–391.
Trut, L.N. (1999) Early canid domestication: the farm-fox experiment. *American Scientist* 87, 160–169.
Vigne, J.-D., Briois, F., Zazzo, A., Willcox, G., Cucchi, T. *et al.* (2012) First wave of cultivators spread to Cyprus at least 10,600 years ago. *Proceedings of the National Academy of Sciences of the United States of America* 109, 8445–8449.
Vila, C., Savolainen, P., Maldonado, J.E., Amorim, I.R., Rice, J.E. *et al.* (1997) Multiple and ancient origins of the domestic dog. *Science* 276, 1687–1689.

Wastlhuber, J. (ed.) (1991) *History of Domestic Cats and Cat Breeds*. American Veterinary Publications, Goleta, California.

Wayne, R.K. (ed.) (2001) *Consequences of Domestication: Morphological Diversity of the Dog*. CAB International, Wallingford, UK.

Webster, A.J.F. (2002) Rendering unto Caesar: welfare problems in Belgian Blue cattle. *The Veterinary Journal* 163, 228–229.

Wilkinson, G.T. (ed.) (1984) *Diseases of the Reproductive System*. Blackwell Scientific Publications, Oxford, UK.

Zou, Q., Wang, X., Liu, Y., Ouyang, Z., Long, H. *et al.* (2015) Generation of gene-target dogs using CRISPR/Cas9 system. *Journal of Molecular Cell Biology* 7, 580–583.

8 Methods to Increase Fish Production: Welfare and Sustainability Implications

FELICITY HUNTINGFORD[1,*], JIMMY TURNBULL[2] AND SUNIL KADRI[3]

[1]*Institute of Biodiversity, Animal Health and Comparative Medicine, University of Glasgow, Glasgow, UK;* [2]*Institute of Aquaculture, University of Stirling, Stirling, UK;* [3]*Aquaculture Innovation, Edinburgh, UK*

A Brief Introduction to Aquaculture

What aquaculture is and why it is important

Aquaculture is the farming of aquatic organisms, including finfish, molluscs, crustaceans and plants. Here we concentrate on intensification in finfish aquaculture, but similar issues arise, for example, in prawn culture (Little *et al.*, 2016). Finfish are cultured for many purposes: for the aquarium trade, for restocking wild populations and for food, the latter being the subject of this chapter. Of more than 35,000 species of finfish (hereafter 'fish'), some 350 species are farmed for food worldwide, but production is dominated by a few groups, predominantly freshwater (Figure 8.1a).

Wild fisheries have been in decline, and now more than half of fish produced globally have been farmed (Fig. 8.1b). As a source of affordable and healthy food, aquaculture plays an important role in nutrition security (Tidwell and Allen, 2001). Aquaculture is also an important source of household income and employment in developed and, particularly, developing countries (Klinger and Naylor, 2012; Little *et al.*, 2016); in 2014, 18.75 million people relied on aquaculture as a source of income (FAO, 2014). Additionally, fish culture can provide a variety of ecosystem services (wastewater treatment, for example) and can help rebuild depleted wild fish populations by relieving fisheries pressure. In the right conditions, rearing fish in culture can reduce contaminants in fish flesh; for example, cleaned up fish meal and fish oil from contaminated natural sources can be turned into healthy feed for farmed fish (Cheng *et al.*, 2016).

What intensive aquaculture means

Global aquaculture is one of the fastest growing agriculture sectors. Over the last 50 years, production of farmed fish has increased at a rate of about 8% per year, to a volume

*Address for correspondence: Felicity.Huntingford@glasgow.ac.uk

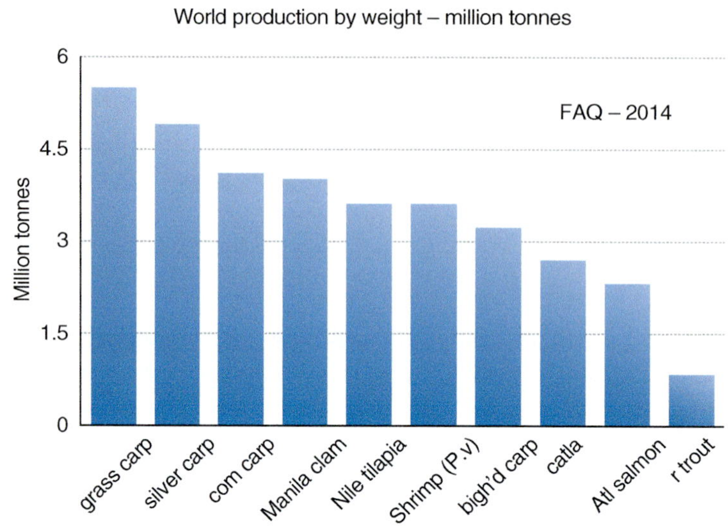

Fig. 8.1a. Annual production of key farmed finfish by weight. Salmonids replace carp as the dominant species in terms of production value (US$18 million per year).

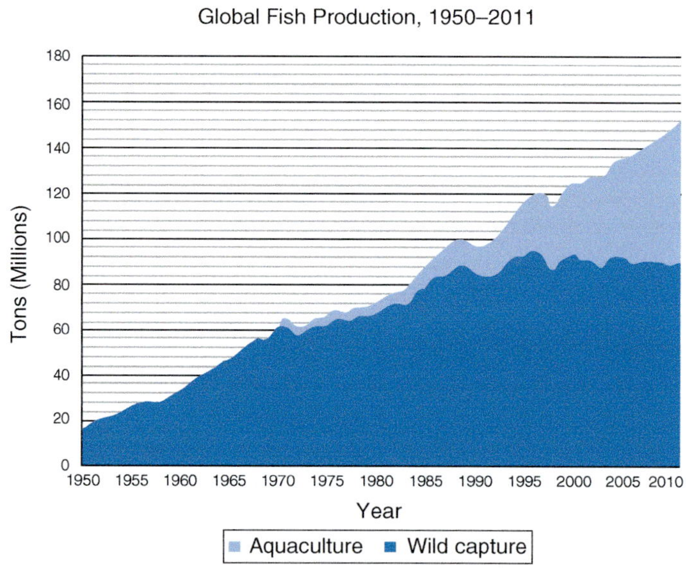

Fig. 8.1b. Tonnes of fish produced by capture fisheries and aquaculture from 1950–2011 (FAO, 2014; http://www.fao.org/figis).

of more than 60 million tonnes in 2010 (Fig. 8.1b), and since 2012 has outstripped beef production (Klinger and Naylor, 2012; Little *et al.*, 2016).

This striking increase has been achieved partly through extension to new species and locations, but mainly through a process of intensification (increasing weight of

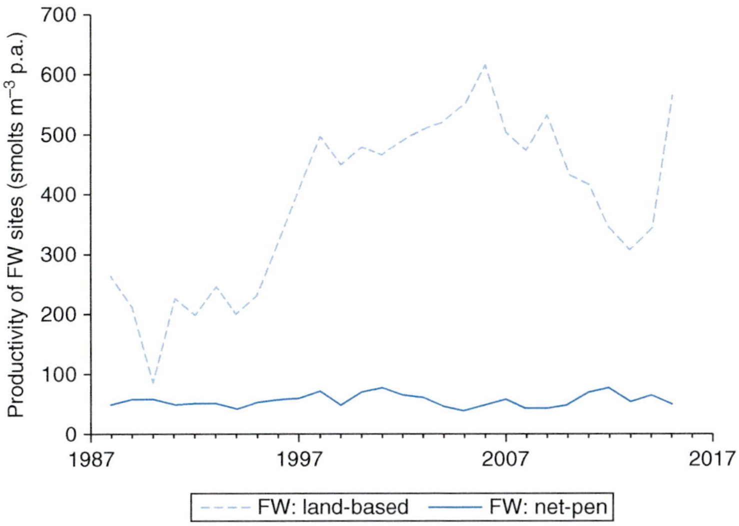

Fig. 8.2. Productivity of Scottish farmed Atlantic salmon in the freshwater (FW) phase from 1987 to 2014. For land based systems, productivity more than doubled during this period (Ellis *et al.*, 2016).

edible flesh produced per unit of space). For example, in Scottish land based Atlantic salmon culture, since *c.*1990 there has been a sixfold increase in the number of juvenile fish produced per m^3 of water (Fig. 8.2). Modern fish culture systems range from extensive natural ponds that require little management, through semi-intensive ponds with supplementary feeding, to various intensive systems in which fish are entirely dependent on added feed (Jobling *et al.*, 2010; Klinger and Naylor, 2012). Globally, 60% of farmed fish are still produced in extensive or semi-intensive systems, but there has been a broad shift from largely subsistence to intensive market-oriented production (Diana *et al.*, 2013).

Special features of finfish aquaculture in the context of intensification

Physiologically, fish are much like mammals and birds, for example having similar stress responses (Jobling, 2012), but some special characteristics, several related to living in water, make them different when it comes to intensification (Table 8.1). Being relatively recent, intensification in aquaculture has coincided with unprecedented technological advances that have been embraced by an innovative and adaptable industry (Klinger and Naylor, 2012). Recent intensification also means that, while some domestication has taken place (Huntingford *et al.*, 2012), this is much less marked than in farmed birds and mammals. In welfare terms, farmed fish may be less well adapted to intensive culture than animals that have been domesticated for millennia.

Table 8.1. Special features of fish compared with birds and mammals that impact on intensification of aquaculture.

Special characteristic	Implications
Compared with mammals and birds, fish naturally produce huge numbers of eggs (e.g. approx. 8000 per spawning in a 12lb female Atlantic salmon) and natural mortality levels are very high, especially in early life history stages.	Survival in the wild is very low for many fish species, especially those with small eggs. There is an argument for assessing mortality against the maximum possible rather than 100%, whilst maintaining the aspiration to improve.
Many species have complex life histories, with marked changes in habitat and form at critical points.	Diverse optimal husbandry conditions apply for culture of a single species.
• Fish can manufacture protein particularly efficiently. • Being ectotherms, fish do not need to expend energy on thermoregulation. • Being supported by water, fish do not need a large bony skeleton or to expend energy maintaining posture. • Fish show continuous growth.	Fish can generate a higher yield of edible flesh per unit of feed input than can terrestrial animals.
Mammals, birds and fish are all intimately exposed to the environment through their huge respiratory surfaces, but in fish there is no buffering prior to contact with the gills.	Fish health and welfare are particularly compromised by poor water quality, but, conversely, improved water quality can lead to major improvements in health and welfare.
Many farmed fish species naturally spend their lives in dense schools. Farmed birds tend to be flocking species, but natural densities are lower.	The higher stocking density associated with intensive culture is not necessarily detrimental, if combined with good water quality and access to food.

How Intensive Aquaculture has Been Achieved

Measures and actions for aquaculture intensification

Table 8.2 outlines the broad measures on which aquaculture intensification has been based and the various actions through which these have been achieved; how these actions are implemented and what they mean for fish welfare are discussed below ('Analysis of the Implications of Aquaculture Intensification for Fish Welfare'). Given the great diversity of farmed fish species, the measures responsible for intensification are strongly sector specific, and we make an important if imprecise distinction between those aspects of intensification that are in use for most intensively farmed species, those that are in use for a subset of species and those that are feasible in a research context but not in commercial use. In the section referred to above we use a series of icons (Table 8.2) to remind the reader of this distinction.

Table 8.2. Measures and actions for aquaculture of intensification. These are loosely classified in terms of their prevalence in systems with some degree of intensification, as follows (with logo used in text, and different fonts to identify each).

Used in most cases: Used in a subset of cases: *Feasible in a research context, but not in use in production systems:*

Intensification measure	Actions for implementation
CONTROL OVER THE PHYSICAL ENVIRONMENT	• **Improved design of cages, tanks and ponds** • Oxygenation/control of gases in water • Control of water temperature • Water recirculation and filtering • Water quality monitoring systems • Predator exclusion
INCREASED STOCKING DENSITY	• **Improved design of cages, tanks and ponds** • Oxygenation/ **control of gases in** water • Water recirculation • Water quality monitoring systems
FASTER GROWTH	• **Improved feed management** • **Increased use of manufactured feed** • Selective breeding for fast growth • Use of triploids • Use of monosex populations • *Use of growth hormone transgenic fish*
HEALTH MANAGEMENT	• Use of antimicrobial treatments • Use of vaccines • Food-based treatment for endo- and ecto-parasites • External treatment for parasites • Selective breeding for disease resistance
CONTROL OF REPRODUCTION: INDUCING MATURATION IN BROODSTOCK	• **Providing optimal physical and social conditions for maturation** • Hormonal induction of breeding
CONTROL OF REPRODUCTION: PREVENTING MATURATION IN ON-GROWING FISH	• **Avoiding optimal physical and social conditions for maturation** • Selective breeding for late maturation • Use of monosex populations • Use of triploids

A brief comment on markets and supply chains

Partly because of intensification, high quality, moderately priced fish of a range of species are now a readily and reliably obtainable commodity (FAO, 2014). More salmon and tilapia are being eaten than ever before, all over the world and not just where they are produced. In some countries, at least, consumers prefer to eat fish that has been farmed sustainably with respect to fish welfare and the environment (Young, 2010; Little *et al.*, 2016), a strong motivation for quality assurance on these issues. Finally, an increasingly international market, dependent on increasingly costly technologies and with increasingly complex regulation has led consolidation of seafood production (both capture fisheries and aquaculture) into a few large enterprises involved at all levels of the supply chain (Little *et al.*, 2016).

Aquaculture Intensification, Sustainability and Fish Welfare

Sustainable aquaculture

The term sustainability is used in different ways (Hansen, 1996); according to the UN, sustainable development 'meets the needs of the present without compromising the ability of future generations to meet their own needs' (www.un-documents.net/our-common-future.pdf). To be sustainable, intensive aquaculture must balance the benefits of producing fish for the growing human population against costs in terms of possible damage to the environment and of impaired fish welfare (Garnet *et al.*, 2013). The welfare implications of intensive aquaculture are the main topic of this chapter, but key ecosystem issues (use of limited food resources, spread of disease between wild and farmed fish and the impact of escapees on natural populations) are discussed briefly where relevant.

Aquaculture intensification and welfare

There is controversy about what fish welfare means, particularly about whether it is best defined in terms of how fish function or of how they feel (Huntingford and Kadri, 2014). The latter definition hinges on the extent to which fish are sentient, a difficult question, currently being addressed by neurobiologists, behaviour biologists and welfare scientists. At present, very little is known about how the actions that underpin intensification are experienced by the fish concerned. Realistically, welfare of farmed fish is mainly measured by how well they function, including survival, growth, health status and stress physiology. Such measures do not capture all aspects of fish welfare, but are useful when used correctly (at the population level, reduced survival is one of the most robust indications of deteriorating welfare) and they tell us that, in general, intensification has improved fish welfare. Survival in Atlantic salmon farming has increased markedly (Kristensen *et al.*, 2012), in the case of seawater production in Scotland rising from 50% in 1987 to 80% in 2013 (Ellis *et al.*, 2016). The well-being of their stock are matters of strong concern for fish farmers, and the aquaculture industry has been proactive in developing technologies to improve welfare, protection of which is included in industry guidelines for best practice (e.g. Scottish Salmon Producers' Organisation, 2014).

Analysis of the Implications of Aquaculture Intensification for Fish Welfare

This section considers all the intensification measures and actions in Table 8.2, looking at positive and negative effects on fish welfare, mitigation measures available in the case of adverse effects and, where relevant, implications for ecosystem health.

Increased control over the physical environment

How this is achieved

Almost all the improvements in control over the physical environment listed in Table 8.2 involve technological advances, often including mechanization and computerized monitoring and control of operations (Ellis *et al.*, 2016). Good water quality is critical for fish health and welfare (Table 8.1) and some of the most important factors in the successful intensification of aquaculture relate to increasingly effective water management.

Implications for fish welfare and mitigation measures

The impacts of better control of the physical environment on the welfare of intensively farmed fish are complex, but in general are positive, since the aim is to provide fish with appropriate, species-specific environmental conditions, including an ample supply of clean, well aerated water at the correct temperature. Such improvements have played a large part in the increased survival of farmed Atlantic salmon associated with intensification. Increasing technological complexity may mean increased vulnerability to system failure, but with rigorous monitoring and robust control processes in place, fish are largely protected from such failure.

In some respects, increased control over the physical environment means more interference with farmed fish; many husbandry practices are stressful and can pose risks of injury (Noble *et al.*, 2012), so they could impact negatively on welfare. One response has been to focus aquaculture on strains that are relatively resistant to stress, due either to inadvertent partial domestication (Huntingford *et al.*, 2012) or to targeted selective breeding for low-stress responsiveness, which has been successful for a variety of species (e.g. rainbow trout – Quillet *et al.*, 2014; European sea bass – Vandeputte *et al.*, 2016). In addition, the aquaculture industry has developed low-stress, hands-off systems for some common aquaculture practices (Lines *et al.*, 2001). Several commercially available systems exist for estimating the size of free-swimming farmed fish. The VICASS (AKVA Group, Norway) and AM-100 systems (AQ1 Systems, Hobart) reconstruct size from stereoscopic images while VAKI (Reykjavik) use optical sensors to model fish size from data collected as fish swim through a square frame; the Biometrics system (Biometrics, Norway) uses acoustic signals reflected from swim bladders. Size grading normally involves capturing fish and confining them before passing them through a grid, often in air; passive grading allows fish in sea cages to swim voluntarily through an underwater grid, sometimes in response to simple directional stimuli (Fig. 8.3).

Arguably, the technology of intensification, including such hands-off systems, may distance farmers from fish, removing opportunities for monitoring health and welfare during routine husbandry. Here, intensification has been accompanied by improved technology and resources for routine monitoring of fish in production systems. Video filming is used to reveal the physical status and behaviour of fish, and sonar and echo integration is used to allow distribution of large numbers of fish to be visualized (Figure 8.4). Such information helps to ensure both good production and good welfare.

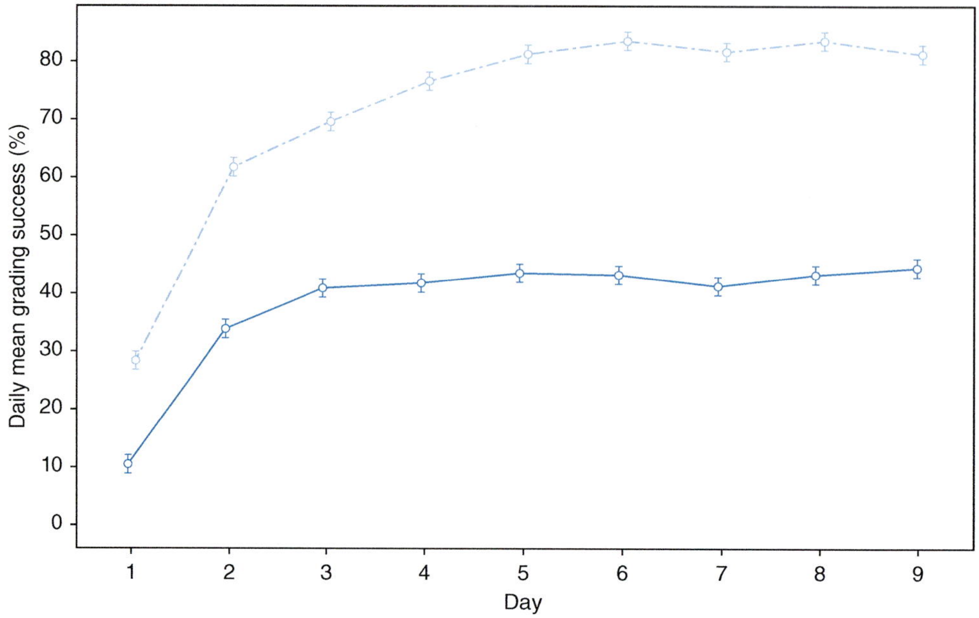

Fig. 8.3. Self-grading system in turbot. Mixed-sized groups of turbot were placed at one end of a tank divided by a transverse grid through which fish of a given size, or smaller, could swim. The figure shows for nine successive days the percentage of fish, of a size that could pass through the grid into the graded section, that did so, either with no additional stimulus (continuous line) or with an additional light placed above the graded section during the daytime, and the grid coloured white on the non-graded side and black on the graded side (broken line). Error bars = 95% confidence intervals. Self-grading is highly effective with the combination of light and grid colour (Bogner *et al.*, 2017).

Increased stocking density

How this is achieved

The initial stages of intensification have always involved increasing stocking density (weight of fish per volume of water), but this has not always continued. Stocking density in Scottish Atlantic salmon initially increased from a relatively low starting point, but was reduced somewhat as adverse consequences became apparent. Where stocking density has increased, improved water management, along with improvements in the design of fish-holding units, have been important, for example development of self-cleaning tanks and of more robust cages that can be used in exposed locations with higher water flow (Price *et al.*, 2015).

Implications for fish welfare

Many farmed fish species live naturally in social groups or schools (Table 8.1), which provide a variety of benefits, so welfare is not automatically compromised by high densities. Atlantic salmon smolts make their seaward migration in shoals of approx.

30 fish (Davidsen *et al.*, 2005), but, given optimal water quality, can be held at much higher densities without adverse effects on growth, feed conversion efficiency or stress physiology (Calabrese *et al.*, 2017). Between 1999 and 2006, survival after smolt transfer in Norwegian salmon farming was positively associated (slightly but significantly) with increasing production intensity (including stocking density – Kristensen *et al.*, 2012). In other cases, perhaps involving inadequately managed systems, high stocking density has adverse effects on welfare, even when water quality is high. In Nile tilapia, stocking densities in the range 200–800 fish/m^3 are associated with lower growth, poorer food conversion efficiency and more variation in size and food intake (Azaza *et al.*, 2013). There is evidence of reduced welfare at both very high and very low stocking densities for several farmed species, but the relationship is highly confounded, by environmental and social conditions and with feeding regimes (Turnbull *et al.*, 2005).

Mitigation of negative effects on welfare

The best way of avoiding adverse effects of inappropriate stocking density is to ensure that the optimal density is known for a given species/age/rearing system and is achieved reliably on working farms. In this context, the Atlantic salmon farming industry uses specific water flow (volume of water/kg of fish/min.) as a practical index of welfare-friendly stocking density in relation to water quality. For example, evidence of stress in post-smolts, for example, becoming apparent at specific flow rates of less than 0.3 l/kg/min. (Sveen *et al.*, 2016).

Negative effects of high stocking density can be counteracted by various manipulations that encourage fish to spread out, reducing the actual density that they experience. Submerged lights prevent Atlantic salmon in sea cages congregating at excessively high densities (Fig. 8.4). Encouraging sustained swimming by exposing a characid fish (*Brycon*

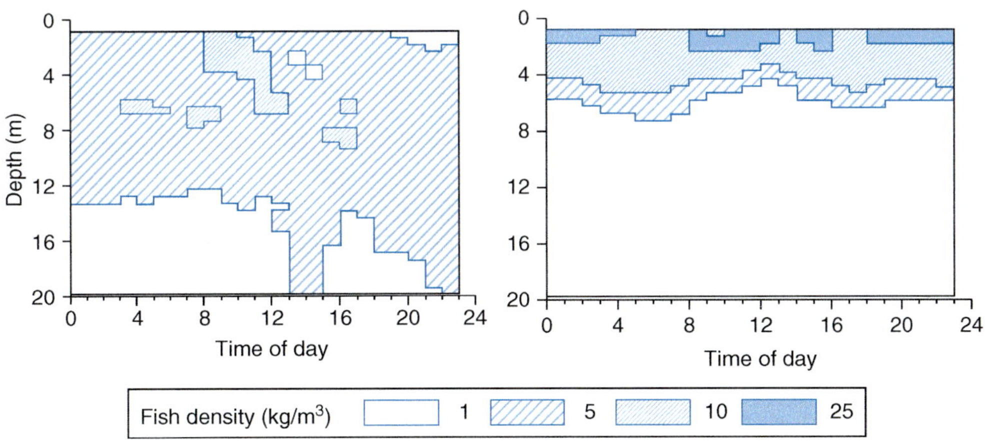

Fig. 8.4. Mitigating the welfare effects of high stocking density. Depth distribution of Atlantic salmon in a fully stocked sea cage across 24 hours in February with (LHS) and without (RHS) submerged lights. Fish are spread more or less throughout the cage with submerged lights, but concentrated in the surface areas without lights (Juell *et al.*, 2003).

amazonicus) to water currents and promoting sustained swimming at 1 body length/s mitigates the stressful effects of high stocking density (Arbelas-Rojas *et al.*, 2017).

Faster growth

How this is achieved

Successful aquaculture intensification always involves increasing growth rates (Fig. 8.5a). Numerous scientific studies show that growth can be enhanced by manipulating hormonal processes, but such manipulations are not used in commercial fish production, because other ways of generating fast growth are sufficiently effective.

Growth rates and welfare in general

In general, spontaneously fast growth in farmed fish suggests that holding conditions are good, which is why good growth is often used as a welfare indicator (Huntingford and Kadri, 2014). However, there is no reason to think that fast growth in and of itself is beneficial for welfare, or the converse. Wild fish often experience periods when they do not feed or grow, due to natural anorexia or perhaps because food is in short supply, and they have an excellent capacity for compensatory growth (Ali *et al.*, 2003). In nature, fast growth involves a variety of costs. These mainly become evident at breeding, so are not particularly relevant to aquaculture, where most fish are harvested before they mature. However, rapid growth in on-growing Atlantic salmon is associated with changes in the mineral composition of the otoliths, which decreases hearing sensitivity in these fish and so may impair welfare (Reimer *et al.*, 2017). Apart from possible negative effects of fast growth *per se*, the specific actions used to enhance growth (Table 8.2) may have their own positive or negative implications for fish welfare.

Feed management

MODERN FEED MANAGEMENT SYSTEMS AND IMPLICATIONS FOR FISH WELFARE Sophisticated, scientifically informed feed management strategies have been critical for aquaculture intensification (Jobling, 2010b). Computerized feed delivery systems aimed at delivering appropriate rations with minimal waste (often with video monitoring to ensure that food is not monopolized) have been critical for aquaculture intensification. Feeders designed specifically to match delivery to current appetite are particularly effective in this context (Attia *et al.*, 2012). By ensuring that fish have the right amount of food at the right time (allowing for species, age, size, reproductive status and environmental conditions), good feed management promotes welfare.

Increased use of manufactured feed

THE IMPORTANCE OF MANUFACTURED FEED Manufactured feeds based on the known nutritional requirements of the fish concerned have been essential for intensification, with total

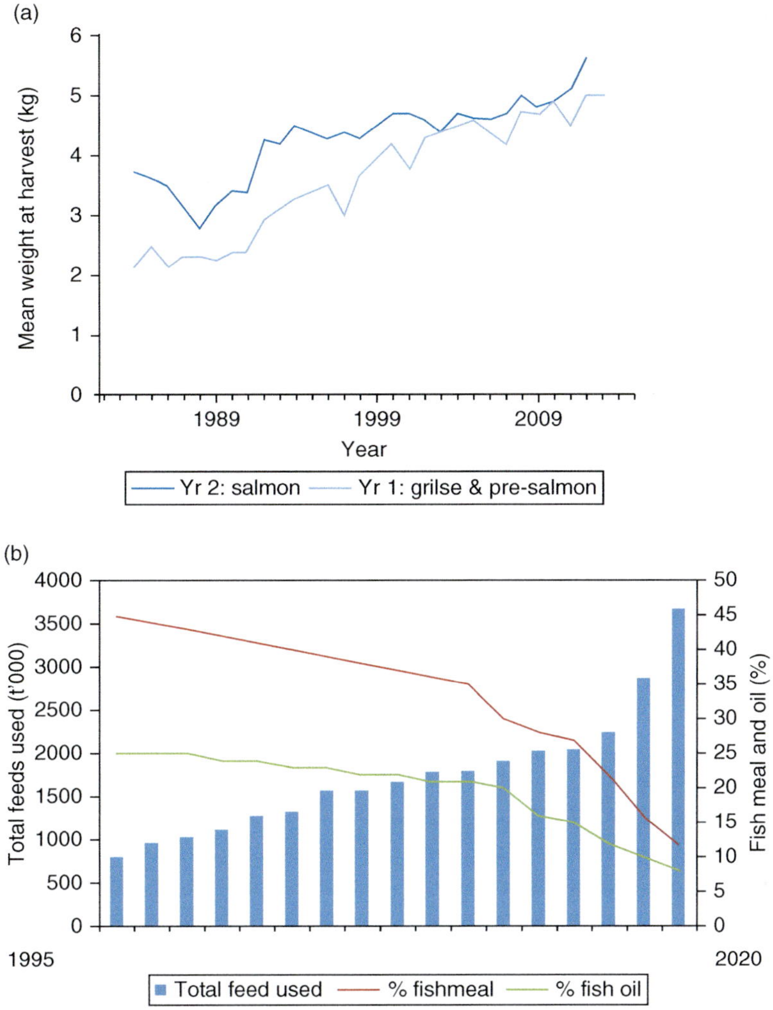

Fig. 8.5. (a) Increased growth rates during intensification in Scottish Atlantic salmon aquaculture between 1984 and 2012, reflected in weight at harvest after 1 and 2 years at sea (Ellis *et al.*, 2016). (b) Declining use of reduction fisheries products in Atlantic salmon aquaculture between 1995 and 2020 (projected) (Bostock *et al.*, 2010).

feed production increasing from 7.6 million tonnes in 1995 to 27.1 million tonnes in 2007 (Edwards, 2015 – Fig. 8.5b).

ECOSYSTEM ISSUES: USE OF FISHMEAL Historically, manufactured fish feed has made significant use of fish meal (FM) and fish oil (FO), derived from small marine fish, which contain key nutrients needed for the health and welfare of both farmed fish and the humans that eat them. FM and FO are used in many branches of agriculture and in the nutraceutical industry (which markets food-derived products with special health benefits) and there is a real potential for overfishing stocks of such forage fish, with knock-on detrimental consequences for the marine ecosystems

(Klinger and Naylor, 2012; Diana *et al.*, 2013; Lekang *et al.*, 2016). In response to competition from the other sectors and concerns about ecosystem impacts, a major research and development effort has led to dramatic falls in the use of reduction fisheries products across the aquaculture industry (Fig. 8.5b). This has been achieved by more efficient feed management (between 1995 and 2015, feed utilization efficiency increased by approx. 25% in all the major groups of farmed fish (Little *et al.*, 2016)), and by a successful search for other sources of nutrients for farmed fish (Box 8.1).

IMPLICATIONS FOR FISH WELFARE If the species- and age-specific nutritional needs of fish are fully known and feed can be manufactured that meets these needs, their use must be good for the health and welfare of farmed fish. On the other hand, manufactured feeds can have adverse effects if they fail to meet the nutritional needs of the fish, perhaps because these are not fully known or because new feed ingredients are being tried. Many species grow well and keep healthy on feed containing plant material, but for carnivorous fish, such material (typically containing high levels of fibres and non-starch polysaccharides) may induce inflammation of the gastro-intestinal tract (Francis *et al.*, 2001). Even nutritionally optimal manufactured feed usually looks and may smell different from natural food, and so may fail to stimulate feeding, particularly in young fish at first feeding (Jobling *et al.*, 2012).

MITIGATION OF NEGATIVE EFFECTS Negative effects of plant material in fish feed can be reduced by pre-treating such material with exogenous enzymes to break down non-starch polysaccharides and improve digestibility (Castillo and Gatlin, 2015; Dalsgaard *et al.*, 2016). Addition of live microbial feed supplements can improve digestion and assimilation of plant-based nutrients by carnivorous fish and prevent intestinal inflammation, at least under experimental conditions (Romarheim *et al.*, 2010). Inherited differences in ability to digest plant-derived feeds means that carnivorous fish could be selectively bred for good growth on such diets, while maintaining good

Box 8.1. Some sources of nutrients used effectively for at least partial replacement of reduction fisheries products in manufactured feed for intensive aquaculture.

- Processing trimmings from farmed fish and land animals.
- Various invertebrates, including zooplankton, polychaetes and a variety of insects (e.g. locusts, termites and dipteran larvae (Henry *et al.*, 2015)).
- Plants, most notably soya (*Glycine max*) and brassica such as false flax (*Camelina sativa* (Klinger and Naylor, 2012)).
- Cultured single celled organisms such as yeast (Klinger and Naylor, 2012) and the bacterium *Methylobacterium extorquens*, which grows rapidly on gas-derived methanol and contains naturally occurring, beneficial carotenoids (Tlusty *et al.*, 2017).

intestinal condition (e.g. rainbow trout – Vernold *et al.*, 2012). Failure of farmed fish to recognize pellets at first exposure can be mitigated by appropriate management, including addition of natural feeding stimulant to manufactured feed (found in shellfish, for example), which promotes intake of plant-derived feeds (for example, turbot – Nagel *et al.*, 2014; sunshine bass – Barry *et al.*, 2017).

Selective breeding for fast growth

BREEDING FOR FAST GROWTH Targeted breeding programmes have produced dramatic effects in several species of farmed fish, resulting in 10–20% faster growth per generation of selection (Klinger and Naylor, 2012; Diana *et al.*, 2013). Modern molecular tools can increase the effectiveness of such programmes, for example by providing markers to identify fast growers, while avoiding traits linked to fast growth in nature that are undesirable in aquaculture, such as early maturation (see below – 'Control of reproduction') (Dunham *et al.*, 2014; Ye *et al.*, 2015).

IMPLICATIONS FOR FISH WELFARE Traditional selection for growth in aquaculture would automatically have selected for survival as well, so in several farmed species (Atlantic salmon and Nile tilapia, for example), fast growth carries with it increased survival and resistance to various diseases (Diana *et al.*, 2013; Klinger and Naylor, 2013). Scientific studies of traits that covary with fast growth in selected strains give variable results. In growth-selected channel catfish (Peterson *et al.*, 2008) and European sea bass (Vandeputte *et al.*, 2016), body size is negatively correlated to post-stress cortisol levels. Here selection for fast growth may have favoured fish with low stress responsiveness. The opposite is the case for growth-selected rainbow trout (Weber and Silverstein, 2007). Positive genetic correlations between fast growth and the incidence of vertebral deformities have been reported for sea bream, among other species (Garcia-Celdran *et al.*, 2015).

MITIGATION OF NEGATIVE EFFECTS A better understanding is needed of the conditions in which selective breeding for fast growth brings adverse effects, so that such conditions can be avoided, perhaps with the help of molecular markers. For example, information on susceptibility to deformities could inform selective breeding for fast growth (Garcia-Celdran *et al.*, 2015; Lee-Montero *et al.*, 2015). The incidence of deformities in fast-growing fish can also be prevented by use of diets with supplementary minerals (Lu *et al.*, 2013).

Increasing growth by manipulating reproductive biology

TRIPLOIDS In general, growth is faster if fish are prevented from maturing, and for some species, triploid fish, which have three rather than the normal two sets of chromosomes and are effectively sterile, are farmed to improve growth (Tiwary *et al.*, 2004;

Ye *et al.*, 2015). Techniques for producing triploids and possible implications for welfare are discussed below ('Control of reproduction').

MONOSEX POPULATIONS In nature, growth rates are often different in males and females, because size is more important for fitness in one or other sex. Male tilapia and channel catfish naturally grow faster than do females; the converse is true in crucian carp and vundu, another catfish (Tarranger *et al.*, 2010; Martinez *et al.*, 2014). In such cases, growth rates among farmed fish can be increased by culturing only the faster-growing sex (e.g. tilapia – Mair and Little, 1991; rainbow trout and salmon – Jungalwalla, 1991; Pennell and Barton, 1996).

HOW MONOSEX POPULATIONS ARE PRODUCED Monosex populations can be produced by hand sorting prior to maturity and, in species such as sea bass (see below), by manipulation of rearing temperature (Singh, 2013). Mostly, though, they are produced by early exposure to sex hormones (androgens or oestrogens depending on whether males or females are required), followed by breeding programmes to produce permanently all-male or all-female strains for human consumption (Mei *et al.*, 2015).

WELFARE IN MONOSEX POPULATIONS Mechanisms of sex determination are highly variable among fish, depending on sex chromosomes in some species (e.g. Nile tilapia) and environmental conditions in others (water temperature in the case of European sea bass). Even in species with chromosomal sex determination, gender is plastic and chromosomal sex can be completely overridden by early environmental conditions, under the control of androgens (causing testes to develop) and oestrogens (promoting ovarian development – Martinez *et al.*, 2014). Although changing sex is a complex issue in humans, many species of fish are sequential hermaphrodites, with either females turning into males or the converse (Fleming and Huntingford, 2012). So for fish, sex change, with all its hormonal, morphological and behavioural correlates, is a natural process. Inducing sex change in young fish by early hormone treatment taps into natural mechanisms and there is no reason to think that this, in itself, will have negative consequences for welfare.

Some indicators suggest that welfare may be better in fish held in monosex groups, but this depends on species and circumstances. In Nile tilapia, males survive better and grow faster and more uniformly in monosex compared to mixed-sex groups (Omasaki *et al.*, 2016). On the other hand, in Mozambique tilapia, various measures of specific and non-specific immunity and resistance to bacterial disease are all lower in monosex compared to mixed-sex groups (Binuramesh *et al.*, 2006).

Transgenic fish

GROWTH HORMONE (GH) ENHANCED FISH An alternative approach for increasing growth rates is to genetically engineer fish to over-express genes that naturally promote growth (Ye *et al.*, 2015). GH transgenic strains are available for various farmed species, including salmonids (Rasmussen *et al.*, 2007), carp (Zhong *et al.*, 2012) and tilapia (Fujimura and Kocher, 2011) and all show markedly higher growth rates (Tibbetts *et al.*, 2013). At the time of writing, only transgenic Atlantic salmon are licensed for use in the human food chain (in the USA) and no transgenic fish are in commercial production. In some parts of the world, the public have a strongly negative perception of genetic engineering and sectors of the aquaculture industry avoid transgenic fish and any association with transgenic technology. In addition, there would be serious concerns about possible impact of GH transgenic escapees on wild populations. It is therefore unlikely that use of GH transgenic will ever be the solution of choice for achieving fast growth in farmed fish.

IMPLICATIONS FOR WELFARE Potential welfare implications of the use of transgenic fish have been well researched. On the plus side, GH transgenic fish show good protein utilization and retention and, in some cases, improved immune function and disease resistance (e.g. Rasmussen and Morrisey, 2007). Set against this, increased appetite in GH transgenic fish could cause welfare problems if they are not able to feed to satiation (Kim *et al.*, 2015), though this can be avoided by increasing rations. Transgenic Nile tilapia have more skeletal deformities than normal fish, because they need more calcium and phosphorus than normal fish, and this can be avoided by mineral supplements (Lu *et al.*, 2013).

Health management

Disease in aquaculture

Aquaculture has problems with viral, bacterial, endoparasitic and ectoparasitic diseases (Sommerset *et al.*, 2005; Richards, 2014; Sahoo *et al.*, 2016) and a variety of strategies have been used to bring such diseases under control. Since ill health is both a cause and an index of poor welfare, in general terms, reducing the incidence of disease must be good for the welfare of farmed fish. Certainly, failure to treat farmed fish due to lack of diagnosis or lack of effective treatments can seriously compromise welfare. However, in specific cases actions used to improve the health of intensively farmed fish may themselves have adverse effects and some of these are discussed below.

Antimicrobial drugs

USE OF ANTIBIOTICS IN AQUACULTURE AND IMPLICATIONS FOR WELFARE A variety of antimicrobial medicines have been used in aquaculture and these have been effective in controlling many serious bacterial diseases, although evolution of antimicrobial resistance is a problem here as in other sectors (Miranda *et al.*, 2013; McNair, 2015; Sahoo *et al.*, 2016). Antimicrobial drugs can have side effects for the treated fish, for example by disturbing bacterial fauna (Tapia-Paniaga *et al.*, 2015). Use of probiotics (live microbial feed supplements that improve gut microbial balance) are reported to reduce the negative effects of antibiotics on intestinal microbiota diversity, as well as directly protecting fish against disease (Akhter *et al.*, 2015; Sahoo *et al.*, 2016). It is worth noting that clear evidence on the effectiveness of probiotic supplements in working farms is lacking. In response to various problems, antibiotic use in some aquaculture sectors has declined significantly, for example in intensive salmon culture (Fig. 8.6a), where antibiotics have largely been replaced by vaccination.

Vaccines

VACCINES FOR FARMED FISH A growing number of serious bacterial and viral diseases in aquaculture can be controlled by vaccines, which are mostly injected into the body cavity (Sommerset *et al.*, 2005; Yanong, 2015). Vaccination of juvenile Atlantic salmon against the bacterial disease furunculosis was introduced in Scotland in the mid-1980s; by 1996, 95% of fish were being vaccinated and prevalence had fallen dramatically (Ellis *et al.*, 2016).

IMPLICATIONS FOR WELFARE Vaccine delivery, which usually involves capture and handling as well as skin puncture, is stressful, and this is mitigated by mild anaesthesia. Vaccination may have unwanted side effects, including abdominal adhesions (Fraser *et al.*, 2014b), probably associated with immune-stimulants (adjuvants) that are added to vaccines and increase efficiency (Tafalla *et al.*, 2013). The incidence of adverse side effects is recorded as part of an extensive monitoring programme and the resulting data are used to inform continuous development of more humane vaccination procedures. Vaccination can now be carried out by machines, some using image analysis to locate the best vaccination site, suction to lift the abdominal wall away from underlying organs, and pressure sensors to detect blockage or blunting of the needle. Despite this sophistication, continual human monitoring is still required and more research is needed to reduce the side effects of adjuvants, while still promoting immune responses (Sommerset *et al.*, 2005; Drangsholt *et al.*, 2011; Tafalla *et al.*, 2013).

Selective breeding for disease resistance

EXPLOITING INHERITED VARIATION IN DISEASE RESISTANCE Successful selective breeding has improved disease resistance in several intensively farmed species (salmonids – Yanez *et al.*, 2016; tilapia – Diana *et al.*, 2013). Mortality in Atlantic salmon dropped by 50% following several generations of selection for resistance to pancreatic necrosis (Wetten *et al.*, 2007). Resistant strains have contributed to a consistent decline in disease outbreaks, although it should be noted that long generation times in fish compared to pathogens makes selective breeding slow compared with the rate at which new pathogens emerge.

IMPLICATIONS FOR WELFARE The mechanisms that protect against disease are complex and closely linked to other functional systems, so selection for disease resistance will have ramifying consequences. The evidence concerning traits that covary with selected disease resistance is contradictory, depending on fish species and pathogen. For

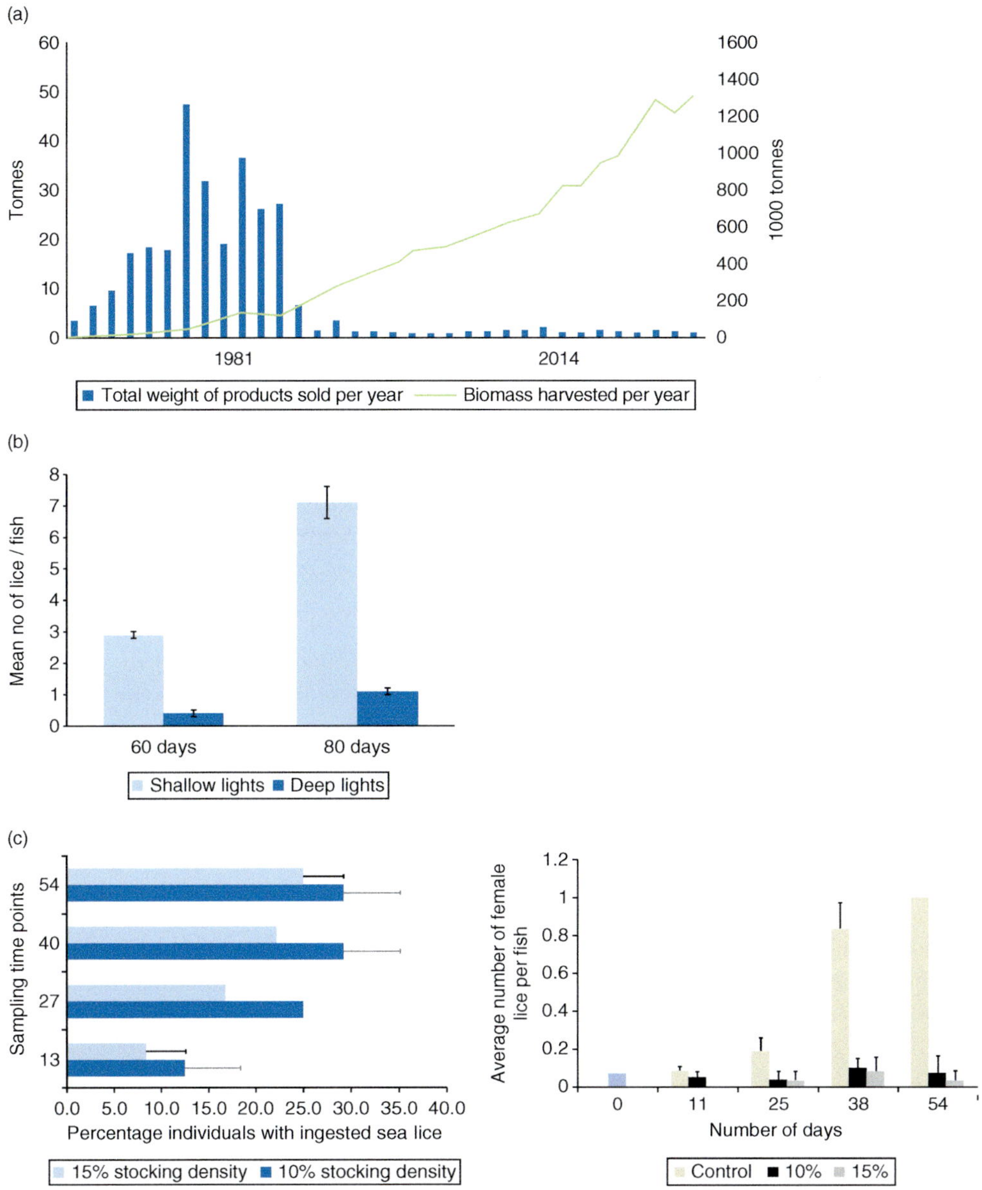

Fig. 8.6. (a) Total weight of antimicrobial products sold for use in farmed fish in Norway and biomass harvested from 1981 to 2014 (Norwegian Veterinary Institute, 2016). (b) Using lights to keep salmon away from infective sea lice. Mean (+SE) juvenile lice per fish in post-smolt Atlantic salmon in cages with submerged lights at depths of 1.5 m (shallow) and 10 m (deep) approx. 60 and 80 days after the lights were installed. Densities of fish in the top 4m of the cage and lice levels were both lower in the deep light condition (Frenzl *et al.*, 2014). (c) Using lumpfish to remove sea lice from Atlantic salmon. *Left*: mean (SD) percentage of lumpfish with sea lice in their stomachs; *Right*: mean (SD) number of female lice per fish from 13 to 54 days after lumpfish were stocked into salmon cages at densities of 10% and 15%. By the end of the trial, about 25% of lumpfish had been eating lice and infection levels were strikingly lower in salmon co-housed with lumpfish at both densities, compared to control fish (Imsland *et al.*, 2014).

example, in European sea bream, inherited resistance to pasteurellosis (a bacterial disease) is positively genetically linked to inherited differences in size, suggesting that disease resistance is associated with good growth (Antonello *et al.*, 2009). In contrast, there is a negative genetic correlation between resistance to Salmon Rickettsial Syndrome (another bacterial disease) and weight at harvest in Coho salmon (Yanez *et al.*, 2016). Carefully designed breeding programmes that take account of other important traits while selecting for disease resistance, possibly informed by use of molecular markers, could mitigate any such negative effects (Das and Sahoo, 2014).

The special case of salmon lice

SALMON LICE INFESTATIONS IN FARMED FISH AND HOW THESE ARE CONTROLLED One pathogen of farmed salmonids that continues to be a major source of concern for both fish welfare and environmental protection is the salmon louse. This ectoparasite attaches to the fish and feeds on mucous, skin and blood, damaging the skin; depending on louse intensity, this can increase risk of infection by other pathogens, disturb osmoregulation and impair swimming (Revie *et al.*, 2009; Torrisen *et al.*, 2013), which all compromise welfare.

Use of some highly effective organophosphate drugs for sea louse control is prohibited on environmental grounds and parasite resistance has evolved to successive alternative treatments (McNair, 2015). Treating sea louse infestations with chemicals is highly regulated (Revie *et al.*, 2009) and the aquaculture industry has supported an intense research and development effort to find other solutions (Box 8.2; Figs 6b and 6c). Some of these (for example, physically removing lice or warming the water to get rid of them) could themselves have adverse effects on individual fish, in the short term at least, and need to be specifically evaluated for any such effects.

The various approaches to salmon lice control are implemented through pest management strategies that combine several integrated actions. These have been effective in controlling sea louse infestation in farmed salmonids, so that normally the number of sea lice per fish rarely exceeds the threshold level at which health is compromised (Revie *et al.*, 2009).

Lice levels on farmed fish are monitored closely, to allow any problems to be detected and treated early. For example, the 2017 Scottish Salmon Producers' Health Management Report has identified six active farming regions (out of 28) with lice counts above the critical level of two adult females per fish, so there are challenges in some, but not all, areas.

ECOSYSTEM ISSUES: CROSS-INFECTION WITH WILD FISH There is concern that wild salmonids may acquire sea lice infections from farmed fish and that this may be a major contributor to the decline of wild stocks. There is convincing evidence that cross-infection between farmed and wild fish does occur, though just how important this has been in stock declines, compared for example to overfishing and habitat degradation, is not yet clear. In any event, salmon farmers and their regulators rightly take a strongly precautionary approach to the problem of preventing transfer from farmed wild salmonids (Harvey, 2008; Revie *et al.*, 2009). All the procedures for reducing lice infestations in farmed fish (Box 8.2) will also reduce the chances of salmon farms

Box 8.2. Some strategies for the control of sea lice, both established (normal font) and in development (italicized).

General management actions (Revie *et al.*, 2009):

- Joint disease management areas for coordinated louse control e.g. http://www.gov.scot/Topics/marine/Fish-shellfish/FHI/managementagreement
- Fallowing regimes, leaving a rotated subset of sites un-stocked to break the 'parasite's' life cycle
- Shortening production cycle, reducing the time that potential hosts spend in sea cages
- Siting farms to avoid areas of high infection risk, identified by louse dispersal models

Reducing contact between fish and infective larvae:

- Enclosed cages that prevent access of larvae to fish (Nilsen *et al.*, 2017)
- *Using plant extracts to mask chemicals in salmon skin that attract larval lice (O'Shea et al., 2017)*
- Keeping salmon away from the surface, where larvae congregate, for example by using underwater lights (Fig. 8.6b)

Chemotherapeutic treatment:

- The main chemotherapeutic agent against sea lice is emamectin benzoate (or SLICE®)
- *Helixir – Archimedes screw bath for administration of chemotherapeutants*

Alternative treatments:

- Cold-water cleaner fish (lumpfish remove ectoparasites from the skin of larger fish and are effective in reducing lice levels in salmon cages (Fig. 8.6c)
- Temperature adjusted seawater (Thermolicer and Optilicer)
- Seawater under pressure to wash lice off (Flatsetsund delouser and Hydrolicer)
- Soft brushes and seawater flushing (Skamik)
- *Selective breeding for resistance to lice is viable and could remove the need for chemical treatment in 10 generations (Gharbi et al., 2015)*

acting as a source of infestation for wild fish. Regular surveillance of lice levels in wild as well as farmed fish is used to monitor current risk and to inform treatment programmes (Revie *et al.*, 2009). Additional steps to reduce the probability of cross-infection include positioning salmon cages away from the migration paths of wild conspecifics, targeted fallowing of farms along key migratory corridors (Harvey, 2008; Revie *et al.*, 2009), and moving cages offshore when wild smolts are migrating (Penston *et al.*, 2011).

Control of reproduction

Stimulating and inhibiting maturation

Effective intensification requires control of the whole life cycle (as opposed to collecting brood stock or fry from the wild) and this means being able to bring cultured fish into full breeding condition when required. In fish being grown for food, growth slows down if fish mature, energy being diverted from production of muscle to gonads, compromising production. The aquaculture industry uses scientific understanding of the environmental conditions that initiate maturation in fish and hormones to control reproduction in both brood stock and on-growing fish (Tarranger *et al.*, 2010; Fleming and Huntingford, 2012).

Optimal environmental conditions for maturation

DETERMINANTS OF MATURITY IN FISH In nature, environmental conditions, particularly water temperature and photoperiod, create the circumstances in which fish may mature. Whether fish experiencing such conditions do mature depends on their reaching a threshold size and/or level of energy reserves at critical times. To bring potential brood stock into full reproductive condition, farmers expose fish with appropriate growth histories and nutritional status to the optimal combination of temperature and photoperiod (Tarranger *et al.*, 2010; Fleming and Huntingford, 2012). In contrast, farmers prevent maturation by 'tricking' fish into responding as if conditions are wrong for breeding, usually by manipulating photoperiod (Tarranger *et al.*, 2010; Good and Davidson, 2016). Maturation can also be prevented by using short-term feed restriction to ensure that growth rates and body condition are low at critical times, lost production being made good by subsequent compensatory growth (Tarranger *et al.*, 2010; Fleming and Huntingford, 2012). This approach works in, for example, Atlantic salmon (Rowe *et al.*, 1990 and yellowtail (Miura *et al.*, 2014).

IMPLICATIONS FOR WELFARE Age of maturation is naturally variable in many fish species. Wild Atlantic salmon may spend up to five years feeding and growing at sea, but a significant proportion mature at a small size after just one year, which is bad news for aquaculture. The proportion of fish adopting these different life history strategies is shaped by natural selection in relation to local environmental conditions (Johnston *et al.*, 2014). Bringing fish into full reproductive condition by providing optimal conditions for breeding, or preventing maturation by doing the opposite, both tap into natural systems that adjust reproductive state to external environmental condition and/or current energy reserves. Consequently, there is no reason to think that such procedures compromise the welfare of the fish concerned, provided that, in the case of feed restriction, the period of restriction is brief.

Hormonal control of breeding

REPRODUCTIVE HORMONES IN FISH AND IMPLICATIONS FOR WELFARE The hormonal control of reproduction in fish is very well understood. Briefly and simply, once maturation is triggered by the appropriate conditions, gonadotropic releasing factors (GnRF) secreted in the brain stimulate production of gonadotropic hormones (GTHs) in the pituitary. GTHs are released into the bloodstream and picked up by the gonads, where they stimulate production of germ cells and gonadal hormones (Tarranger *et al.*, 2010).

Although it is possible to supress maturation by hormonal manipulation, this strategy is not used in commercial aquaculture, other effective methods being available. In the case of broodstock management, however, treatment with GnRF and GTH is used to induce maturation in many farmed fish species. Promoting maturation artificially by hormonal manipulation could potentially have adverse effects if reproduction (which requires a lot of energy) is induced in fish that do not have sufficient reserves. However, this is unlikely to be the case, since brood stock nutrition is very carefully managed (Tarranger *et al.*, 2010).

Selective breeding for late maturation

BREEDING FOR LATE MATURATION AND IMPLICATIONS FOR WELFARE Selective breeding for delayed maturation has been successful in a few farmed species (Tarranger *et al.*, 2010). A possible complication is that in nature, early maturation is often linked to fast growth, so selection for late maturation may be targeting slow-growing fish. This need not be the case; strains of Atlantic salmon having been successfully selected for a combination of fast growth and late maturation (e.g. Gjerde, 1984) and late-maturing strains are now extensively used in salmon aquaculture (www.fao.org; Ellis *et al.*, 2016). Modern molecular tools can potentially be used to improve the effectiveness of selection for late maturation, providing genetic markers for crosses that will optimize age of maturation and growth (Gutierrez *et al.*, 2014). As discussed above, age of first breeding is variable in many fish species, late maturation being favoured by natural selection under certain environmental conditions, relating particularly to temperature regimes and food supply. In a sense, artificial selection for delayed maturation mimics this natural process and there is no reason to expect adverse effects on the welfare of the fish concerned.

Triploids

PRODUCING AND FARMING TRIPLOID FISH As already discussed, triploid fish are sometimes used in the finfish culture because, being essentially sterile, they grow fast. Triploids are produced by subjecting newly shed eggs to temperature or pressure shock, preventing the usual exclusion of one set of chromosomes at cell division and so generating fish with three sets of chromosomes after fertilization (Tarranger *et al.*, 2010; Benfey, 2016). Both male and female triploids are normally functionally sterile, though triploid males can develop gonads and may try to spawn (Fjelldal *et al.*, 2014). Triploids have been produced successfully for many species of fish (Tarranger *et al.*, 2010), but apart from rainbow trout, few are used commercially. Triploid Atlantic salmon are farmed commercially in Tasmania, because dark water colour makes it difficult to use lights to prevent early maturation (Jungalwalla, 1991).

IMPLICATIONS FOR WELFARE Triploidy is common in fish and diploid and triploid individuals can coexist within natural populations. Levels of triploidy can be as high as 16% in some populations of wild *pond loach,* an Asian farmed species in which the same female can produce both diploid and triploid offspring (Zhang and Arai, 1999). The fish genome is in a sense adapted to functioning at different ploidy levels and, in general, triploids produced for aquaculture look broadly normal and function well. In some species, life history stages and conditions, they survive better and grow faster than diploids (Tarranger *et al.*, 2010; Benfrey, 2016). Triploid Atlantic salmon make the challenging transition from fresh to seawater normally (Taylor *et al.*, 2007) and show normal responses to anaesthetics used during fish husbandry (Fraser *et al.*, 2014a). Triploid Atlantic salmon and rainbow trout are less aggressive than diploids, which may promote welfare in all-triploid groups (Tiwary *et al.*, 2004; Benfrey, 2016).

Several negative effects of triploidy have been identified in salmonids. For example, compared to diploid fish, triploid Atlantic salmon have shorter intestines relative to their size, which may compromise digestive efficiency (Peruzzi *et al.*, 2015), maintain homeostasis less well following stress (Cnaani *et al.*, 2014; Fraser *et al.*, 2015a), show more abdominal adhesions following vaccination and grow relatively poorly in seawater (Fraser *et al.*, 2014b). The most consistent effect of triploidy, with the most likely negative impact on welfare, is an increased frequency of skeletal abnormalities (Tiwary *et al.*, 2004; Tibbetts *et al.*, 2013). These include deformed vertebrae (Fig. 8.7) and shortened, misaligned jaws (Fraser *et al.*, 2015b; Amoroso *et al.*, 2016), which potentially compromise swimming and feeding. Such deformities are common because triploids need more phosphorus and histidine to support their faster growth and incidence of deformities can be reduced by appropriate diets (Fig. 8.7; Fjelldal *et al.*, 2016). Possibly because they have a higher resting metabolic rate, triploids do not perform well at high temperatures (Tarranger *et al.*, 2010) and jaw deformities can be reduced in triploid Atlantic salmon by incubating eggs at temperatures of 6 rather than 8 or 10°C (Fraser *et al.*, 2015b).

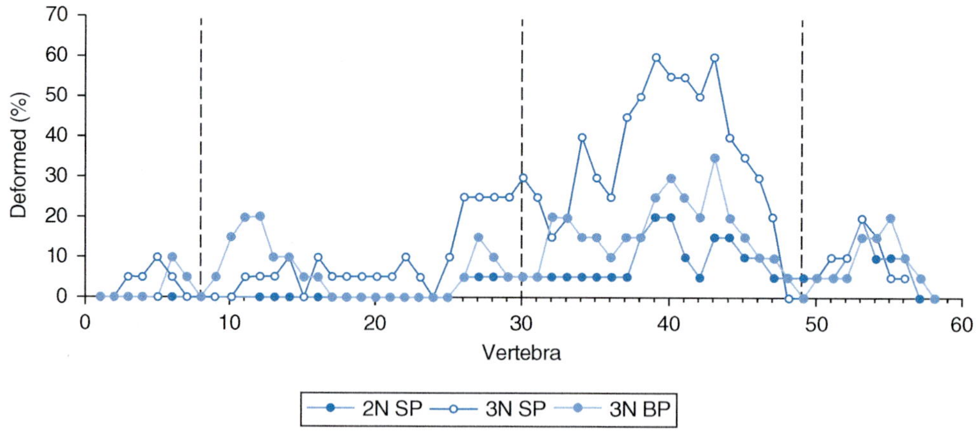

Fig. 8.7. Distribution of deformities along the vertebral column (0 = head) in diploid Atlantic salmon (2N) and in triploid fish (3N) reared on standard (SP) and mineral-supplemented (BP) diets. On the standard diet, deformities are significantly more common in triploid fish, but their frequency is reduced in triploid fish fed a mineral-enriched diet (Smedley *et al.*, 2016).

ECOSYSTEM ISSUES: IMPACT OF FARM ESCAPEES ON WILD POPULATIONS Regardless of any beneficial effects on growth, the use of triploids in aquaculture is likely to increase as a means of protecting native stocks from interbreeding with farm escapees. Despite the best efforts of farmers, farmed fish do escape into the wild, during transport, through holes in nets or when cages are damaged by storms. This raises concern about the welfare of the individual fish that escape, since their chances of finding food and avoiding predators in the wild are likely to be slim, especially in strains selected for fast growth. On the other hand, poor survival in escaped fish is good for the ecosystem if it reduces potential impact of escapees on wild populations, a topic of considerable concern (Diana *et al.*, 2013; Ellis *et al.*, 2016). Most seriously, interbreeding between wild and farmed fish could disrupt the genetic make-up of locally adapted populations, especially in salmonids, which show clear local population structuring. Genes from farmed salmon have been identified in many wild populations (Glover *et al.*, 2013) and, over time and in small populations, this can cause genetic change (Glover *et al.*, 2012). The aim for responsible finfish aquaculture should be to prevent any escapes, and the aquaculture industry has taken effective steps to achieve this (Fig. 8.8), for example through better management and improved cage design, including stronger, sometimes double, nets and the use of closed cages (Diana *et al.*, 2013; Price *et al.*, 2015; Lekang *et al.*, 2016).

Unless all aquaculture is carried out on land in closed recirculation systems, which is unfeasible, escape can never be completely prevented, so the only sure way of avoiding introgressive hybridization is to farm sterile fish. At present, this means using triploids, which can be produced on a large scale for most farmed species (Tarranger *et al.*, 2010; Benfey, 2016). Intensive research is currently directed at other ways of producing sterile fish for aquaculture, a promising development for the near future being the use of molecular tools to eliminate developing germ cells. A maternal sterility construct has been developed for zebrafish that selectively destroys the primordial germ cells, producing 'lineage-ending females' (Wong and Zohar, 2014). Large numbers of sterile female zebra fish can be produced by immersion in a bath containing a compound molecule that passes into the developing embryos and disrupts one of the genes that normally promote germ cell development (Wong and Zohar, 2014, 2015). To date, such approaches have been used effectively only in zebra fish, but trials are underway in some farmed species (Su *et al.*, 2014), and, given the stakes involved, are likely to find their place in the aquaculture of the future.

Conclusions and Future Trends

Aquaculture intensification and fish welfare

Some of the actions that allow intensification of aquaculture may seem strange and problematic to humans, but are not necessarily unnatural for fish; these include high densities, periods without food, ploidy manipulations and sex change. In broad terms, the available simple welfare indicators show that intensification has been beneficial for the health and welfare of farmed fish. Nevertheless, many actions for intensification can have specific adverse effects on welfare; for the most part, these have been identified and steps have been/are being taken to mitigate them.

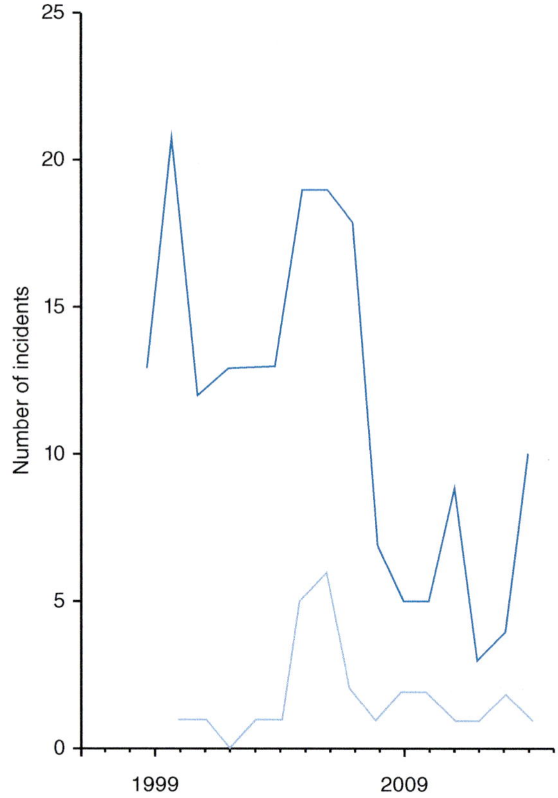

Fig. 8.8. Incidents of fish escaping from freshwater and seawater Scottish Atlantic salmon farms between 1999 and 2009. The number of escape incidents in seawater has fallen markedly; the number of incidents in freshwater has been low throughout this period (Ellis *et al*. 2016).

What the future of aquaculture might involve

The aquaculture of the future will have to tackle several challenges simultaneously (producing more fish; meeting water requirements; securing fish-feed supply; enhancing disease control; reducing waste; prevention of escapes), while at the same time protecting fish welfare. The human population is inevitably set to increase, at least until 2050, and an estimated 50% more food will be needed. Aquaculture will play an increasingly important role in food security, so fish production must increase, but against a background of increasing public concern about fish welfare and environmental protection. All this will happen at a time when the effects of climate change are likely to be increasingly apparent, making water a precious resource and lands for new agriculture limited, particularly in low-lying coastal zones, where much aquaculture is concentrated.

To meet these challenges, the industry will have at its disposal powerful and rapidly developing technologies, from engineering, electronics and computer science to molecular biology. Trying to look into a crystal ball, we expect to see a continuation and expansion of existing trends, including:

- *Geographic range and variety of farmed species.* An intensive programme of research is underway aimed at identifying suitable new species for aquaculture and at developing appropriate husbandry systems for rearing them, and this will surely continue in the future. If such research identifies species that can readily be farmed in a welfare-friendly, environmentally sustainable way, or concerns species that are to be farmed because wild stocks are declining, they may find their way into production. Arguably, however, as with terrestrial agriculture, in the longer term, the bulk of intensively farmed fish will likely come from a relatively small number of species that can be grown economically in many parts of the world. Given current market and production trends, in seawater these will probably include sea breams, European sea bass, amberjacks and barramundi (Asian sea bass) and possibly Atlantic cod. Freshwater aquaculture is likely to involve rainbow trout and several species of tilapia, carp, catfish and basa. Among species that migrate between fresh and sea water, Atlantic salmon are likely to remain a dominant aquaculture species.
- *Use of a wider range of production systems.* Developments are likely to include increasingly sophisticated recirculation systems, as well as closed and offshore cages. Use of production based on the recycling principles of traditional fish culture, but with the benefits of modern technology, is also likely to increase. In modern multi-trophic aquaculture systems pellet-fed fish are co-cultured with, for example, shellfish that feed on their faeces and wastes, and macroalgae, which use dissolved minerals and carbon dioxide from both up-stream species. All these developments will reduce the release of wastes into the environment.
- *Arrival/expansion of big data.* The aquaculture industry already produces and manages prodigious amounts of data, driven by large farmed fish populations and the need to monitor fish and their environment, using rapidly advancing sensor technology. This can only increase, offering both a challenge and an opportunity.
- *Expanding use of molecular technologies.* Potentially, genetic engineering has many uses in the aquaculture of the future. For example, carnivorous fish could be engineered to synthesisze the health-giving, highly unsaturated fatty acids that they must currently obtain from their diet, further reducing the need for fish oils in manufactured feed. More realistically, given consumer resistance to eating species that have themselves been genetically modified, sustainable sources of these key nutrients could come from genetically engineered single-cell organisms and plants, both of which have already been engineered to mass-produce key fatty acids, and which promote good, healthy growth in carnivorous fish.
- *New approaches to disease control.* In the near future, nanoparticle technology offers the potential for improving the effectiveness and minimizing the side effects of antibiotics and vaccines through highly targeted drug delivery. Nanoparticles also offer new approaches to disease control; for example, the antibacterial effects of zinc oxide nanoparticles arise, in part, through physical disruption of bacterial cell walls. Another promising development on the horizon is the use of bacteriophages, viruses that naturally infect and kill specific bacteria and can be used to control bacterial diseases in farmed fish.
- *Better understanding of the welfare of farmed fish.* At present, no tools are available for determining how fish experience the various treatments they receive in intensive production systems, but with increasing interest in and understanding of

Box 8.3. Latin names of the species mentioned in this chapter.

- Amberjacks: *Seriola* spp.
- Atlantic cod: *Gadus morhua*
- Atlantic salmon: *Salmo salar*
- Barramundi: *Lates calcarifer*
- Basa: *Pangasius bocourti*
- Channel catfish: *Ictalurus punctatus*
- Coho salmon: *Onchorhynchus kisutch*
- Common carp: *Cyprinus carpio*
- Crucian carp: *Carassius carassius*
- European sea bass: *Dicentrachus labrax*
- Gilthead sea bream: *Sparus aurata*
- Lumpfish: *Cycopterus lumpus*
- Mozambique tilapia: *Oreochromis mossambicus*
- Nile tilapia: *Oreochromis niloticus*
- Pond loach: *Misgurnus anguillicaudatus*
- Rainbow trout: *Onchorhynchus mykiss*
- Sunshine bass: hybrid between white and striped bass, *Morone chrysops* and *M. saxatilis*
- Turbot: *Scophthalmus maximus*
- Vundu: *Heterobranchus longifilis*
- Yellowtail: *Seriola quinqueradiata*
- Zebra fish: *Danio rerio*

cognition and sentience in fishes, such tools will come. It is impossible to predict what they will tell us about the mental states of fish that are functioning well or badly in intensive production systems, but the results will surely be interesting, and here, too, we see both a challenge and an opportunity.

References

Akhter, N., Wu, B., Memon, A.M. and Mohsin, M. (2015) Probiotics and prebiotics associated with aquaculture: a review. *Fish & Shellfish Immunology* 45, 733–741.

Ali, M., Nicieza, A. and Wootton, R.J. (2003) Compensatory growth in fishes: a response to growth depression. *Fish and Fisheries* 4, 147–190.

Amoroso, G., Cobcroft, J.M., Adams, M.B., Ventura, T. and Carter, G.C. (2016) Concurrence of lower jaw skeletal anomalies in triploid Atlantic salmon (*Salmo salar* L.) and the effect on growth in freshwater. *Journal of Fish Diseases* 39, 1509–1521.

Antonello, J., Massault, C., Franch, R., Haley, C., Pellizzari, C. *et al.* (2009) Estimates of heritability and genetic correlation for body length and resistance to fish pasteurellosis in the gilthead seabream. *Aquaculture* 298, 29–35.

Arbeláez-Rojas, G.A., Moraes, G., Nunes, C.S. and Fabrizzi, F. (2017) Sustained swimming mitigates stress in juvenile *Brycon amazonicus* reared in high stocking densities. *Pesquisa Agropecuaria Brasília* 52, 1–9.

Attia, J., Millot, S., Di-Poi, C., Begout, M.-L., Noble, C. *et al.* (2012) Demand feeding and welfare in farmed fish. *Fish Physiology and Biochemistry* 38, 112–125.

Azaza, M.S., Assad, A., Maghrbi, W. and El-Cafsi, M. (2013) The effects of rearing density on growth, size heterogeneity and inter-individual variation of feed intake in monosex male Nile tilapia *Oreochromis niloticus* L. *Animal* 7,1865–1874.

Barry, K.J., McClure, R.L. and Trushenski, J.T. (2017) Sea clam-derived feeding stimulants enhance acceptability and intake of reduced fish meal, soy-based sunshine bass feeds. *North American Journal of Aquaculture* 79, 115–122.

Benfey, T.J. (2016) Effectiveness of triploidy as a management tool for reproductive containment of farmed fish: Atlantic salmon (*Salmo salar*) as a case study. *Reviews in Aquaculture* 8, 264–282.

Binuramesh, C., Prabakaran, M., Steinhagen, D. and Michael, R.D. (2006) Effect of sex ratio on the immune system of *Oreochromis mossambicus* (Peters). *Brain Behaviour and Immunity* 20, 300–308.

Bogner, M., Zwicker, S., Bogner, D. and Slater, M. (2017) Influence of feeding sequence, light and colour on the performance of a self-grading system designed for turbot (*Scophthalmus maximus*). *Aquaculture Engineering* 77, 1–8.

Bostock, J., McAndrew, B., Richards, R., Jauncey, K., Telfer, T., Lorenzen, K., Little, D., Ross, L., Handisyde, N., Gatward, I. and Corner, R. (2010) Aquaculture: global status and trends. *Philosophical Transactions of the Royal Society of London* B365, 2897–2912.

Calabrese, S., Nilsen, T.O., Kolarevic, J., Ebbesson, L.O.E., Pedrosa, C. *et al.* (2017) Stocking density limits for post-smolt Atlantic salmon (*Salmo salar* L.) with emphasis on production performance and welfare. *Aquaculture* 468, 363–370.

Castillo, S. and Gatlin, D.M. (2015) Dietary supplementation of exogenous carbohydrase enzymes in fish nutrition: a review. *Aquaculture* 435, 286–292.

Cheng, K., Wagner, L., Moazzami, A.A., Gomez-Requeni, P., Vestergren, A.L.S. *et al.* (2016) Decontaminated fishmeal and fish oil from the Baltic Sea are promising feed sources for Arctic char (*Salvelinus alpinus* L.): studies of flesh lipid quality and metabolic profile. *European Journal of Lipid Science and Technology* 118, 862–873.

Cnaani, A., McLean, E. and Hallerman, E.M. (2014) Effects of growth hormone transgene expression and triploidy on acute stress indicators in Atlantic salmon (*Salmo salar* L.). *Aquaculture* 420–421, S124–S133.

Dalsgaard, J., Knudsen, K.E.B., Verlhac, V., Ekmann, K.S. and Pedersen, P.B. (2016) Supplementing enzymes to extruded, soybean-based diet improves breakdown of non-starch polysaccharides in rainbow trout (*Oncorhynchus mykiss*). *Aquaculture Nutrition* 22, 419–426.

Das, S. and Sahoo, P.K. (2014) Markers for selection of disease resistance in fish: a review. *Aquaculture International* 22, 1793–1812.

Davidsen, J., Svenning, M.-A., Orell, P., Yoccoz, N., Dempson, J.B. *et al.* (2005) Spatial and temporal migration of wild Atlantic salmon smolts determined from a video camera array in the sub-Arctic River Tana. *Fisheries Research* 74, 210–222.

Diana, J.S., Egna, H.S., Chopin, T., Peterson, M.S., Cao, L. *et al.* (2013) Responsible aquaculture in 2050: valuing local conditions and human innovations will be key to success. *BioScience* 63, 255–262.

Drangsholt, T.M., Bjarme, G., Odegard, J., Fridell, F. and Bentsen, H.N. (2011) Quantitative genetics of vaccine-induced side effects in farmed Atlantic salmon. *Aquaculture* 318, 316–324.

Dunham, R.A., Taylor, J.F., Rise, M.L. and Liu, Z. (2014) Development of strategies for integrated breeding, genetics and applied genomics for genetic improvement of aquatic organisms. *Aquaculture* 420–421, S121–S123.

Edwards, P. (2015) Aquaculture environment interactions: past, present and likely future trends *Aquaculture* 447, 2–14.

Ellis, T., Turnbull, J.F., Knowles, T.G., Lines, J.F.A. and Auchterlonie, N.A. (2016) Trends during development of Scottish salmon farming: an example of sustainable intensification? *Aquaculture* 458, 82–99.

FAO (Food and Agriculture Organization) (2014) The state of world fisheries and aquaculture. Available at: http://www.fao.org/figis (accessed 26 January 2018).

Fjelldal, P.G., Wennevik, V., Fleming, I.A., Hansen, T. and Glover, K.A. (2014) Triploid (sterile) farmed Atlantic salmon attempt to spawn with wild females. *Aquaculture Environment Interactions* 5, 155–162.

Fjelldal, P.G., Hansen, T.J., Lock, E.-J., Wargelius, A., Fraser, T.W.K. *et al.* (2016) Increased dietary phosphorus prevents vertebral deformities in triploid Atlantic salmon (*Salmo salar* L.). *Aquaculture Nutrition* 22, 72–90.

Fleming, I. and Huntingford, F. (2012) Reproductive behaviour. In: Huntingford, F., Jobling, M. and Kadri, S. (eds) *Aquaculture and Behavior*. Wiley-Blackwell, Oxford, UK, pp. 286–321.

Francis, G., Makkar, H.P.S. and Becker, K. (2001) Anti-nutritional factors present in plant-derived feed ingredients and their effects in fish. *Aquaculture* 199, 197–227.

Fraser, T.W.K., Mayer, I., Skjaeraasen, J.E., Hansen, T. and Fjelldal, P.G. (2014a) The effect of triploidy on the efficacy and physiological response to anesthesia with MS 222 and isoeugenol in Atlantic salmon post-smolts. *Aquaculture International* 22, 1347–1359.

Fraser, T.W.K., Hansen, T., Mayer, I., Skjæraasen, J.E., Glover, K.A., Sambraus, F. and Fjelldal, P.G. (2014b) The effect of triploidy on vaccine side-effects in Atlantic salmon. *Aquaculture* 433, 481–490.

Fraser, T.W.K., Vindas, M.A., Fjelldal, P.G., Winberg, S., Thörnqvist, P-O, Øverli, O., Skjæraasen, J.-E., Hansen, T.J. and Mayer, I. (2015a) Increased reactivity and monoamine dysregulation following stress in triploid Atlantic salmon (*Salmo salar*). *Comparative Biochemistry and Physiology, Part A* 185, 125–131.

Fraser, T.W.K., Hansen, T., Fleming, M.S. and Fjelldal, P.G. (2015b) The prevalence of vertebral deformities is increased with higher egg incubation temperatures and triploidy in Atlantic salmon *Salmo salar* L. *Journal of Fish Diseases* 38, 75–89.

Frenzl, B., Stien, L.H., Cockerill, D., Oppedal, F., Richards, R.H.. *et al.* (2014) Manipulation of farmed Atlantic salmon swimming behaviour through the adjustment of lighting and feeding regimes as a tool for salmon lice control. *Aquaculture* 424–425, 183–188.

Fujimura, K. and Kocher, T. (2011) Tol2-mediated transgenesis in tilapia (*Oreochromis niloticus*). *Aquaculture* 319, 342–346.

Garcia-Celdran, M., Ramis, G., Manchado, M., Estevez, A., Afonso, J.M., Maria-Dolores, E., Penalver, J. and Armero, E. (2015) Estimates of heritabilities and genetic correlations of growth and external skeletal deformities at different ages in a reared gilthead sea bream (*Sparus aurata* L.) population sourced from three broodstocks along the Spanish coasts. *Aquaculture* 445, 33–41.

Garnett, T., Appleby, M.C., Balmford, A., Bateman, I.J., Benton, T.G. *et al.* (2013) Sustainable intensification in agriculture: premises and policies. *Science* 341, 33–34.

Gharbi, K., Matthews, L., Bron, J., Roberts, R., Tinch, A. and Stear, M. (2015) The control of sea lice in Atlantic salmon by selective breeding. *Journal of the Royal Society Interface* 12, article no: 20150574.

Gjerde, B. (1984) Response to individual selection for age at sexual maturity in Atlantic salmon. *Aquaculture* 38, 229–240.

Glover, K.A., Quintela, M., Wennevik, V., Besnier, F., Sørvik, A.G.E. and Skaala, O. (2012) Three decades of farmed escapees in the wild: a spatio-temporal analysis of Atlantic salmon population genetic structure throughout Norway. *PLOS ONE* 7, e4129.

Good, C. and Davidson, J. (2016) A review of factors influencing maturation of Atlantic salmon, *Salmo salar*, with focus on water recirculation aquaculture system environments. *Journal of the World Aquaculture Society* 47, 605–632.

Gutierrez, A.P., Lubieniecki, K.P., Fukui, S., Withler, R.E., Swift, B. and Davidson, W.S. (2014) Detection of quantitative trait loci related to grilsing and late sexual maturation in Atlantic salmon (*Salmo salar*). *Marine Biotechnology (New York)* 16, 103–110.

Hansen, J.W. (1996) Is agricultural sustainability a useful concept? *Agricultural Systems* 50, 117–143.

Harvey B. (2008) Science and sea lice: What do we know? BC Pacific Salmon Forum report. Available at: http://www.pacificsalmonforum.ca/pdfs-all-docs/ScienceandSeaLiceFinalFeb22-08.pdf (accessed 26 January 2018).

Henry, M., Gasco, L., Piccolo, G. and Fountoulaki, E. (2015) Review of the use of insects in the diet of farmed fish: past and future. *Animal Feed Science and Technology* 203, 1–22.

Huntingford, F.A. and Kadri, S. (2014) Defining, assessing and promoting the welfare of farmed fish. In: Mellor, D.J. and Bayvel, A.C.D. (eds) *Animal Welfare: Focussing on the Future*. World Organisation for Animal Health Scientific and Technical Review 33(1), 233–244.

Huntingford, F., Kadri, S. and Jobling, M. (2012) Introduction: aquaculture and behaviour. In: Huntingford, F., Jobling, M. and Kadri, S. (eds) *Aquaculture and Behavior*. Wiley-Blackwell, Oxford. UK, pp. 1–35.

Imsland, A.K., Reynolds, P., Eliassen, G., Hangstad, T.A., Foss, A., Vikingstad, E. and Elvegård, T.A. (2014) The use of lumpfish (*Cyclopterus lumpus* L.) to control sea lice (*Lepeophtheirus salmonis* Krøyer) infestations in intensively farmed Atlantic salmon (*Salmo salar* L.). *Aquaculture* 424–425, 18–23.

Jobling, M. (2010a) Fish culture: feeds and feeding. In: Le Francois, N.R., Jobling, M., Carter, C., Blier, P.U. and Savoie, A. (eds) *Finfish Aquaculture Diversification*. CAB International, Wallingford, UK, pp. 61–87.

Jobling, M. (2010b) Fish culture: the rearing environment. In: Le Francois, N.R., Jobling, M., Carter, C., Blier, P.U. and Savoie, A. (eds) *Finfish Aquaculture Diversification*. CAB International, Wallingford, UK, pp. 33–60.

Jobling, M. (2012) Fish in aquaculture environments. In: Huntingford, F., Jobling, M. and Kadri, S. (eds) *Aquaculture and Behavior*. Wiley-Blackwell, Oxford, UK, pp. 36–64.

Jobling, M., Alanärä, A., Kadri, S. and Huntingford, F. (2012) Feeding biology and foraging. In: Huntingford, F., Jobling, M. and Kadri, S. (eds) *Aquaculture and Behavior*. Wiley-Blackwell, Oxford, UK, pp. 121–149.

Johnston, S.E., Orell, P., Pritchard, V.L., Kent, M.P., Lien, S., Niemela, E., Erkinaro, J. and Primmer, C.R. (2014) Genome-wide SNP analysis reveals a genetic basis for sea-age variation in a wild population of Atlantic salmon (*Salmo salar*). *Molecular Ecology* 23, 3452–3468.

Juell, J.-E., Oppedal, F., Boxaspen, K. and Tarranger, G.L. (2003) Submerged light increases swimming depth and reduces fish density of Atlantic salmon in production cages. *Aquaculture Research* 34, 469–477.

Jungalwalla, P.J. (1991) Production of non-maturing Atlantic salmon in Tasmania. *Canadian Technical Reports in Fisheries and Aquatic Science* 1789, 47–71.

Kim, J.-H., Leggatt, R.A., Chan, M. and Volkoff, H. (2015) Effects of chronic growth hormone overexpression on appetite regulating brain gene expression in Coho salmon. *Molecular and Cellular Endocrinology* 413, 178–188.

Klinger, D. and Naylor, R. (2012) Searching for solutions in aquaculture: charting a sustainable course. *Annual Review of Environmental Resources* 37, 247–276.

Kristensen, T., Haugen, T.O., Rosten, T., Fjellheim, A., Atland, A. and Rosseland, B. (2012) Effects of production intensity and production strategies in commercial Atlantic salmon smolt (*Salmo salar*) production on subsequent performance in the early sea stage. *Fish Physiology and Biochemistry* 38, 273–282.

Lee-Montero, I., Navarro, A., Negrin-Baez, D., Zamorano, M.J., Berbel, C. *et al.* (2015) Genetic parameters and genotype-environment interactions for skeletal deformities and growth traits at different ages on gilthead seabream (*Sparus auratus* L.) in four Spanish regions. *Animal Genetics* 46, 164–174.

Lekang, O.I., Salas-Bringas, C. and Bostock, J.C. (2016) Challenges and emerging technical solutions in on-growing salmon farming. *Aquaculture International* 24, 757–766.

Lines, J.A., Tillett, R.D., Ross, L.G., Chan, D., Hockaday, S. and McFarlane, N.J.B. (2001) An automatic image-based system for estimating the mass of free-swimming fish. *Computers and Electronics in Aquaculture* 31, 151–168.

Little, D.C., Newton, R.W. and Beveridge, M.C.M. (2016) Aquaculture: a rapidly growing and significant source of sustainable food? Status, transitions and potential. *Proceedings of the Nutrition Society* 75, 274–286.

Lu, J., Yoshizaki, G., Endo, M. and Takeuchi, T. (2013) Effect of dietary high amount of calcium and phosphorus on reducing the prevalence of morphological deformities in GH-transgenic Nile tilapia. *Fisheries Science* 79, 647–658.

Mair, G.C. and Little, D.C. (1991) Population control in farmed tilapias. *NAGA – The ICLARM Quarterly* 14, 8–13.

Martinez, P., Vinas, A.M., Sanchez, L., Doaz, N., Ribas, L. and Piferrer, F. (2014) Genetic architecture of sex determination in fish: application to sex ratio control in aquaculture. *Frontiers in Genetics* 5, article 340.

McNair, C.M. (2015) Ectoparasites of medical and veterinary importance: drug resistance and the need for alternative control methods. *Journal of Pharmacy and Pharmacology* 67, 351–363.

Mei, J. and Gui, J.-F. (2015) Genetic basis and biotechnological manipulation of sexual dimorphism and sex determination in fish. *Science China Life Sciences* 58, 124–136.

Miranda, C.D., Tello, A. and Keen, P.L. (2013) Mechanisms of antimicrobial resistance in finfish aquaculture environments. *Frontiers in Microbiology* 4, article 233.

Miura, C., Yoshihara, Y., Shimizu-Yamaguchi, S., Hayashi, D., Hamada, K. *et al.* (2014) Controlled feeding alleviates the reduced growth associated with spawning in farmed yellowtail (*Seriola quinqueradiata*). *Aquaculture* 424, 10–17.

Nagel, F., von Danwitz, A., Schlachter, M., Kroeckel, S., Wagner, C. and Schulz, C. (2014) Blue mussel meal as feed attractant in rapeseed protein-based diets for turbot (*Psetta maxima* L.). *Aquaculture Research* 45, 1964–1978.

Nilsen, A., Nielsen, K.V., Biering, E. and Bergheim, A. (2017) Effective protection against sea lice during production of Atlantic salmon in floating enclosures. *Aquaculture* 466, 41–50.

Noble, C., Jone, C.N., Damsgaard, B., Flood, M., Midling, K., Roque, A., Saether, B.-S. and Cottee, S.U. (2012) Injuries and deformities in fish: their potential impact upon aquacultural production and welfare – summary. *Fish Physiology and Biochemistry* 38, 61–83.

Norwegian Veterinarian Institute (2016) Use of antibiotics in Norwegian Aquaculture. NVI report 22. Norwegian Veterinarian Institute, Oslo.

Omasaki, S.K., Charo-Karisa, H., Kahi, A.K. and Komen, H. (2016) Genotype by environment interaction for harvest weight, growth rate and shape between monosex and mixed sex Nile tilapia (*Oreochromis niloticus*). *Aquaculture* 458, 75–81.

O'Shea, B., Wadsworth, S., Marambio, J.P., Birkett, M.A., Pickett, J.A. and Mordue, A.J. (2017) Disruption of host-seeking behaviour by the salmon louse, *Lepteophtheirus salmonis*, using botanically-derived repellents. *Journal of Fish Diseases* 40, 495–505.

Pennell, W. and Barton, B.A. (1996) *Principles of Salmonid Culture. Developments in Aquaculture and Fisheries Science*, volume 29. Elsevier, Amsterdam.

Penston, M.J., McBeath, A.J.A. and Millar, C.P. (2011) Densities of planktonic *Lepeophtheirus salmonis* before and after an Atlantic salmon farm relocation. *Aquaculture Environment Interactions* 1, 225–232.

Peruzzi, S., Hagen, O. and Jobling, M. (2015) Gut morphology of diploid and triploid Atlantic salmon (*Salmo salar* L.). *Aquaculture International* 23, 1105–1108.

Peterson, B.C., Small, B.C., Waldbieser, G.C. and Bosworth, B.G. (2008) Endocrine responses in fast- and slow-growing families of channel catfish. *North American Journal of Aquaculture* 70, 240–250.

Price, C., Black, K.D., Hargrave, B.T. and Morris, Jr, J.A. (2015) Marine cage culture and the environment: effects on water quality and primary production. *Aquaculture Environment Interactions* 6, 151–174.

Quillet, E., Krieg, F., Dechamp, N., Hervet, C., Berard, A. *et al*. (2014) Quantitative trait loci for magnitude of the plasma cortisol response to confinement in rainbow trout. *Animal Genetics* 45, 223–234.

Rasmussen, R. and Morrisey, M. (2007) Biotechnology in aquaculture: transgenics and polyploidy. *Comprehensive Reviews in Food Science and Food Safety* 6, 2–16.

Reimer, T., Dempster, T., Wargelius, A., Fjelldal, P.G., Hansen, T. *et al*. (2017) Rapid growth causes abnormal vaterite formation in farmed fish otoliths. *Journal of Experimental Biology* 220, 2965–2969.

Revie, C., Dill, L., Finstad, B. and Todd, C.D. (2009) Sea Lice Working Group Report. NINA Special Report 39.

Richards, G.P. (2014) Bacteriophage remediation of bacterial pathogens in aquaculture: a review of the technology. *Bacteriophage* 4(4), e975540. DOI: 10.4161/21597081.2014.975540.

Romarheim, O.H., Øverland, M., Mydland, L.T., Skrede, A. and Landsverk, T. (2010) Bacteria grown on natural gas prevent soybean meal-induced enteritis in Atlantic salmon. *Journal of Nutrition*. DOI: 10.3945/jn.110.128900.

Rowe, D.K. and Thorpe, J.E. (1990) Suppression of maturation in male Atlantic salmon (*Salmo salar* L.) parr by reduction in feeding and growth during spring months. *Aquaculture* 86, 291–313.

Sahoo, T.K., Jena, P.K., Patel, A.K. and Seshadri, S. (2016) Bacteriocins and their applications for the treatment of bacterial diseases in aquaculture: a review. *Aquaculture Research* 47, 1013–1027.

Scottish Salmon Producers' Organisation (2014) *Scottish Salmon Farming: Growing a Sustainable Industry*. Scottish Salmon Producers' Organisation.

Singh, A.K. (2013) Introduction of modern endocrine techniques for the production of monosex populations of fishes. *General and Comparative Endocrinology* 181, 146–155.

Smedley, M.A., Clokie, B.G.J., Migaud, H., Campbell, P., Walton, J., Hunter, D., Corrigan, D. and Taylor, J. (2016) Dietary phosphorous and protein supplementation enhances seawater growth and reduces severity of vertebral malformation in triploid Atlantic salmon (Salmo salar L.). *Aquaculture* 451, 357–368.

Sommerset, I., Krossøy, B., Biering, E. and Frost, P. (2005) Vaccines for fish in aquaculture. *Expert Reviews of Vaccines* 4, 89–101.

Su, B., Peatman, E., Shang, M., Thresher, R., Grewe, P. *et al*. (2014) Expression and knockdown of primordial germ cells genes, *vasa, nanos* and *dead end* in common carp (*Cyprinus carpio*) embryos for transgenic sterilisation and reduced sexual maturity. *Aquaculture* 420–421, 572–584.

Sveen, L.R., Timmerhaus, G., Torgersen, J.S., Ytteborg, E., Jorgensen, S.M. *et al*. (2016) Impact of fish density and specific water flow on skin properties in Atlantic salmon (*Salmo salar*) post-smolts. *Aquaculture* 464, 629–637.

Tafalla, C., Bogwald, J. and Dalmo, R.A. (2013) Adjuvants and immunostimulants in fish vaccines: current knowledge and future perspectives. *Fish & Shellfish Immunology*. DOI: 10.1016/j.fsi.2013.02.029.

Tapia-Paniaga, S.T., Vida, S., Lobo, C., Carcia de la Banda, I., Esteban, M.A., Balebona, M.C. and Morinigo, M.A. (2015) Dietary administration of the probiotic SpPdp11: effects on the intestinal microbiota and immune-related gene-expression of farmed *Solea senegalensis* treated with oxytetracycline. *Fish and Shellfish Immunology* 46, 449–458.

Tarranger, G.L., Carrillo, M., Schulz, R.W., Fontaine, P., Zanuy, S. *et al.* (2010) Control of puberty in farmed fish. *General and Comparative Endocrinology* 165, 483–515.

Taylor, J.F., Needham, M.P., North, B.P., Morgan, A., Thompson, K. and Migaud, H. (2007) The influence of ploidy on seawater adaptation, acute stress response and immune function following seawater transfer in non-smolting rainbow trout. *General and Comparative Endocrinology* 152, 314–325.

Tibbetts, S.M., Wall, C.L., Barbosa-Solomieu, V., Bryenton, M.D., Plouffe, D.A., Buchanan, J.T. and Lall, S.P. (2013) Effects of combined 'all-fish' growth hormone transgenics and triploidy on growth and nutrient utilization of Atlantic salmon (*Salmo salar* L.) fed a practical grower diet of known composition. *Aquaculture* 406–407. 141–152.

Tidwell, J.J. and Allen, G.L. (2001) Fish as food: aquaculture's contribution. Ecological and economic impacts and contributions of fish farming and capture fisheries. *EMBO Reports* 2, 958–963.

Tiwary, B.K., Kirubagaran, R. and Ray, A.K. (2004) The biology of triploid fish. *Reviews in Fish Biology and Fisheries* 14, 391–402.

Tlusty, M., Rhyne, A., Szczebak, J.T., Bourque, B., Bowen, J.L., Burr, G., Marx, C.J. and Feinberg, L. (2017) A transdisciplinary approach to the initial validation of a single cell protein as an alternative protein source for use in aquafeeds. Available at: https://peerj.com/articles/3170/ (accessed 26 January 2018).

Torrissen, O., Jones, S., Asche, F., Guttormsen, A., Skilbrei6, O.T. *et al.* (2013) Salmon lice – impact on wild salmonids and salmon aquaculture. *Journal of Fish Diseases* 36, 171–194.

Turnbull, J., Bell, A., Bron, J., Adams, C.E. and Huntingford, F.A. (2005) Stocking density and welfare of cage farmed Atlantic salmon: application of a multivariate analysis. *Aquaculture* 243, 1–4, 121–132.

Vandeputte, M., Porte, J.D., Auperin, B., Dupont-Nivet, M., Vergnet, A. *et al.* (2016) Quantitative genetic variation for post-stress cortisol and swimming performance in growth-selected and control populations of European sea bass (*Dicentrarchus labrax*). *Aquaculture* 455, 1–7.

Vernold, F.F., Penn, M.H., Krogdahl, A. and Overturf, K. (2012) Severity of soybean meal induced distal intestinal inflammation, enterocyte proliferation rate, and fatty acid binding protein (Fabp2) level differ between strains of rainbow trout (*Oncorhynchus mykiss*). *Aquaculture* 364–365, 281–292.

Weber, G.M. and Silverstein, J.T. (2007) Evaluation of a stress response for use in a selective breeding programme for improved growth and disease resistance in rainbow trout. *North American Journal of Aquaculture* 69, 69–79.

Wetten, M., Aasmundstad, T., Kjøglum, S. and Storset, A. (2007) Genetic analysis of resistance to infectious pancreatic necrosis in Atlantic salmon (*Salmo salar* L.). *Aquaculture* 272, 111–117.

Wong, T.T. and Zohar, Y. (2014) Production of reproductively sterile fish: a mini-review of germ cell elimination technologies. *General and Comparative Endocrinology* 221, 3–8.

Wong, T.T. and Zohar, Y. (2015) Production of reproductively sterile fish by a non-transgenic gene silencing technology. *Scientific Reports* 5, 15822. DOI: 10.1038/srep15822.

Yanez, J.M., Bangera, R., Lhorente, J.P., Barria, A., Oyarzun, M., Neira, R. and Newman, S. (2016) Negative genetic correlation between resistance against *Piscirickettsia salmonis* and harvest weight in Coho salmon (*Onchorhynchus kisutch*). *Aquaculture* 459, 8–13.

Yanong, R.P.E. (2015) *Use of Vaccines in Finfish Aquaculture*. Available at: http://edis.ifas.ufl.edu/fa156 (accessed 26 January 2018).

Ye, D., Zhu, Z.Y. and Sun, Y.H. (2015) Fish genome manipulation and directional breeding. *Science China: Life Sciences* 58, 170–177.

Young, J.A. (2010) Organic and ecolabelling. In: Le Francois, N.R., Jobling, M., Carter, C., Blier, P.U. and Savoie, A. (eds) *Finfish Aquaculture Diversification.* CAB International, Wallingford, UK, pp. 556–566.

Zhang, Q.Q. and Arai, K. (1999) Distribution and reproductive capacity of natural triploid individuals and occurrence of unreduced eggs as a cause of polyploidization in the loach, *Misgurnus anguillicaudatus*. *Ichthyological Research* 46, 153–161.

Zhong, C.R., Song, Y.L., Wang, Y.P., Li, Y.M., Liao, L.J. *et al.* (2012) Growth hormone transgene effects on growth performance are inconsistent among offspring derived from different homozygous common carp (Cyprinus carpio L.). *Aquaculture* 356, 404–411.

9 Welfare Concerns in Genetically Modified Laboratory Mice and Rats

Nikki Osborne,[1,*] David Morton[2] and Jan-Bas Prins[3]

[1]*Responsible Research in Practice, Horsham, UK;* [2]*University of Birmingham, UK;* [3]*University of Leiden, The Netherlands*

The last 40 years or so has seen the emergence of scientific advances in genetics that are having significant public impact and raising serious ethical concerns. Since the discovery of the structure of DNA by Crick and Watson, followed by the associated advances in our ability to understand better our genetic make-up, our genetic defects and associated diseases, concerns have been raised. This concern has been further increased particularly by our ability to manipulate the genomes of animals to eliminate and to model some harmful human diseases, as well as the potential to promote gene enhancement for agricultural objectives. This chapter describes the development of genetic modification techniques in animals and looks at some of the ethical issues arising, particularly for research animals, i.e. laboratory mice and rats.

The Development of GM Rodents

> Genetic engineering is an old practice, which has recently added transgenic technology to its traditional armamentarium of procedures. Selective breeding, the most widely used form of genetic engineering techniques, is in many respects more powerful than transgenic technology. Transgenic technology as a genetic engineering tool should therefore be regarded in the proper perspective. It is rapid, in the sense that genes from widely disparate species can be brought together in a single generation, but it is limited by the technical reality that relatively few traits can be modified in any single experiment.
>
> (Gordon, 1997)

Originally, spontaneous mutations were identified as a valuable source of mouse models to discover novel genes and functions relevant to human disorders. These models are molecularly similar to mutations in the human genome, and therefore often produce phenotypes that more closely resemble those that are characteristic of human disease than do genetically engineered mutations. Spontaneous mutations are, however, by their very nature unpredictable and relatively few in number. Thus the scientific desire for animal-intensive, large-scale analysis of spontaneous genetic mutations has traditionally been limited to large mammalian genetics institutes (Davisson *et al.*, 2012). It is here that the desire to create new genetic mutations arose, resulting in the development of other strategies collectively known as 'forward genetic' approaches.

*Corresponding author e-mail: nikki@responsibleresearchinpractice.co.uk

This approach relies upon scientific developments to enable researchers to initiate mutagenic events on demand in mice to create genetic mutations that can be detected using phenotypic screens. In this way, genetically modified (GM) mice with a genetic trait can be identified and studied (Doyle *et al.*, 2012). Ethylnitrosourea (ENU) has, and is, still being used as a chemical mutagen to create mutagenic lesions in the murine genome that are transmitted to offspring. Following the detection of a phenotype, a thorough analysis of the genome can be undertaken to find the underlying genetic mutation(s) and their mode of inheritance. 'Reverse genetics' is the opposite approach whereby a gene or genes of interest are identified first, then their function is determined by analysing the phenotypic effects detectable in mice containing genetically modified sequences within these genes.

To date, the genome of the mouse has been the most modified of all the mammalian species for the simple fact that mouse genetics is a longstanding and well funded area of research. The genetic homology (shared ancestry) between the laboratory mouse and humans is a major driver for this. In January 2015, the Mouse Genome Database at the Jackson Laboratory reported 17,055 mouse–human homologs, genes related by descent, and 18,461 mouse–rat homologs (Dolan *et al.*, 2015). This includes both 'orthologs' – related genes in different species that result from a shared ancestry – and 'paralogs' – genes that result from gene duplication events within a species. Indeed. current understanding is that the protein coding regions of *Homo sapiens* and *Mus musculus* genomes are, on average, 85% identical – some genes are 99% identical, whilst others are just 60% identical (http://www.genome.gov/10001345/). This implies a high degree of homology between these species but it should be realized that a substantial number of mouse genes are regulated in different ways from similar genes in humans. These differences are not random, but appear to be clustered along certain signalling pathways, such as in genes regulating the immune system (Carninci, 2014; Yue *et al.*, 2014). Another driver for the mouse becoming a preferred model organism is the availability of well characterized inbred strains. These display a high level of genetic homology between individual animals, thus making it easier to identify genetic mutations of interest because of the naturally low level of genetic variation present within each strain. When combined with the technical ease, the fact that mice can be housed, bred and cared for at a low cost, relative to other larger species; are small and easy to handle; and have very simple dietary, housing and care requirements lends to their research appeal.

Gene modification

There are at least four approaches to introduce genetic modification into the genome: DNA microinjection; virus mediated gene transfer; embryonic stem (ES) cell gene transfer; and the more recently developed gene editing technology. The first reports on the successful introduction of foreign DNA into both somatic and germ cells of mammalian species date back to the late 1970s. It was discovered that introduction of DNA-sharing homology with an endogenous locus into a cell's nucleus could induce recombination using the host's DNA repair machinery. This resulted in the transfer of information from an exogenous (other organisms) DNA sequence to the endogenous (host organisms) chromosomal target. This technique became known as 'gene targeting'. Later results demonstrated the repair of double strand DNA breaks through homology directed repair pathways. An alternative 'emergency' DNA repair pathway called non-homologous end joining (NHEJ), whereby the break ends are directly ligated without the need for a homologous template, also exists, resulting in insertion and deletion ('indel') mutations.

Jeanisch was the first to report on a second approach, to introduce genetic modifications (virus mediated gene transfer) using the integration of murine leukemia virus (MuLV) into both somatic and germ cells (Jaenisch, 1976). By dissecting the retroviral life cycle it became possible to genetically engineer these viruses to carry exogenous genes. These recombinant viruses could then be used to infect pre-implantation embryos. However, this never really developed into a routine procedure with wide application, unlike the extensively used technique of directly injecting DNA into the pronucleus of fertilized oocytes (Brinster *et al.*, 1981; Palmiter and Brinster, 1986). The first successful attempts at microinjection used a recombinant plasmid composed of segments of herpes simplex virus and simian virus 40 viral DNA inserted into the bacterial plasmid pBR322, which was injected into the pronuclei of fertilized mouse oocytes. This led to offspring carrying the foreign DNA in most of its cells as was reported in 1980 (Gordon *et al.*, 1980). Soon after, other reports followed (for review see Palmiter and Brinster, 1986). These transgenic (TG) lines were recognized as important models to dissect biological processes in health and disease. This technology also developed because of advancements in mammalian embryology and cell culture technology. Thus embryonic stem (ES) cell gene transfer to genetically transform the mammalian germline developed as a third approach. The ES cells can be isolated from the inner cell mass of a blastocyst and cultured under specific conditions to maintain their unique characteristic. They then resume a normal programme of development once inserted into the cavity of another blastocyst by injection and differentiate into all cell types of the body including germ cells (Evans and Kaufman, 1981; Martin, 1981). The technology of genetic modification of cells in culture by homologous recombination of host DNA by donor gene constructs, discovered by Smithies and others, made it possible to modify ES cells before introducing them into the cavity of blastocysts (Smithies *et al.*, 1985; Thomas *et al.*, 1986).

Knockouts

The technique to select modified ES cells from the pool of unmodified ES cells in a culture dish was developed by Mansour and others (Mansour *et al.*, 1988). It is mostly used for the creation of knockout animals to model human diseases. In these animals a specific gene or genes are modified such that they are defective and are no longer expressed. Until very recently, the generation of knockout animals was restricted to mice, since only germline- competent ES-cell lines from murine origin were available, and initially only from one genetic background, the 129/SvJ strain (Brook and Gardner, 1997). Since most research uses mice with a C56BL/6 or C56BL/6N genetic background, the genetic modification requires backcrossing to introduce it onto the B6 or any other relevant genetic background of choice through several generations of crossing animals carrying the genetic modification with unmodified, wild-type animals with the preferred genetic background. Commonly, 3–10 generations of backcrossing are needed; the resultant animals are called congenic – they differ in only one locus and a linked segment of chromosome from the wild-type animals. The exact number of backcross generations required is dependent on the genetic background and method that is applied to select the most appropriate male animals for the next generation. The rapid elimination of heterozygosity occurs only in regions of the genome that are not linked to the donor allele, which, of course, is maintained by selection in a state of heterozygosity throughout the breeding protocol. Unfortunately, genomic linkages cause the retention of a significant length of chromosome flanking the mutated locus, which is called the differential chromosomal segment. Even for congenic lines at the same backcross generation, the length of this segment can vary greatly because of the inherently random distribution of crossover sites (1995/2008; http://www.informatics.jax.org/silver/index.shtml). However, the establishment of ES cells from C56BL/6 origin made it possible to create knockout mice on the much favoured B6 genetic background (for review see Seong *et al.*, 2004). Repeated backcrossing for each required genotype is therefore not necessary, saving animals and time.

At this stage of the 'knockout' technology the knockout gene(s) was absent from the zygote stage onwards and therefore deleted from all cells of the body. Some knockout models proved to be lethal at the embryonic stage whereas other knockout animals did develop. However, the absence of the knocked out gene(s) in all tissues of the body resulted in complex phenotypes, especially in those cases where the normal 'wildtype' gene was expressed in multiple cell lineages. As a consequence, the GM mouse was not always replicating the human condition for which the model was intended in the first place. Technological advances enabled the introduction of recombination tools discovered in bacteria and yeasts into mammalian cells, the Cre-*lox* and FLP-*FRT* mediated recombination gave rise to 'conditional' and 'inducible' knockout animals (reviewed in Lewandoski, 2001). This was a leap forward enabling a gene to be knocked out in a specific cell lineage at any chosen moment during the lifetime of the animal and made a significant contribution to the refinement of the GM mouse models to replicate human conditions.

Knock-ins

The generation of knock-in models, to gain function from genetic mutations, was made possible by a more sophisticated use of existing strategies employed in the gene targeting efforts. Specifically, gene targeting vectors previously designed to mediate the deletion of gene sequences were crafted to mediate the one-to-one replacement of sequences so that defined base sequence changes could be engineered into the genetic locus of interest. These experimental strategies took advantage of the methodologies used to create conditional knockout mice to make sure that only the targeted sequence changes of interest remained while any other introduced sequences, like selection markers, were deleted. Despite representing the most difficult strategy to develop a gene targeted mouse, these knock-in models have proved very informative, allowing the introduction of specific genetic aberrations identified as biologically relevant in earlier *in vitro* and *in vivo* studies, or indeed patients. Thus, these 'next generation' knock-in models have become the 'workhorses' of hypothesis driven studies whose goals are to define gene function and to integrate these definitions into broader models to explain organismal biochemistry and physiology. In many ways these developments represent a significant leap forward in our understanding of gene function and its role in both health and disease (Doyle *et al.*, 2012). GM mouse models of increasing complexity then followed, like compound (multiple) transgenic/knock-in conditional lines of mice, used to replicate the unique patterns of gene expression occurring in many human diseases. A detailed review of genetic engineering in mice was recently published (Bouabe and Okkenhaug, 2013).

Gene editing

In more recent years the gene editing approach has taken off. Several designer endonuclease platforms were developed including Zinc Finger Nucleases (Porteus and Carroll, 2005; Urnov *et al.*, 2010), TALENs (Bogdanove and Voytas, 2011; Scharenberg *et al.*, 2013) and CRISPR (Doudna and Charpentier, 2014) (for a review see Certo and Morgan, 2016). These systems are all used in the same way; they cleave the DNA at the targeted locus and the cell subsequently repairs the break by NHEJ or by homologous recombination. This is by no means an error-free process and may lead to deletions or the introduction of a frame shift leading to a dysfunctional gene, i.e. a knockout. When a homologous repair template is delivered, together with the endonuclease system, specific changes to the endogenous gene can be made. It has been demonstrated that it is possible, in a single step, to produce complex multigene knockouts with simultaneous homology directed repair (Wang *et al.*, 2013; Yang *et al.*, 2013). It is this aspect that has generated much excitement. This capability brings with it the promise of being able, in a single step, to create GM rodents containing multiple genome edits. Previously this has required the creation of animals with single or double genetic mutations that can subsequently be bred. Since these gene editing techniques are not dependent on species-specific cell systems like ES-cells, they can also be used across species. Thus scientists wanting to study the effect of gene alterations are no longer restricted to working with mice. There are already increasing numbers of zebra fish being used in biomedical research as well as other less sentient species such as nematodes, so only time will tell if the mouse continues to be researchers' model of choice.

Gene modification, phenotypes and harm

The resultant phenotype of a genetic modification is dependent on how critical the function of the modified gene or genes is for the normal development and function of the organism, and on the type of modification. A genetic modification that is constitutively present is more likely to result in a developmental phenotype than a modification that is inducible, and can be triggered at any time point during the lifetime of the organism. Similarly, the deletion of a gene that is critical for the normal functioning of the organism is more likely to result in a severe phenotype than the deletion of a non-critical gene. To date, however, the function of many genes is still unknown, let alone the function of DNA sequences labelled as non-coding. The scale at which GM mutants, which are generated to address a specific research question, are phenotyped is very often limited by the expertise and interest of the individual investigator. However, the systematic broad-based phenotypic screens by consortia of mouse clinics complements these efforts with phenotyping of large numbers of different GM mutant strains. These efforts provide a basis for the characterization of relationships between gene and function, i.e. associated phenotype. At the same time the phenotyping data coming from these consortia allow an assessment to be made of the scale of potential welfare issues accompanying the widespread generation of GM animals. The EUMODIC consortium developed and validated methodologies for phenotyping of knockouts through the pipeline comprising 20 disease-oriented platforms. In 2015, the consortium reported phenotyping results of 449 mutant mouse alleles representing 320 unique genes, of which half had no functional annotation. The consortium captured data from over 27,000 mice and found that 83% of the mutant lines were phenodeviant with, in 65% of the cases, one gene influencing two or more apparently unrelated phenotypes. Furthermore, there were significant differences in phenotype annotations according to the degree of similarity between alleles for each trait (Hrabe de Angelis *et al.*, 2015). The goal of the International Mouse Phenotyping Consortium (IMPC) is to generate a catalogue of gene function by systematically generating and phenotyping a genome-wide collection of gene knockouts in mice. IMPC has created around 5000 new knockout lines. The consortium identified 410 lethal genes during the production of the first 1751 unique gene knockouts, which amounts to about 23% of the genes targeted so far. Furthermore, they observed instances of phenotypes that displayed incomplete penetrance, including variable lethality (sub-viability) (Dickinson *et al.*, 2016). These efforts to generate a genome-wide catalogue of gene function, taken together with the type of GM modification technique used, will aid efforts to make a more informed prospective welfare assessment possible and to narrow the attention to specific phenotypes to arise based on the known function(s) of the modified gene(s).

SOCIETAL, ETHICAL AND WELFARE CONCERNS

General Ethical Concerns[1]

A fundamental question is whether it is ethically permissible to use animals (such as rodents) that are sentient beings and, as such, have an intrinsic value,[2] as 'tools' purely for human benefit, and whether that use extends to the use of animals for research. There are many arguments about whether animals have rights that preclude that use but, currently, the global consensus is that it is permissible. Consequently, our starting point is that animals can be used but there are limits to that use. This utilitarian position is usually qualified by a statement to the effect that the likely harms done to animals have to be in some way proportionate to the potential benefits of the research, e.g. low potential benefit cannot justify severe harm. Such a 'harm–benefit' analysis requires some form of assessment of both the harms and the benefits, and that can be very contentious, particularly in the area of GM where the research is very speculative. Nevertheless, these assessments are often part of any ethics authorization. In the following section we touch on some of the inherent issues that apply to the genetic alteration of laboratory rodents.

Genetic modification

Since the late 1990s there has been increased press and public/consumer interest in the genetic modification of anything biological. This includes everything from plants and animals (vertebrates and invertebrates), to enzymes and cell lines. The context frequently varies both in terms of culture and geography, i.e. where in the world the research is taking place and the location where the GM organism will ultimately exist (more on this later). Other concerns involve more detailed specifics such as the species involved (this chapter will only discuss mice and rats), or indeed the biological process or pathways to be altered. There is a great deal of variation in terms of the purpose for which an organism is being genetically modified, but in terms of laboratory mice and rats, this is ultimately for human benefit. The exact nature of these benefits will vary, but can include fundamental aims such as increasing our knowledge of human and animal physiology, behaviour, health, welfare and disease progression, to more applied purposes such as testing and developing novel treatments or refining research methods, techniques or models to improve the reproducibility and translatability of research results.

Public surveys

Societal concerns over genetic modification in animals are most often founded in ethics, and are notoriously difficult to pinpoint at any given time so it is perhaps unsurprising that there is very little, if any, data collected that records concerns regarding transgenic, or genetically modified, rodents specifically. In a recent survey of 4726 US citizens published by the Pew Research Centre, 68% of respondents were somewhat or very worried about gene editing to give babies a much reduced disease risk (Funk *et al.*, 2016). This survey is about gene editing for human enhancement, but is relevant because its realization is dependent upon ongoing research using mice and rats. To get an idea of European perspectives regarding gene editing we can look at the European Commission's Eurobarometer surveys on Biotechnology, the most recent of which was published in 2010 (TNS, 2010). In this survey of 26,671 Europeans across 33 countries, 53% thought biotechnology and genetic engineering would have a positive effect 'on our way of life in the next 20 years'. This overall figure, whilst positive, is not, however, an indication of unequivocal support across all member states. Indeed, a closer look at the figures reveals a definite split in the number of countries reporting a positive response ranging from 77% to 39%. Interestingly, 53% of Europeans agreed with the statement that 'mixing human and animal genes is unacceptable even if it helps medical research for human health'. However, 57% approved (when regulated by strict laws) the statement: 'Scientists can put human genes into animals that will produce organs and tissues for transplant into humans, such as pigs for transplants, or to replace pancreatic cells to cure diabetes.'

The nuances in how the different survey questions are framed may affect public survey responses, but also provide some insight into the factors that influence societal opinions regarding genetic modification. In this context, three factors influencing public survey responses are: (i) how tightly such research is regulated; (ii) what the intended benefit of the research is; and (iii) what potential risks are associated with the research (Frewer, 2013). Societal opinions are highly dependent upon local cultural and ethical factors that underlie questions such as: (i) Is there a 'good/ethical reason for genetically altering rodents of any species? (ii) Does the specific method/technique used to genetically alter rodents alter the ethics of doing so? (iii) Is it right to use rodents, that are sentient beings and, as such, have an intrinsic value, as 'research tools' purely for human benefit? The answers to both these sets of questions are often interlinked as we see when we consider the concerns that are most frequently cited by survey respondents or scientific reports within the mainstream press.

The first of these is the question: Is it safe to edit genes? Some will argue that humans have been 'editing' the genes of animals using selective breeding for hundreds of years and so the increasing scientific development of more precise gene editing tools is just a natural progression from this. It cannot be denied that selective breeding has led to the domestication of many species including mice and rats. However, many consider genetic engineering, whether by established methods such as microinjection or the more recent development of genome editing tools, to have taken selective breeding a step further. For many, editing genomes in ways that are simply not physically possible through natural mating, or through assisted reproductive techniques, is a step into the unknown. This opinion is often expressed as 'It isn't natural' or 'I don't understand it', therefore 'I don't like it'. This deontological style dialogue, when an individual judges the ethics of the situation, i.e. should it be done at all, based upon their appraisal of the morality of the action, can also present itself as a more moral objection or theologically based argument centred around the opinion that 'humans were put on this earth to look after the animals and so should not do anything that may harm them or the earth which we share', or that 'animals were created by an entity greater than man (e.g. God), and so humans should not meddle lest there be unforeseen dangers for us all'.

If we focus for a moment on whether it is possible to provide an evidence-based answer to the question 'Is it safe to edit genes?', at the present time a definitive yes/no answer is not possible. There is no specific evidence that genetic modification or genome editing techniques pose a specific safety risk to humans, animals or the environment, but there is also little definitive evidence to indicate that there is definitely no risk either. Indeed, the advent of gene drive techniques to create novel, genetically modified organisms has given rise to renewed concerns regarding the safety of such technology being expressed both within the broadsheet and scientific press. Gene drive is a technique that biases inheritance to spread a gene or a modified gene rapidly through a population or even an entire species (Bohannon, 2015). Thus, what we can say at this point is that there are some outstanding questions that have yet to be resolved including whether the genomes of genetically modified rodents are any less stable (i.e. subject to an increased mutation rate) than those of non-GM rodents, and whether genetic modifications are as targeted or complete as they may at first appear. Questions regarding the potential impact on the environment or wild/domesticated populations, should GM animals ever escape or be released, are also asked, but are not relevant in this context because legislation regulating genetically modified organisms (GMOs) prevents their release from the laboratory setting. There is, however, variation in how the genetic modification of animals, including rodents, is regulated as will become apparent throughout this chapter.

Animal impact and animal welfare

Another societal concern often cited by public survey respondents is 'What will the likely impact of this technology be in terms of risks to human/animal health and welfare and the environment?' In a review of ethical issues, including welfare concerns associated with the genetic modification of animals, Ormandy *et al.* (2011) discuss the invasiveness of procedures, the large number of animals required to produce each genetically modified founder animal, and unanticipated welfare concerns as key issues of public concern. In terms of procedural harms, this includes killing animals as well as surgical and invasive non-surgical methods, many of which are not unique to GM animals but are typically required for their production. With regards to the large numbers of animals required to produce each GM founder animal, this varies considerably between methods and species and is the result of variable success rates at each stage in the production process. Both these concerns have benefited from technological developments that refine the production process, and the incidence of unanticipated welfare concerns is no different. Until the discovery of genome editing tools, scientists have been limited, to a greater or lesser extent, depending on the methodology used, in their ability to precisely control the site at which foreign DNA is incorporated into the animal's own genome. Thus it is possible that as gene modification technology progresses, this 'waste' can be reduced, and with it the level of societal concern relating to animal welfare may diminish.

If we focus purely on mice and rats, the biggest potential impact is if quality of life is reduced for any period of time. Large numbers of mice will also be killed as part of the process of creating a novel GM mouse. For example, before the advent of genome editing tools, approximately 112–224 mice would be used during the production of a single founding transgenic mouse (Ittner and Gotz, 2007). Some founder animals may cost fewer lives, but others cost many more. This figure reflects the sheer scale of the enterprise required to produce novel GM mice and serves to underline the natural inefficiencies intrinsic to the process. Mice will be killed to supply sufficient embryos for microinjection. Some embryos won't survive past the microinjection phase; others will fail to develop normally post-genetic modification, and so will never be transferred into surrogate mothers. Some GM embryos will fail to develop *in utero* and so will be reabsorbed by the surrogate mothers; others will die at later times before birth or soon after. The surrogate mothers used to gestate and give birth to modified embryos are commonly killed post weaning, and many of the resulting offspring will also be killed as soon as they are identified as not carrying the desired genetic alteration. All of this adds up to an intrinsic wastage that is improving, but far from a 100% success rate.

Thus, to some, the large-scale production of GM rodents can appear wasteful, but to others this will seem a calculated risk worth taking. There is an argument that even if there is nothing to distinguish the resulting GM mouse from their wild-type littermates, this in itself is now known (a benefit) and with very little perceived harm to the mouse involved. This is when it becomes important to look at the big picture and consider the cost to other animals killed during the creation of each GM founder. This is one reason why the big mutant mouse projects started – to generate a collection of GM mice in the most efficient way that the research community could then access and use to answer their research questions. The consortia are also open to requests from researchers to make GM mice with alterations in their particular gene of interest. On the surface this sounds good; after all, it demonstrates that there is a scientific need or interest in using that particular GM line. But in reality it would be very naïve to believe that the creation of every single new GM rodent line, whether by the big projects or by individual research groups, has been subject to a full harm–benefit analysis, and herein lies a potentially serious ethical issue.

Animal numbers

The management of GM mouse colonies and the numbers of animals involved is another challenge, requiring knowledge and competence in different areas.

The generation of GM founder animals is followed by breeding according to specific schemes aimed at producing sufficient animals for phenotyping and to establish a genetically stable line. The line must then be propagated to preserve the genetic integrity of the line whilst generating sufficient GM animals for use in scientific procedures, i.e. experiments (Lambert, 2009). Any improvement in the efficiency of creating and subsequent breeding of novel GM rodents is welcomed, but it is possible that improved efficiencies may have another consequence. A reduction in costs and technical challenges of producing novel genome edited animals could drive increased demand for such animals, thus cancelling out any potential reduction in the overall numbers. The number of animals used to create and breed GM rodents is already a concern for many.

In the UK, information on the number of GM animals used in scientific procedures has been published since 1995, and in 2012 the number of scientific procedures conducted involving GM animals exceeded the number of scientific procedures using non-GM animals for the first time (Home Office, 2013). Since then the creation and breeding of GM rodents (predominantly mice) has been a regular feature of press releases relating to the annual UK statistics on animal use in scientific procedures. The latest statistics to be released relate to 2015, when the UK conducted 2.06 million procedures for the purpose of creating or breeding genetically modified animals. Of this figure, 1.78 million, or 87%, involved mice (86%) and rats (1%) (Home Office, 2016; EC, 2013). An additional 247,000 scientific procedures for experimental purposes also involved the use of genetically modified mice and rats, meaning that, in 2015 alone, around 2 million GM mice and rats were either created, bred or used for a scientific purpose in the UK. Requirements to report GM animal numbers varies around the world, and as mice, rats, birds and fish are not covered by the US Animal Welfare Act there are no statistics available for these species. However, mice and rats are included within the scope of the European Directive 2010/63/EU on the Protection of Animals Used for Experimental and Other Scientific Purposes. The Commission to the Council and the European Parliament publishes statistics on the number of animals used for experimental and other scientific purposes in the 27 member states of the European Union. The latest data released relates to 2011, when only the UK, Denmark, The Netherlands and Sweden stated in the commentary accompanying the statistics that the numbers reported include GM mice and rats (EC, 2013). Thus it is not always clear what information countries record. Australia and Canada also publish relevant data.

The big mutant mouse projects also have to consider how best to ensure that the creation/production side of things matches up with phenotyping capacity. Without some knowledge of what effect, if any, the genetic mutation has, it can prove difficult to move GM mice out of their production facilities and into the research community. Thus the rate and number of GM mice being created and bred by the big projects can be self-limiting due to the availability of resources such as funding, staff and the cage space available for housing such animals. In this context, production rates are more reflective of each facility's ability to identify phenotypic traits and move GM lines out into the research community rather than an indication of definitive scientific benefit. In an attempt to ensure scientific benefits are maximized, it has become good practice to archive GM lines, but this ethical fail-safe is often more ideological than it is practical. There is also an obligation to preserve GM lines from which results have been published. This requires the cryopreservation of sperm, embryos and/ or ovaries, and also facilitates the sharing of GM lines. This is why many GM lines are now maintained and available from repositories. For example, the International Mouse Phenotyping Consortium (IMPC) has generated and phenotypically characterized 5000 knockout mouse lines (Dickinson *et al.*, 2016; Raess *et al.*, 2016). Other renowned resources for mouse GM lines and information are the Jackson Laboratory (https://www.jax.org/) in the USA, Infrafrontier (https://www.infrafrontier.eu/) in Europe, and Riken (http://en.brc.riken.jp/) in Japan. For information on the rat, the Rat Resource & Research Center (http://www.rrrc.us/) in the USA and the Rat Genome Database (http://rgd.mcw.edu/) are valuable resources. Archive facilities have, however, faced uncertain funding commitments, and so most centralized repositories are not-for-profit services run on a cost recovery model. As such, few have the capacity to accept archive material for which there is no definite research demand because costs are recovered by charging for their supply. Thus having big centres creating novel GM mice by the most efficient means, on the face of it appears ethical, but how ethical is it, in practice, to create potentially huge numbers of GM rodents for which the actual scientific benefits are not always clear?

Methods of genetic modification

If we move on to think about other impacts, there are many, but again this varies between the different methods of genetic modification. ENU mutagenesis, for example, causes the males to become very unwell, such that they require a recovery period of several weeks before they are in sufficient health to breed and produce offspring. The targeted and specific nature of genome editing tools means that it should be possible to reduce the incidence of unexpected adverse effects in offspring caused by unwanted genetic modifications. It does not automatically follow that the survival rates of genome edited offspring will be better, nor does it necessarily follow that there will be any improvement in the long-term health and welfare of genome edited rodents, but improvements in both are possible. Another more obvious impact is the genetic modification of rodents, specifically to model the onset and progression of a specific disease (e.g. cystic fibrosis, Parkinson's disease) or health compromising condition (e.g. cancer). For these animals the intention of the genetic modification is specifically to compromise their health and welfare, but the actual impact this has in practice will, again, vary depending on the desired scientific outcome and experimental endpoints. With this in mind, the 2015 UK statistics recorded for the first time an assessment of the actual severity (denoting intensity and duration) of suffering an animal experienced as the result of an entire scientific procedure. The report states that 127,000 procedures with the purpose of creating or breeding GM animals caused moderate or severe suffering, whilst 806,000 caused mild suffering (Home Office, 2016). If we think about whether the genetic modification of animals is likely to directly impact the health and welfare of humans, or indeed the environment, then in terms of rodents, specifically, there is circumstantial evidence to support this. In reality, a 'precautionary principle' has been applied, given that there is little evidence that humans and the environment would not be affected. If we consider whether the genetic modification of rodents is likely to indirectly impact the health and welfare of humans, then there is an argument that GM rodents, especially mice, have enabled research to be undertaken to improve our knowledge and understanding of human health and welfare that may not have otherwise been possible. Thus, in this context, a positive impact is conceivable, even if it is not easily measurable.

Benefits and disbenefits of genetic modification of rodents

This raises another societal concern: 'How will I know what benefits have arisen as a result of genetically altering mice or rats and can I choose to avoid those benefits if I wish to?' The short answer is that the public will not know what benefits have arisen unless the research community as a whole engages with the public to share this information with them. Transgenic technologies illustrate this point well, having traditionally been developed using animals, but without any significant acknowledgment of this animal use. Whether intentional or not, this diminishes the intrinsic value subconsciously attributed to the life of each GM rodent or, indeed, the animals killed during its creation. In this way, a cycle develops whereby the responsibility for, and the ethical costs of, each animal's life are lost, become accepted, then meaningless, until it reaches a point at which they can become forgotten entirely. This then brings us to consider an underlying ethical question that simply does not arise outside of the context of animal research: 'Is it right to use rodents, that are sentient beings and, as such, have an intrinsic value, as "research tools" purely for human benefit?' This question, of course, applies to all animal research, but relies upon a utilitarian assessment of what society judges it is permissible to do under certain restrictive conditions and within certain limits of human gain. This point becomes important when considering the statistic that 65% of the public feel either 'not at all' or 'not very well' informed about the use of animals in scientific research in the UK (https://www.ipsos.com/sites/default/files/publication/1970-01/sri-public-attitudes-to-animal-research-2016.pdf). When we consider that this is the statistic for the UK, where the number of animals used is reported annually by the government and receives general press coverage, one can only imagine how the public in some other countries may feel.

There are indications that this is changing, and, indeed, a 2015 study (Hamlyn *et al.*, 2015) conducted on behalf of a consortium of UK research funders on the 'factors affecting public engagement by researchers' revealed that a lack of support and time constraints were two of the major factors limiting researchers' efforts in this regard. In the UK, specific efforts to improve the communication of animal use in research resulted in a *Concordat on Openness on Animal Research in the UK* (UAR, 2014). Similar 'transparency' initiatives have also been launched in other European countries including Spain (COSCE, 2016), Belgium (EARA, 2016) and Germany (https://www.mpg.de/10722421/PM-Allianz-Tierversuche-verstehen.pdf). We will have to wait and see whether these efforts will reduce the frequency with which society asks researchers questions such as: 'Why do scientists need to genetically alter animals?' and 'What other options are there?' There is, however, a point worth reflecting on here, which is: Could the scientific benefits gained through research involving GM rodents have been obtained without genetically modifying these animals, or in fact without using animals at all? Such questions also remind us of a general public uneasiness regarding genetic modification that was first triggered by the introduction and subsequent banning of GM crops/food within Europe in the 1990s. Since then there has been some urgency to discuss and debate the responsible use of such technology, but as yet very little action has been taken on this point. This needs to be recognized, given this recent episode in scientific history shows us that if society does not understand genome editing technology and any associated risks, then there is a high chance that they will reject the products of such research. Thus the development and application of gene editing technologies could be considered unethical in the current climate, given that it is unclear whether such activities and their resulting advances would ever receive public support.

Translational research

So to try to address these questions, there are a number of different 'scientific needs' that researchers cite as to why they genetically alter mice. For example 'to improve animal models such that the results translate better into human subjects' or 'to demonstrate that it is possible to treat genetic defects before birth'. In reality, this desire to create new and improved, or 'better', GM rodent models often simply results in a new addition to a growing list of existing animal models without actually replacing those already in use. In the case of the 'forward genetics' approaches mentioned earlier, for example ENU mutagenesis, the 'need' is to contribute to an 'academic' aim to further human knowledge. In terms of what other options exist, this can be difficult to identify and will depend on the scientific purpose. Sometimes, but not always, research using *in vitro* systems may have been exhausted or need to be progressed *in vivo* before approval can be sorted for clinical testing. Indeed, good use can be made of *in vitro* technologies such as cells or non-sentient species especially to study conserved genomic regions. There will also be some work that can be conducted using samples collected from human patients, but the supply of this material is limited and it is not always readily accessible, and can require complex consent processes. These are, however, the kind of issues that should be discussed when reviewing a research funding or project licence application. Requirements for this will vary between countries, but implementation of the '3 Rs' principles of humane experimental technique – Replacement, Reduction and Refinement (Russell and Burch, 1959) – is enshrined within EU Directive 2010/63 and its subsequent translation into national legislation within all European member states.

An issue we have not yet touched on is whether the results of studies involving GM rodents translate well into a clinical setting and help inform the care and treatment of human patients. This is something that is increasingly being challenged for all animal models, for a whole host of reasons. There are very many factors that impact on the reliability and usability of data generated using any animal model, be they GM rodents or not, starting with the relevance and applicability of the very research question being investigated. Other critical considerations include the experimental design methods, models and statistical analysis used. There is a growing awareness of publication bias caused by the increased likelihood of only positive results being shared or published and therefore skewing the publication record. The poor quality of research reporting is another contributing factor because it can make replicating or validating other researchers' work very difficult. Thus with a growing number of GM rodents in existence, the scientific justification for a reverse genetics approach to produce a GM mouse for every known gene in the mouse genome is diminishing

Application of Ethical Frameworks

The 3 Rs (Replacement, Reduction and Refinement), mentioned above is the most commonly used ethical framework for the use of animals in research and it can be applied to the use of GM animals. The first R (Replacement) should first be reviewed (e.g. systematic reviews) before using GM technologies on living animals to make sure that essentially similar work has not been carried out before. Studies should be made on *in vitro* technologies on cells, organs, computer modelling etc., and non-sentient species (especially for research that may involve highly conserved genomic regions). However, often only certain effects may be studied such as mechanisms of molecular and cell–cell interactions, but this still leaves the question of what happens in whole organisms with their complex interacting integrated organ systems. The other two Rs (Reduction and Refinement) come into play after Replacement has been considered, when it has been established that animals have to be used; and, of course, that the question is worth trying to answer. Inadvertent losses of animals through technical failures or experimental limitations have been a significant ethical concern. It is also possible to reduce losses through improved husbandry and housing (Robinson, 2003), and many of these improvements come from refining techniques to accommodate the changed biology of the animals due to constitutive expression, or after it has been induced in conditional GM animals. These environmental and husbandry adaptations can markedly affect the quality of life for the animals, particularly their relatively short life experiences, and their importance cannot be underestimated (Hawkins *et al.*, 2011). Finally, it is important to remember that even after the application of the 3 Rs, and the application of positive welfare measures, the question still remains as to whether GM should be done at all. This is the point at which the harm–benefit analysis should be carried out and considered in the context of local societal perspectives, before a final decision is made.

A note on the popularization of some GM and mutant animals

The breeding of 'fancy mice' is a popular hobby for many around the world, involving the selective breeding of (spontaneous mutant) mice that may be hairless or display a variety of coat colours, patterns or textures, as well as other physical attributes such as short tails or enlarged ears. There is also a commercial market for a trade in GM animals (to date, fish and cats) that carry the jellyfish aequorin gene, which makes them glow under UV light. Some of these mutations have become popular in the fur and feather fancier trade. However, the question of whether animals should be exploited in this way through complex scientific techniques simply for profit is debatable. But what is permissible and impermissible, and on what basis, become important questions. If it is economically driven, is that bad? If so, how do we regard attempts to patent GM animals, intellectual property, commercial services etc. Are these simply by-products of animal research? If no harm accrues to the animals, does that make it right, or is there some degree of manipulation of nature that makes it unacceptable? If so, where do we draw the line? This is not the place to start to answer these questions.

Moving On

Society is reliant on each and every researcher using GM rodents to ensure that they start with a clear hypothesis regarding the gene or regulatory sequence of interest and its potential function. The most appropriate research method or model for testing this hypothesis, which may or may not be a GM rodent, must then be identified, and the responsibility for phenotyping, registering and annotating any novel GM line fulfilled. There is a general acknowledgement among scientists that some earlier animal and clinical studies have been performed poorly, that due regard has not been paid to the animals concerned, and that there is a need for proper statistical design of all experiments to ensure the significance of the results and the removal of bias. Thus, open and systematic review of all animal research proposals should be encouraged from the time of preparation of project proposals. Proper reporting of tests is essential, and guidelines, such as ARRIVE (Kilkenny *et al.*, 2010), should also become implemented as standard practice. There are also Minimum Information in the reporting of Biological and Biomedical Investigations (MIBBI) reporting standards, including ones for genotyping experiments, mouse phenotyping procedures and many others that are GM-animal relevant (see http://www.biosharing.org for more information). Moreover, further benefits may be gained by including a retrospective review section when reporting work that is devoted to the use, care and impact on animals. This would ensure that others become aware of any inadvertent deleterious and unwanted side effects and failed trial experiments (Morton, 1992), as well as how animal pain and distress was recognized and assessed. Open repositories to publish all data including negative results and supporting information would also enable information to be reused and preserved on a greater scale. This would support the evolving needs for education and training in all aspects of replacement science and implementation of the 3 Rs, from school/university students to established researchers in laboratories. Proper and full dissemination of knowledge is key, and consistent with the current efforts by the European Commission and other research funding organizations. Times are changing, and the principles of 'responsible research and innovation' are becoming firmly embedded whereby 'Responsible Research and Innovation is a dynamic, iterative process by which all stakeholders involved in the R&I practice become mutually responsive and share responsibility for both the outcomes and processes involved' (Owen, 2012). This approach requires the research community to work together with research funders, regulators, educators, business/industry and civil society organizations to meet societal challenges in an ethically acceptable, environmentally sustainable and socially desirable way. To date, the transgenic community as a whole has not been particularly proactive in identifying, acknowledging and engaging with society as we have noted throughout this chapter. This situation is unsustainable and thus unlikely to continue, so perhaps the next generation of transgenic researchers will bring with them the necessary cultural change.

Notes

[1] A general introduction to some of the ethical issues in the human use of animals, as well as some critiques of ways animals have been used, can be found in Orlans *et al.* (1998).

[2] Having intrinsic value infers that it is wrong to take their lives or to cause them to suffer. Sometimes this is expressed as animals having a right to a life and a right not to be caused to suffer.

References

Bogdanove, A.J. and Voytas, D.F. (2011) TAL effectors: customizable proteins for DNA targeting. *Science* 333, 1843–1846.

Bohannon, J. (2015) Biologists devise invasion plan for mutations. *Science* 347, 1.

Bouabe, H. and Okkenhaug, K. (2013) Gene targeting in mice: a review. *Methods in Molecular Biology* 1064, 315–336.

Brinster, R.L., Chen, H.Y., Trumbauer, M., Senear, A.W., Warren, R. and Palmiter, R.D. (1981) Somatic expression of herpes thymidine kinase in mice following injection of a fusion gene into eggs. *Cell* 27, 223–231.

Brook, F.A. and Gardner, R.L. (1997) The origin and efficient derivation of embryonic stem cells in the mouse. *Proceedings of the National Academy of Sciences of the United States of America* 94, 5709–5712.

Carninci, P. (2014) Genomics: mice in the ENCODE spotlight. *Nature* 515, 346–347.

Certo, M.T. and Morgan, R.A. (2016) Salient features of endonuclease platforms for therapeutic genome editing. *Molecular Therapy: The Journal of the American Society of Gene Therapy* 24, 422–429.

COSCE (2016) Acuerdo de transparencia sobre el uso de animales en experimentación científica en España. European Animal Research Association. Available at: http://eara.eu/es/propuesta-cosce/ (accessed 29 January 2018).

Davisson, M.T., Bergstrom, D.E., Reinholdt, L.G. and Donahue, L.R. (2012) Discovery genetics – the history and future of spontaneous mutation research. *Current Protocols in Mouse Biology* 2, 103–118.

Dickinson, M.E., Flenniken, A.M., Ji, X., Teboul, L., Wong, M.D. *et al.* (2016) High-throughput discovery of novel developmental phenotypes. *Nature* 537, 508–514.

Dolan, M.E., Baldarelli, R.M., Bello, S.M., Ni, L., McAndrews, M.S. *et al.* (2015) Orthology for comparative genomics in the mouse genome database. *Mamm Genome* 26, 305–313.

Doudna, J.A. and Charpentier, E. (2014) Genome editing: the new frontier of genome engineering with CRISPR-Cas9. *Science* 346, 1258096.

Doyle, A., McGarry, M.P., Lee, N.A. and Lee, J.J. (2012) The construction of transgenic and gene knockout/knockin mouse models of human disease. *Transgenic Research* 21, 327–349.

EARA (2016) Statement in support of animal research in Belgium and a transparent approach. Available at: http://eara.eu/wp-content/uploads/2016/04/Statement-and-signatories-in-support-of-animal-research-in-Belgium.pdf (accessed 29 January 2018).

EC (2013) Report from the Commission to the Council and the European Parliament – Seventh Report on the Number of Animals used for Experimental and Other Scientific Purposes in the Member States of the European Union. European Commission. COM(2013) 859 final. Available at: http://eur-lex.europa.eu/resource.html?uri=cellar:e99d2a56-32fc-4f60-ad69-61ea-d7e377e8.0001.03/DOC_1&format=PDF (accessed 29 January 2018).

Evans, M.J. and Kaufman, M.H. (1981) Establishment in culture of pluripotential cells from mouse embryos. *Nature* 292, 154–156.

Frewer, L. (2013) Final Report Summary – PEGASUS (Public perception of genetically modified animals – science, utility and society). Available at: http://cordis.europa.eu/result/rcn/58569_en.html (accessed 29 January 2018).

Funk, C., Kennedy, B. and Podrebarac Sciupac, E. (2016) U.S. Public Wary of Biomedical Technologies to 'Enhance' Human Abilities. PewResearchCenter report, 26 July. Available at: http://www.pewinternet.org/2016/07/26/u-s-public-wary-of-biomedical-technologies-to-enhance-human-abilities/ (accessed 29 January 2018).

Gordon, J.W. (1997) Transgenic technology and laboratory animal science. *ILAR Journal* 38, 32–41.

Gordon, J.W., Scangos, G.A., Plotkin, D.J., Barbosa, J.A. and Ruddle, F.H. (1980) Genetic transformation of mouse embryos by microinjection of purified DNA. *Proceedings of the National Academy of Sciences of the United States of America* 77, 7380–7384.

Hamlyn, B., Shanahan, M., Lewis, H., O'Donoghue, E., Hanson, T. and Burchell, K. (2015) Factors affecting public engagement by researchers: a study on behalf of a consortium of UK public research funders. TNS BMRB and Policy Studies Institute. Available at: https://wellcome.ac.uk/sites/default/files/wtp060033_0.pdf (accessed 29 January 2018).

Hawkins, P., Morton, D.B., Burman, O., Dennison, N., Honess, P. *et al.* (2011) A guide to defining and implementing protocols for the welfare assessment of laboratory animals: eleventh report of the BVAAWF/FRAME/RSPCA/UFAW Joint Working Group on Refinement. *Laboratory Animals* 45, 1–13.

Home Office (2013) Statistics of scientific procedures on living animals, Great Britain 2012. Home Office, 16 July. Available at: https://www.gov.uk/government/statistics/statistics-of-scientific-procedures-on-living-animals-great-britain-2012 (accessed 29 January 2018).

Home Office (2016) Statistics of scientific procedures on living animals, Great Britain 2015. Home Office, 20 July. Available at: https://www.gov.uk/government/statistics/statistics-of-scientific-procedures-on-living-animals-great-britain-2015 (accessed 29 January 2018).

Hrabe de Angelis, M., Nicholson, G., Selloum, M., White, J.K., Morgan, H. *et al.* (2015) Analysis of mammalian gene function through broad-based phenotypic screens across a consortium of mouse clinics. *Nature Genetics* 47, 969–978.

Ittner, L.M. and Gotz, J. (2007) Pronuclear injection for the production of transgenic mice. *Nature Protocols* 2, 1206–1215.

Jaenisch, R. (1976) Germ line integration and Mendelian transmission of the exogenous Moloney leukemia virus. *Proceedings of the National Academy of Sciences of the United States of America* 73, 1260–1264.

Kilkenny, C., Browne, W.J., Cuthill, I.C., Emerson, M. and Altman, D.G. (2010) Improving bioscience research reporting: the ARRIVE guidelines for reporting animal research. *PLOS Biology* 8, e1000412.

Lambert, R. (2009) *Breeding Strategies for Maintaining Colonies of Laboratory Mice*. The Jackson Laboratory, Bar Harbor, Maine. Available at: https://www.research.uci.edu/forms/docs/iacuc/JAX-breeding-strategies.pdf (accessed 29 January 2018).

Lewandoski, M. (2001) Conditional control of gene expression in the mouse. *Nature Reviews Genetics* 2, 743–755.

Mansour, S.L., Thomas, K.R. and Capecchi, M.R. (1988) Disruption of the proto-oncogene int-2 in mouse embryo-derived stem cells: a general strategy for targeting mutations to non-selectable genes. *Nature* 336, 348–352.

Martin, G.R. (1981) Isolation of a pluripotent cell line from early mouse embryos cultured in medium conditioned by teratocarcinoma stem cells. *Proceedings of the National Academy of Sciences of the United States of America* 78, 7634–7638.

Morton, D.B. (1992) A fair press for animals. *New Scientist* 134, 28–30.

Orlans, F.B., Beauchamp, T.L., Dresser, R., Morton, D.B. and Gluck, J.P. (1998) *The Human Use of Animals: Case Studies in Ethical Choice*. Oxford University Press, New York.

Ormandy, E.H., Dale, J. and Griffin, G. (2011) Genetic engineering of animals: ethical issues, including welfare concerns. *Canadian Veterinary Journal* 52, 544–550.

Owen, R. (2012) Responsible research and innovation: options for research and innovation policy in the EU. Available at: https://ec.europa.eu/research/innovation-union/pdf/expert-groups/Responsible_Research_and_Innovation.pdf (accessed 29 January 2018).

Palmiter, R.D. and Brinster, R.L. (1986) Germ-line transformation of mice. *Annual Review of Genetics* 20, 465–499.

Porteus, M.H. and Carroll, D. (2005) Gene targeting using zinc finger nucleases. *Nature Biotechnology* 23, 967–973.

Raess, M., de Castro, A.A., Gailus-Durner, V., Fessele, S., Hrabe de Angelis, M. and Consortium, I. (2016) INFRAFRONTIER: a European resource for studying the functional basis of human disease. *Mamm Genome* 27, 445–450.

Robinson, V. (2003) Refinement and reduction in production of genetically modified mice. *Laboratory Animals* 37, 373–375.

Russell, W.M.S. and Burch, R.L. (1959) *The Principles of Humane Experimental Technique*. Methuen, London. Available at: http://altweb.jhsph.edu/pubs/books/humane_exp/het-toc (accessed 6 February 2018).

Scharenberg, A.M., Duchateau, P. and Smith, J. (2013) Genome engineering with TAL-effector nucleases and alternative modular nuclease technologies. *Current Gene Therapy* 13, 291–303.

Seong, E., Saunders, T.L., Stewart, C.L. and Burmeister, M. (2004) To knockout in 129 or in C57BL/6: that is the question. *Trends Genet* 20, 59–62.

Silver, L.M. (1995, rev. 2008) *Mouse Genetics: Concepts and Applications*. The Jackson Laboratory, Bar Harbor, Maine.

Smithies, O., Gregg, R.G., Boggs, S.S., Koralewski, M.A. and Kucherlapati, R.S. (1985) Insertion of DNA-sequences into the human chromosomal beta-globin locus by homologous recombination. *Nature* 317, 230–234.

Thomas, K.R., Folger, K.R. and Capecchi, M.R. (1986) High frequency targeting of genes to specific sites in the mammalian genome. *Cell* 44, 419–428.

TNS (2010) *Eurobarometer 73.1: Biotechnology*. TNS Opinion & Social, Brussels. Available at: http://ec.europa.eu/commfrontoffice/publicopinion/archives/ebs/ebs_341_en.pdf (accessed 29 January 2018).

UAR (2014) *Concordat on Openness on Animal Research in the UK*. Understanding Animal Research, London. Available at: http://concordatopenness.org.uk/ (accessed 29 January 2018).

Urnov, F.D., Rebar, E.J., Holmes, M.C., Zhang, H.S. and Gregory, P.D. (2010) Genome editing with engineered zinc finger nucleases. *Nature Reviews of Genetics* 11, 636–646.

Wang, H., Yang, H., Shivalila, C.S., Dawlaty, M.M., Cheng, A.W., Zhang, F. and Jaenisch, R. (2013) One-step generation of mice carrying mutations in multiple genes by CRISPR/Cas-mediated genome engineering. *Cell* 153, 910–918.

Yang, H., Wang, H., Shivalila, C.S., Cheng, A.W., Shi, L. and Jaenisch, R. (2013) One-step generation of mice carrying reporter and conditional alleles by CRISPR/Cas-mediated genome engineering. *Cell* 154, 1370–1379.

Yue, F., Cheng, Y., Breschi, Y., Vierstra, J., Wu, W. *et al.* (2014) A comparative encyclopedia of DNA elements in the mouse genome. *Nature* 515, 355–364.

10 Cloning, Editing and GMOs for Animal Enhancement

Elisabeth Ormandy*

Animals in Science Policy Institute, Vancouver, Canada

Introduction

The genetic manipulation of domesticated animals (i.e. farm animals, companion animals and animals used for research) has been practised for many decades through the practice of selective breeding (sometimes called classical breeding) – that is, breeding of animals who have desired traits or mutations so that those traits are passed on, and often become more pronounced, in subsequent generations (Snow, 2003). In recent years, genetic manipulation of animals has taken the more direct form of genetic engineering, gene editing and cloning, but what is it that makes genetic engineering different from selective breeding? Breeding typically consists of three main steps: (i) amassing or producing new genetic diversity; (ii) picking out and testing different genotypes of distinguished superior genetic lines; and (iii) the release, dispersal and commercialization of the new progeny (see Gepts, 2002 for a description of these stages in crop breeding). According to Snow *et al.* (2005) the difference between selective breeding and genetic engineering is in the first phase. Selective breeding enhances genetic diversity via sexual crosses, whereas genetic engineering can introduce genes from any source into recipient cells that can then be integrated directly into an organism's genome.

Traditionally, the most common techniques for genetic engineering were direct pronuclear microinjection of a foreign DNA construct (a transgene), transfection with retroviral or episomal vectors, and gene targeting using homologous recombination. However, new techniques have been developed recently that are much more precise and efficient. In particular, the CRISPR/Cas9 (Clustered Regularly Interspaced Short Palindromic Repeats) technique for gene editing has taken the scientific world by storm, as it gives the ability to edit the genes of all species (including humans) (Shen, 2013a). The advent of this technology might shift trends in the use of animals in research; for example, the CRISPR technique has recently been used to create the first gene edited primates (Shen, 2014) as well as 'primate models' of affective disorders like autism (Cyranoski, 2016).

Cloning is the replication of certain cell types from a 'parent' cell, or the replication of a certain part of the cell or DNA to propagate a certain desirable genetic trait. There are three types of cloning: DNA cloning, therapeutic cloning and reproductive cloning (National Human Genome Research Institute, 2016). In reproductive cloning, researchers remove a mature somatic cell (such as a skin cell) from an animal they wish to copy. The DNA of the donor animal's somatic cell is then transferred into an egg cell (oocyte) that has had its DNA-containing nucleus removed. The egg develops

*E-mail: elisabeth@animalsinscience.org

 Are We Pushing Animals to Their Biological Limits? (eds T. Grandin and M. Whiting)

into an early-stage embryo, which is implanted into an adult female, who then gives birth to an animal that has the same genetic make-up as the somatic cell donor. Thus, cloning is a type of genetic manipulation that is not intended to alter an animal's characteristics, but to make a genetically identical copy.

There are myriad intended applications of genetically engineered, gene edited, or cloned animals – from disease models in research to cloned pets, and from disease resistant farm animals to animal organ donors. While genetic manipulation can be considered to 'enhance' animals in different ways, all practices that alter the genetic material of animals (whether through selective breeding, genetic engineering, or cloning) bring with them ethical issues, some of which relate to animal welfare. Indeed, there are lessons we can learn from some of the undesired effects of selective breeding that have taken a toll on our domesticated animals in terms of their well-being.

Furthermore, the issues that arise from the use of new technologies like genetic engineering, gene editing and cloning need to be considered by all stakeholders to ensure that all parties are aware of the ethical issues at stake and can make a valid contribution to the current debate regarding the genetic manipulation of animals. It is important to try to reflect societal values within scientific practice and emerging technology, especially publicly funded efforts that aim to provide societal benefits, but that may be deemed ethically contentious. This chapter will discuss selective breeding, genetic engineering and gene editing, and cloning of animals, and some of the ethical challenges that can arise with each. In doing so, several key examples of each approach to genetic manipulation are highlighted: pedigree dog breeding and inbreeding of lab mice (selective breeding), xenotransplantation and disease resistant farm animals (genetic engineering and gene editing), and pet cloning and the revival of extinct species (cloning). While there has been a lot of criticism related to the genetic alteration of various species, there is attention given to cases where the genetic manipulation of animals might be used to solve some of the welfare issues associated with current practices involving domesticated animals. The chapter closes with a discussion about societal attitudes towards the creation and use of genetically engineered (GE) animals (including cloned animals) and the potential road blocks that negative perceptions might create to using genetic engineering or cloning techniques to enhance animal welfare.

Selective Breeding for Animal Enhancement

Selective breeding is the term used to describe the practice of breeding together two animals that have desired characteristics so that subsequent generations might possess those traits to a greater degree. This practice has been used for the breeding of farm animals, companion animals and research animals for many years (Snow, 2003). If we take dairy cattle as an illustrative example, genetic selection pressures have been put on these animals (particularly the Holstein Freisen) to increase their milk yield and productivity. Dairy cows are now super-producers: milk yield per cow has more than doubled in the last 40 years, and many cows produce more than 20,000 kg of milk per lactation (Oltenacu and Broom, 2010). However, while this might be applauded as a form of animal enhancement, selective breeding of dairy cattle has also come at some unanticipated animal welfare costs. As a result of being selectively bred for high milk yield, many dairy cows now suffer infertility (Nebel and McGilliard, 1993; Pryce *et al.*, 1999), mastitis and digestive diseases (Mäntysaari *et al.*, 1991; Jones *et al.*, 1994; Lescourret *et al.*, 1995), increased incidence of lameness (Alban *et al.*, 1996) and other so-called 'production diseases' that can result in reduced lifespan due to the heavy metabolic load placed on the animals. And dairy cattle, while used here as an illustrative example, are by no means alone in facing welfare costs due to the genetic selection for high productivity (Rauw *et al.*, 1998).

Due to the animal welfare costs incurred by selectively breeding farm animals for high production levels, it has been recommended that researchers and producers turn to a different approach to breeding that uses a variety of genetic selection pressures to reverse some of the welfare costs (Phillips, 1997; Simm, 1998). As noted by Sandøe *et al.* (1999), 'selection for diverse traits is now more common in the dairy industry, with the development of selection indices such as ITEM (Index of Total Economic Merit)'. In a similar vein, Oltenacu and Broom (2010) recommend the expansion of the Profitable Lifetime Index to include mastitis resistance and fertility. These are examples of how selective breeding can be used to maintain productivity at the same time as addressing some of the key animal welfare issues that have been created by a sole focus on genetic selection for high levels of production. Use of broader selective breeding goals ensures that breeding efforts are not solely focused on production parameters, but can also include animal welfare (and other) considerations, without sacrificing productivity.

Another key example of how selective breeding has been used to 'enhance' animals is pedigree dog breeding. Selective breeding (including inbreeding) has been used to select for desired traits in different breeds of dogs – these are often aesthetic traits that are favoured by national kennel club associations. The result in many cases is a victory of fashion over function, with many pedigree dog breeds having quite serious and often painful welfare issues, such as brachycephalia, syringomyelia, and hip dysplasia (Asher *et al.*, 2009). Furthermore, the inbreeding of pedigree dogs has led to welfare complications, and inbred dogs have a predisposition for congenital diseases such as hypothyroidism, cataracts, Von Willebrand's disease, progressive retinal atrophy, factor VII deficiency, and retinal detachment and glaucoma (Summers *et al.*, 2009). Again, such genetic selection pressures can be overcome by avoiding inbreeding and reclaiming some genetic diversity in our companion dogs by breeding for traits related to temperament and genetic predisposition for disease or disorder, rather than aesthetics (Rooney and Sargan, 2008; British Veterinary Association, 2015).

Inbreeding is also a practice that has long been used for the selective breeding of lab mice strains (Tanooka *et al.*, 2001; Witmer *et al.*, 2003; Yoshiki and Moriwaki, 2006), with the first inbred strain (DBA mice) being created over 100 years ago (Stevens *et al.*, 2007). All lab mice are likely descended from a small number of progenitor domestic mice (*Mus musculus domesticus*), and while the inbreeding of mice yields genetic uniformity that allows for more accurate and repeatable experiments (Stevens *et al.*, 2007), it has caused certain welfare issues to arise; for example, some mouse strains are deaf by the time they reach adulthood (Zheng *et al.*, 1999), the commonly used C57BL/6 strain of mice are deficient in pineal melatonin (which plays an important role in maintaining the circadian rhythm) (Ebihara *et al.*, 1986), and C3H mice carry a recessive retinal degeneration mutation (Sidman and Green, 1965). However, these so-called spontaneous mutations that arise from inbreeding can hold value for research, and individual animals who carry a spontaneous mutation are often selectively bred to create new mutant mouse lines. For example, whole colonies of diabetic mice (non-obese diabetic, or NOD, mice) and rats (the Biobreeding, or BB rat) used in research have been bred after diabetes spontaneously occurred in the population (Yang and Santamaria, 2006) – indeed, several inbred strains from new major mutations are released every year (Casellas, 2011). Major mouse supplier Jackson Laboratory now maintains more than 7500 genetically defined strains of mice (this includes genetically engineered mice) (Jackson Laboratory, n.d.), and there are close to 500 inbred mouse strains used in biomedical research (Stevens *et al.*, 2007).

Using selective breeding to solve welfare issues: the breeding of polled cattle

Nearly all dairy cattle (80%) are dehorned to avoid injuries among herd mates and increase safety for the farmer (Cozzi *et al.*, 2015; Carlson *et al.*, 2016). A review by Stafford and Mellor (2005) reveals that all methods of dehorning and disbudding cause pain to calves – this is demonstrated through a range of physiological and behavioural measures. It is also becoming clear that use of a local anaesthetic alone does not fully mitigate this pain and does not provide adequate post-operative pain relief (von Keyserlingk *et al.*, 2009). However, some cows possess the polled gene, which means that they are naturally born without horns. Polledness is controlled by a major gene, but the frequency of polledness varies over cattle breeds, and is low in the Holstein breed (the most commonly used breed for dairy production). This means that dairy farmers have a limited choice of bulls that inherit the polled gene and can go on to sire plentiful polled offspring. Furthermore, according to Carlson *et al.* (2016) the use of Holstein sires has been impeded by their lower estimated breeding value for milk production. Due to the welfare concerns associated with dehorning, a breeding programme to increase the frequency of the polled gene in the dairy herd is desirable. In an article by Windig *et al.* (2015) the authors illustrate how breeding high genetic merit polled Holstein cows has become a realistic possibility. Thus, selective breeding to enhance dairy cattle by putting selection pressure on the polled gene is an illustrative example of how genetic manipulation of animals through selective breeding can be used to solve current welfare issues. However, Windig *et al.* (2015) recommend that caution be exercised to avoid high relatedness and inbreeding levels (which can cause undesired mutations to arise). It is, in part, these obstacles of high relatedness and inbreeding that have spurred the use of genetic engineering to create hornless cows, rather than relying on selective breeding (Carlson *et al.*, 2016).

While selective breeding can be celebrated as a practice that has refined and enhanced our domesticated animals in certain desirable ways, it is clear that it has also been the cause of some serious welfare issues in current generations of animals. The argument has been made that genetic engineering is merely an extension of historic selective breeding practices, and therefore genetic engineering is ethically sound. However, this argument seems to ignore the fact that selective breeding is not always an ethically sound practice in the first place, as evidenced by the welfare issues that have arisen by breeding animals solely for their desired traits. As such, caution should be exercised when trying to logically argue that genetic engineering is ethically sound simply because we have already been genetically manipulating animals via selective breeding for many years.

Genetic Engineering and Gene Editing for Animal Enhancement

Several terms are used to describe genetically engineered (GE) animals: genetically modified, genetically altered, genetically manipulated, transgenic and biotechnology derived, amongst others. In the early stages of genetic engineering, the primary technology used was transgenesis – literally meaning the transfer of genetic material from one organism to another. However, with advances in the field, new technology has emerged that does not necessarily require transgenesis: recent applications allow for the creation of GE animals via the deletion of genes, or the manipulation of genes already present. According to the Food and Drug Administration (FDA) of the USA:

> [G]enetic engineering generally refers to the use of tools of modern technology and molecular biology to specifically introduce or alter characteristics or traits in organisms. Scientists can use these tools to introduce new genetic material, or delete existing genetic material to introduce intended new or altered traits or characteristics.
>
> (Food and Drug Administration, 2015)

More recently the term 'gene edited' has been introduced to refer to animals that are created using much more precise genetic manipulation techniques, like CRISPR (Clustered Regularly Interspaced Short Palindromic Repeats) technology.

According to Hackett *et al.* (2014), gene edited animals can be used in three distinct areas: (i) improved animal models of human disease that provide reliable pre-clinical information regarding the safety of new drugs and medical devices; (ii) animals designed to harbour patient-specific organs, tissues and cells for transplantation that will not induce adverse immune responses; and (iii) improved animal genomes adapted to local conditions to produce food more efficiently.

All GE and gene edited animals are created in a research environment before the end application is reached, so it is worth exploring trends in the creation and use of GE animals in research to set the stage for a discussion on some of the various applications of GE animals that are either currently in use, or have been proposed.

Trends in the creation and use of genetically engineered animals

The creation and use of GE animal models for research has increased rapidly over the past couple of decades (Ormandy *et al.*, 2009). Some of the well documented issues that are presented with the creation and use of GE animals in the laboratory context include: (i) unanticipated welfare concerns when new genetically engineered animals are created; (ii) invasiveness of procedures to achieve the genetic alteration of interest; (iii) high numbers of animals needed to achieve genetic alteration of interest; and (iv) whether ethical limits can be placed on genetic engineering (Robinson *et al.*, 2003; Ormandy *et al.*, 2013a) – though with the advent of more precise gene editing techniques, issues with large numbers of animals being required might be overcome. The creation and use of GE animals might also pose issues of how to record and report national research animal statistics, which has been discussed elsewhere in a Canadian context (Ormandy *et al.*, 2010; Ormandy *et al.*, 2013), as well as creating competition between researchers and promoting a culture of confidentiality (Ormandy *et al.*, 2013a).

Methods for creating GE animals are becoming more sophisticated and efficient. Traditional methods, such as pronuclear microinjection, were renowned for being unpredictable and inefficient because of their reliance on random gene integration, as well as the high incidence of mosaicism (Niemann and Kues, 2007). This meant that large numbers of animals were required as 'founder' animals to achieve the genetic alterations of interest, which created many animals who were surplus to requirements because they did not carry the required genetic alteration. However, newly developed techniques, such as gene targeting by homologous recombination (Capecchi, 1989), and gene editing using TALENs (Joung and Sander, 2013) and zinc-finger nucleases (Porteus and Carroll, 2005), allow for much more precise, less wasteful approaches.

The recent queen of gene editing techniques is the CRISPR (Clustered Regularly Interspaced Short Palindromic Repeats) system. As noted by Shen (2013a), 'CRISPR has exploded in popularity in recent years, with genetic engineers, neuroscientists and even plant biologists viewing it as a highly efficient and precise tool.' This technique utilizes an immune strategy used by bacteria to identify foreign DNA and cut it into pieces. Cas9 – a DNA-cutting enzyme – locates its target with the help of a guiding RNA sequence that researchers can now engineer to pinpoint any desired gene in any species (including humans). The CRISPR technique has been used to edit the genome of a variety of species, including zebra fish, frogs, rats, rabbits, pigs and monkeys (Hsu *et al.*, 2014; Sander and Joung, 2014). In addition to being able to make changes in differentiated somatic cells of animals, CRISPR technology (as well as other genetic engineering methods) can be used to change the DNA in the nuclei of reproductive cells (or germ cells) that pass genetic information from one generation to the next. As a result, it is now possible to carry out genetic alterations in fertilized animal eggs or embryos, thus altering the genetic make-up of every differentiated cell in an organism and ensuring that the changes will be passed on to the animal's offspring. An additional advantage of gene editing techniques like CRISPR is that they allow for the introduction or removal of a number of genes at a time (*The Economist*, 2015a). This is important since most disorders are not caused by the dysfunction of just one gene.

Furthermore, technologies like CRISPR use something called a 'gene drive' – this is a gene that uses gene editing techniques to copy itself from one chromosome to another. Essentially, engineering the CRISPR system itself into a creature's genome makes it possible for an organism to edit its own genes (*The Economist*, 2015a). Offspring typically inherit only one pair of each chromosome from each parent, so each version of the gene typically gets into only half of the offspring. However, gene drive copies a mutation made by CRISPR on one chromosome to its partner and thereby ensures that all offspring will inherit the edited genome (Caplan *et al.*, 2015; *The Economist*, 2015b). Normally, genes can only spread through a natural population if they confer an advantage. Gene drive is a powerful tool that makes it more likely that an edited trait will be passed on to offspring through sexual reproduction (Caplan *et al.*, 2015). It has been suggested that gene drive be utilized to genetically manipulate wild animals to stop them spreading disease, for example. Gene drives, however, spread faster than natural selection, so they should be able to spread through a population even if it is bad for its predecessors. One major concern, then, is that if an animal escaped from such experiments its gene drive could spread far and wide into natural populations, running the risk of decimating entire species, eliminating a food source for other species, or promoting the proliferation of invasive species (Caplan *et al.*, 2015).

The advent of gene editing technology might also shift trends in the use of animals in research; for example, CRISPR has recently been used to create the first gene edited primates (Shen, 2014) as well as 'primate models' of affective disorders like autism

(Cyranoski, 2016). This might have the effect of increasing the numbers of non-human primates used in research. While some scientists argue that gene edited primates will make better disease models than mice (Shen, 2013b), there is public unease about the use of non-human primates in experiments, so a shift to increasing their use might not be fully publicly acceptable (Ormandy and Schuppli, 2014). Other shifts in species use might include an increase in the use of fish for scientific procedures. While many people tend to think of mice and rats as the predominant species used in research, the advent of new genetic engineering techniques has meant that zebra fish have now become a commonly used species. As noted by Lieschke and Currie (2007) 'Through the 1980s development of zebrafish genetic techniques, such as "cloning", mutagenesis, transgenesis and mapping approaches, underpinned the use of zebrafish to apply invertebrate-style forward genetics to questions of vertebrate development.' As such, the use of zebra fish in research has increased substantially in recent years – fish were the most common lab species in Canada between 2009 and 2011 (CCAC, 2010; CCAC, 2011), and are listed as the most commonly used species in the most recent animal data report (CCAC, 2016) – and the species has now become an indispensable 'animal model', especially in the field of developmental biology (Lieschke and Currie, 2007).

Enhancing research animals with genetic engineering and gene editing

Biomedical applications of GE animals are numerous and include understanding of gene function, and modelling of human disease to either understand disease mechanisms or to aid drug development. Genetic engineering and gene editing has also enabled the production of animal lines that have less genetic variability and more accurately represent the human defects they are used to study (Larson and Schaffer, 2014). More accurate disease models can serve to reduce the numbers of animals needed in a given experiment. However, while this is a laudable goal, the advent of cheaper, more efficient and inexpensive genetic techniques opens up their use to many more labs, which has the potential to lead to an overall increase in the numbers of animals used in research (van Eenennaam, 2015). Recent efforts have focused on developing new GE animal models of conditions such as Alzheimer's disease, amyotrophic lateral sclerosis (ALS), Parkinson's disease and cancer (Ormandy *et al.*, 2011), as well as using gene editing techniques to model affective disorders, such as autism, in primates (Cyranoski, 2016). The advent of gene editing technology means that targeted gene edits are now possible in many more species (as opposed to embryonic cell knockouts, which were typically only successful in mice).

Xenotransplantation: using GE pigs for human therapeutic benefit

Xenotransplantation is the transfer of organs, tissues or cells from one species to another. The use of animal tissues for the treatment of certain human conditions has been carried out for decades (e.g. use of pig heart valves, tissues for ligament reconstruction etc.) (Laurencin and El-Amin, 2008). However, there is an increasing demand to supply organs and tissues to human patients in need. Furthermore, as stated by Ekser *et al.* (2012), 'the provision of tissues such as pancreatic islets and neuronal cells from deceased human donors has never been sufficient'. A lot of progress has been made in xenotransplantation in the past decade due to the increased availability of GE pigs, who have been altered to supply organs that are protected from the human immune response (thus, the recipient of the pig organ does not reject the implant). To refine xenotransplantation and the required genetic alterations, preclinical research has been conducted with transplantation of organs from pigs to non-human primates. So far, the disorders for which xenotransplantation (using GE pig organs, cells or tissues) is a potential therapy have been identified as follows: diabetes mellitus, end-stage cardiac disease, Parkinson's and Huntington's diseases, end-stage renal disease, corneal and neuro-retinal blindness, end-stage hepatic disease, anaemia, end-stage pulmonary disease, cardiac valve replacement, intestinal insufficiency, general surgery and orthopaedic surgery, and multiorgan failure (Ekser *et al.*, 2012).

However, there are some major hurdles to overcome before xenotransplantation can be applied broadly in the human clinical setting. First, issues relating to organ rejection and coagulation dysfunction need to be addressed. To this end, numerous multitransgenic animals have either been produced or are in preparation. Second, physiological compatibility is not well studied. Most work on xenotransplantation has been done with animal recipients, and, to date, the survival time of these recipients has been too short to study longer term physiological compatibility. Third, xenotransplantation might be associated with risk of transmission of microorganisms from the donor animal (typically pigs). This risk can be greatly reduced through the breeding of pathogen free animals; however, porcine endogenous retroviruses (PERVs) represent a special risk (Denner, 2014). In addition to these physical hurdles, there is also the barrier of public perception and people's willingness to accept xenotransplants from animals, let alone GE species. Despite its promise to relieve pressure from the 'organ gap' – that is, the shortage of organs for patients in need of transplant – xenotransplantation has been a matter of policy debate and has prompted negative opinion (Einsiedel and Ross, 2002; Burgess *et al.*, 2007), especially in relation to issues such as individual privacy versus public health protection (Canadian Public Health Association, n.d.).

Genetically engineered farm animals

The first transgenic livestock were reported in 1985 (Hammer *et al.*, 1985; Niemaan and Kues, 2007). Since then, as reviewed by Laible (2009), there is 'an assorted range of agricultural livestock applications [for genetic engineering] aimed at improving animal productivity; food quality and disease resistance; and environmental sustainability'. To date, genetic engineering has been applied to improve the production and growth rate of agricultural animals (Hew *et al.*, 1995; Siedel, 1999), enhance nutritional content of animal-derived products (e.g. Lai *et al.*, 2006), and to help reduce agricultural impacts on the environment (Golovan *et al.*, 2001). The first GE animal to be approved by the FDA for commercial production is the AquAdvantage salmon, which was given the green light for human consumption on 19 November 2015 (Ledford, 2015). Furthermore, the more precise gene editing techniques have already produced pigs and cattle resistant to particular diseases, and polled dairy cows lacking horns, and current research promises to produce chickens who are resistant to heat, beef herds in which only the more profitable male calves are born, and chicken flocks in which only females are needed for production (Cima, 2016).

Effort has also been made to generate GE farm species, such as cows, goats and sheep, that express medically important proteins in their milk or blood. As stated by Dyck *et al.* (2003), 'transgenic animal bioreactors represent a powerful tool to address the growing need for therapeutic recombinant proteins'. The list of products under development includes widely used products such as clotting factors (Gottlieb and Wheeler, 2011), antithrombin (e.g. Morrow, 2009) and human albumin (e.g. Echelard *et al.*, 2009). In February 2009, ATryn® became the first therapeutic protein produced by GE animals to be approved by the Food and Drug Administration (FDA) of the USA (Gottleib and Wheeler, 2011). This product is approved for use as a prophylactic treatment for patients that have hereditary antithrombin deficiency and are undergoing surgical procedures. The FDA has since approved a drug for treating hereditary angioedema that is produced in transgenic rabbits (*Nature Biotechnology News*, 2014) and a recombinant human enzyme drug that replaces a faulty enzyme in people with a rare, inherited condition that prevents the body from breaking down fatty molecules in cells – this drug is produced in transgenic chicken eggs (Becker, 2015).

Researchers have also developed a number of GE farm animals, such as GE goats, capable of producing complex protein-based drugs. Protein-based drugs differ from protein products synthesized in the blood in that they are produced *in vivo* by other organs. This technology is being applied to the development of complex proteins such as monoclonal antibodies (Pollock *et al.*, 1999), polyclonal antibodies (Sullivan *et al.*, 2008), plasminogen activator (e.g. Ebert *et al.*, 1991) human alpha-fetoprotein (Parker *et al.*, 2004), alpha-1-proteinase inhibitor, alpha glucosidase and others (Pollock *et al.*, 1999; Behboodi *et al.*, 2002).

Righting some farm animal welfare wrongs?

While many GE and gene edited farm animals have been created to enhance productivity, efficiency and profit, several applications of GE animals aim to improve animal welfare through increased disease resistance – e.g. mastitis resistant dairy cattle, bovine spongiform encephalopathy resistant cows, and the induction of resistance to viral infection in chickens (Maga and Murray, 2010). This has led to the question of whether there is a risk from *not* using genetically engineered animals (Murray and Maga, 2010).

Although this perspective on the value of GE animals for addressing welfare concerns might be considered by some to be a valuable addition to the conversation about the use of genetic engineering, it results in altering the animal to fit our production environments, rather than altering our production environments so that they better suit animals' needs. As such, it is possible that focusing on GE animals as a potential solution to some farm animal welfare issues is, at best, band-aiding the problem and, at worst, a diversion from a much needed conversation about how to meet the needs of our farm animals in a way that respects their fundamental nature and needs.

Animal Cloning

Animal cloning is a method of asexual reproduction, and results in the birth of one animal (the clone) that is a genetic copy of another animal. If the clone becomes a parent, its children are not clones because they will have been born through sexual reproduction. The cloned animals have no new genes in them; rather they are the same as the animal of which they are a copy. For this reason, cloning is often thought of differently to genetic engineering or gene editing – there is no intention to alter the genome of an animal, only to copy it. However, the process of cloning carries with it some ethical concerns, some of which relate to animal welfare. As such, for the purposes of this chapter cloning will be considered a genetic manipulation.

There are three types of cloning: DNA cloning, therapeutic cloning, and reproductive cloning (National Human Genome Research Institute, 2016). For the purposes of this chapter the term cloning is used to refer to reproductive cloning, as this is the most likely to lead to animal welfare issues. Reproductive cloning is used if the intention is to generate an animal that has the same nuclear DNA as another current or previously existing animal. The process used to generate this type of cloned animal is called somatic cell nuclear transfer (SCNT).

Cloning is still an inefficient process that requires many recipient animals and embryo transfers to produce a cloned individual (Wells, 2005). For example, in a study by Lee *et al.* (2005) in which Afghan hounds were cloned, there were only three pregnancies from embryo transfer to 123 recipients (meaning that pregnancy rates were low), and there were only two pups delivered despite 1095 embryos being transferred in total. Furthermore, one of the two pups was dead within one month after delivery. However, cloning technology might still hold promise, and has been discussed in terms of specific advantages, including: rapid multiplication of desired livestock, animal conservation, multiplication of important research models, and cloning for transgenic applications (Wells, 2005). Cloning is also being used to create genetically identical copies of people's deceased pets.

Cloning of farm animals

Companies in the USA and China are cloning livestock for breeding (not consumption). To date, the livestock species that have been successfully cloned are cattle, pigs, sheep and goats. So far, chickens and other poultry have not been cloned. The advantage of utilizing cloning technology in animal agriculture is that desirable characteristics can be quickly and predictably added to animal herds. Such characteristics include disease resistance, suitability to climate, quality body type, fertility, and market preference (Food and Drug Administration, 2015).

A significant limitation of current cloning technology is the prospect that cloned offspring might suffer some degree of abnormality. Studies have revealed that cloned mammals may suffer from developmental abnormalities, including extended gestation, larger birth weight, inadequate placental formation, and histological effects in organs and tissues. One annotated review highlights 11 different original research papers that documented the production of cloned animals with abnormalities occurring in the developing embryo, and suffering for the new born animal and surrogate mother (Weaver and Morris, 2005). Therefore, despite the reported advantages of using cloning technology in animal agriculture, the Parliament of the European Union recently voted to ban the creation and import of cloned farm animals (Vogel, 2015). Supporters of the ban cited concerns over animal welfare, in particular high mortality rates of cloned offspring (*European Parliament News*, 2015).

De-extinction and conservation of wild species

The cover of the April 2013 edition of *National Geographic* depicted an illustration of a woolly mammoth walking out of a test tube, with the words 'Reviving Extinct Species – We Can, but Should We?' This thought-provoking title poses the most fundamental ethical question about the use of new genetic technologies, and posits that just because we *can* accomplish many different types of genetic manipulation and cloning, it does not necessarily mean that we *should*. Revival of extinct species was a topic I posed to my Ethical Issues in Science students that year, and the overwhelming response from them was that the revival of extinct species was not something that we *should* be doing. Their arguments raised concerns over populations of existing animals being outcompeted (thus causing other species extinctions), and welfare concerns that might arise with the revived species if they no longer have a suitable habitat in which to thrive. However, some students did raise the issue of moral obligations – that is, if a species has been driven to extinction by human actions, is it our moral obligation to bring it back and help that species thrive once more? This is an interesting question, and one that has been raised elsewhere; for example, Shreeve (2013) writes that one argument in favour of species revival is that, 'we should do it because we have an obligation to do it, to right some of the enormous wrongs we have done by driving these co-tenants of the Earth off the planet in the first place'. However, extinct species revival is not a matter for speculation; it is a reality – in 2009, Folch *et al.* published their work on the successful birth of a Pyrenean ibex using nuclear transfer techniques with donor cells obtained from the last female ibex.

In addition to using cloning techniques to revive extinct species, scientists have been proposing cloning technology as a conservation tool ever since the early history of reproductive cloning (e.g. Ryder and Benirschke, 1997; Wells, 2000), and it is now being extensively reviewed (e.g. Holt *et al.*, 2004; Gomez *et al.*, 2009). Species that have either been successfully cloned or are potential candidates include: black-footed ferret, riverine rabbit, Iberian lynx, and the South China leopard (Pina-Aguilar *et al.*, 2009). However, despite these hopes and successes, there is currently poor performance of cloning techniques in wildlife; few cloned offspring are born, and many die shortly after birth. As identified by Pina-Aguilar *et al.* (2009), this poor performance is caused by many obstacles and challenges, including: 'poor knowledge of species reproductive biology, lack of oocytes for cytoplasts source (in most cases interspecific), and suitable embryo recipients of cloned embryos (also in most cases interspecific)'.

The new market for cloned companion animals

The first cloned cat, 'CC', was created in 2002 (Shin *et al.*, 2002), and this achievement was closely followed a few years later by the first cloned dog, 'Snuppy' (Lee *et al.*, 2005). Since these research breakthroughs, pet cloning has become a growing industry, especially in South Korea. Dog breeds that have been cloned since 2005 include: Afghan hounds, toy poodles, beagles, golden retrievers, labrador retrievers and Pekingese (Kim *et al.*, 2012). Early in 2016 the first British couple to clone their pet dog (a boxer called Dylan) went to pick up the cloned puppies from South Korea (Horton, 2016), demonstrating the new global scope of the pet cloning industry. However, while many animal lovers who have gone through the loss of their beloved companions might celebrate the new found ability to have their pets cloned, the practice has been heavily criticized for playing on 'the emotional hopes of animal lovers to make them complicit in the poor treatment of dogs' (Davies, 2012).

This new market for cloned pets sets up the unrealistic expectation that it possible to recreate the exact same dog. Of course, identical nuclear DNA does not make for identical animals (because a cloned dog has different mitochondrial DNA from its genetic donor, and there are also gene–environment interactions to consider); however, many people who pay top dollar for dog cloning do so in the hope that they really will get their dog back (Woestnediek, 2011).

The industry that is being supported when people pay tens of thousands of dollars to get their pet dogs cloned might be considered ethically dubious. As mentioned, the hub of the pet cloning industry is South Korea, a country where the treatment of dogs is not as strictly regulated as in other countries. South Korea has a culture of consuming dog meat, and 2 million dogs are killed annually for their meat. Thus, generally speaking, there is more of an instrumental value placed on dogs in South Korea – they are commodities to be sold for profit and consumption. The cloning of dogs feeds into this culture. In contrast, while North American culture still sees dogs as commodities 'for sale' to a certain degree, the majority of people tend to frown upon puppy mills and dog breeders that do not treat the dogs well. So, as stated by Davies (2012), 'those who would consider having their dogs cloned should examine the current state of the cloning industry and whether people who would be involved in the cloning value dogs as highly as they do'. Moreover, there are millions of dogs that end up in animal rescue shelters every year that need loving homes, and end up being unnecessarily euthanized. The ability to clone a deceased pet may divert pet owners from either obtaining a new dog from a breeder, or fostering or rehoming a dog that desperately needs a home.

Public Attitudes towards Genetic Manipulation of Animals

The genetic manipulation of animals through genetic engineering and cloning has been a topic of vigorous debate amongst the public and policy makers, and as noted by Snow (2003), 'polarized opinions make it hard to discuss scientific questions about [genetically engineered organisms] without delving into the reasons for the passion on both sides of this debate'. Overall, public views toward the creation and use of GE animals tend to be complex, but predominantly negative (Macnaghten, 2001). In his 2001 study, Macnaghten found considerable concern about genetic modification and the uses to which GE animals might be put. He noted people's 'reaction against proposed technology as intrinsically a violation of nature and transgressive of so-called natural parameters'. Other studies have shown people's concern that genetic engineering might lead to unexpected (and potentially bad) consequences; one aspect of the unease about the creation of GE animals is a fear that nature might 'bite back' (Macnaghten, 2004; Birke *et al.*, 2007). An additional concern is that there will be an increase in the numbers of animals used for research due to the inefficient and unpredictable nature of some genetic engineering techniques (Macnaghten, 2004; Schuppli *et al.*, 2004; Ormandy *et al.*, 2009).

A recent Eurobarometer poll on biotechnology indicated that people tend to be divided in their optimism about genetic engineering. Overall, participants were not in favour of genetically engineered food and do not see its benefits, and they had strong reservations about animal cloning in food production (Eurobarometer, 2010). The predominantly negative attitude towards genetic engineering and cloning might present some significant roadblocks to new GE, gene edited or cloned animals ever reaching their intended application. One key example of how public opinion can halt progress is the Enviropig. This is a pig that is genetically engineered so that it does not produce phosphorus – a major agricultural pollutant – in its faeces. The environmental benefits of reducing agricultural pollution are very clear; however, despite years of research to create the Enviropig, there was no commercial market for the pigs due to a lack of public support. Many people simply don't want to consume GE animals.

However, people's support for the creation and use of GE animals tends to vary depending on the intended application, and some studies have shown that some people support the use of GE animals in research if this will increase the chances of successful research that will ultimately lead to human or animal health benefits (Ormandy *et al.*, 2012; Ormandy *et al.*, 2013b). Thus, it seems that there is a tendency for people to be in support of genetic engineering, gene editing and cloning when the animals will be used for research purposes, but not when they will be used in food production.

Summary

There are many proposed applications of genetically engineered, gene edited or cloned animals, and despite public concerns over the potential bad consequences that could result, or concerns about tampering with 'nature', some GE animals have now started to become commercially available. The long-term effects of introducing GE animals into our domestic animal populations remain to be seen; however, advocates of using GE technology to manipulate animal genomes argue that benefits are set to include: increased productivity and disease resistant livestock, more accurate animal 'models' for research, and an abundance of safe organs for transplant into human patients. However, there are lessons to be learned from instances where humans have selectively bred animals for desired traits, and the animal welfare concerns that resulted.

References

Alban, L., Agger, J.F. and Lawson, L.G. (1996) Lameness in tied Danish dairy cattle: the possible influence of housing systems, management, milk yield, and prior incidents of lameness. *Preventive Veterinary Medicine* 29, 135–149.

Asher, L., Diesel, G., Summers, J.F., McGreevy, P.D. and Collins, L.M. (2009) Inherited defects in pedigree dogs. Part 1: Disorders related to breed standards. *The Veterinary Journal* 182, 402–411.

Becker, R. (2015) US government approves transgenic chicken. *Nature News*. Available at: http://www.nature.com/news/us-government-approves-transgenic-chicken-1.18985 (access 28 July 2016).

Behboodi, E., Chen, L., Destrempes, M., Meade, H.M. and Echelard, Y. (2002) Transgenic cloned goats and the production of therapeutic proteins. In: Sibelli, J., Lanza, R., Campbell, K. and West. M. (eds) *Principles of Cloning*. Elsevier Science, USA.

Birke, L., Arluke, A. and Michael, M. (2007) *The Sacrifice: How Scientific Experiments Transform Animals and People*. Purdue University Press, West Lafayette, Indiana.

British Veterinary Association (2015) Screening and responsible breeding are improving dog health, new statistics show. Available at: https://www.bva.co.uk/News-campaigns-and-policy/Newsroom/News-releases/Screening-and-responsible-breeding-are-improving-dog-health,-new-statistics-show/ (access 2 August 2016).

Burgess, J., Stirling, A., Clark, J., Davies, G., Eames, M., Staley, K. and Williamson, S. (2007) Deliberative mapping: a novel analytic-deliberative methodology to support contested science-policy decisions. *Public Understanding of Science* 16, 299–322.

Canadian Public Health Association (n.d.) *Public Consultation on Xenotransplantation*. Available at: http://www.cpha.ca/en/programs/xeno/ethics-1.aspx (accessed 4 August 2016).

Capecchi, M. (1989) The new mouse genetics: altering the genome by gene targeting. *Trends in Genetics* 5, 70–76.

Caplan, A.L., Parent, B., Shen, M. and Plunkett, C. (2015) No time to waste – the ethical challenges created by CRISPR. *EMBO Reports* 16, 1421–1426.

Carlson, D.F., Lancto, C.A., Zang, B., Kim, E.-S., Walton, M., Oldeschulte, D., Seabury, C., Sonstegard, T.S and Fahrenkrug, S.C. (2016) Production of hornless dairy cattle from genome-edited cell lines. *Nature Biotechnology* 34, 479–481.

Casellas, J. (2011) Inbred mouse strains and genetic stability: a review. *Animal* 5, 1–7.

CCAC (2010) *CCAC Animal Data Report 2009*. Available at: http://www.ccac.ca/Documents/Publications/Statistics/Survey_2009.pdf (accessed 29 July 2016).

CCAC (2011) *CCAC Animal Data Report 2011*. Available at: http://www.ccac.ca/Documents/Publications/Statistics/CCAC_Animal_Use_Statistics_2011.pdf (accessed 29 July 2016).

CCAC (2016) *CCAC Animal Data Report 2014*. Available at: http://www.ccac.ca/Documents/AUD/2014-Animal-Data-Report.pdf (access 29 July 2016).

Cima, G. (2016) Gene editing application expanding with advancing technology. *Journal of the American Veterinary Medical Association*. Available at: https://www.avma.org/News/JAVMANews/Pages/160315a.aspx (accessed 29 July 2016).

Cozzi, G., Gottardo, F., Brscic, M., Contiero, B., Irrgang, N. *et al.* (2015) State of the art cattle dehorning in the EU Member States: a quantitative survey of the current practices. *Livestock Science* 179, 4–11.

Cyranoski, D. (2016) Monkeys genetically modified to show autism symptoms. *Nature News*. Available at: http://www.nature.com/news/monkeys-genetically-modified-to-show-autism-symptoms-1.19228 (accessed 21 July 2016).

Davies, L. (2012) Why cloning is a terrible way to bring your pet dog back from the dead. Available at: http://io9.gizmodo.com/5949612/why-cloning-is-a-terrible-way-to-bring-your-pet-dog-back-from-the-dead (accessed 26 July 2016).

Denner, J. (2014) Xenotransplantation – progress and problems: a review. *Transplantation Technologies and Research* 4, 133–143.

Dyck, M.K., Lacroix, D., Pothier, F. and Sirard M.-A. (2003) Making recombinant proteins in animals – different systems, different applications. *Trends in Biotechnology* 21, 394–399.

Ebert, K.M., Selgrath, J., DiTullio, P., Denman, J., Smith, T.E. *et al.* (1991) Transgenic production of a variant of human tissue-type plasminogen activator in goat milk: generation of transgenic goats and analysis of expression. *Bio/Technology* 9, 835–838.

Ebihara, S., Marks, T., Hudson, D.J. and Menaker, M. (1986) Genetic control of melatonin synthesis in the pineal gland of the mouse. *Science* 231, 491–493.

Echelard, Y., Williams, J.L., Destrempes, M.M., Koster, J.A., Overton, S.A. *et al.* (2009) Production of recombinant albumin by a herd of cloned transgenic cattle. *Transgenic Research* 18, 361–376.

The Economist (2015a) *The Most Selfish Genes*. Available at: http://www.economist.com/news/briefing/21661801-giving-bits-dna-power-edit-themselves-intriguing-and-worrying-possibility (accessed 29 July 2016).

The Economist (2015b) *The Age of the Red Pen*. Available at: http://www.economist.com/news/briefing/21661799-it-now-easy-edit-genomes-plants-animals-and-humans-age-red-pen (accessed 29 July 2016).

Einsiedel, E.F. and Ross, H. (2002) Animal spare parts? A Canadian public consultation on xenotransplantation. *Science and Engineering Ethics* 8, 579–591.

Ekser, B., Ezzelarab, M., Hara, H., van der Windt, D.J., Wijkstrom, M., Bottino, R., Trucco, M. and Cooper, D.K.C. (2012) Clinical xenotransplantation: the next medical revolution? *Lancet* 379, 672–683.

Eurobarometer (2010) *Biotechnology Report*. Available at: http://ec.europa.eu/public_opinion/archives/ebs/ebs_341_en.pdf (accessed 4 August 2016).

European Parliament News (2015) EP wants animal cloning ban extended to offspring and imports. Available at: http://www.europarl.europa.eu/news/en/news-room/20150903IPR91517/EP-wants-animal-cloning-ban-extended-to-offspring-and-imports (accessed 29 July 2016).

Folch, J., Cocero, M.J., Chesené, P., Alabart, J.L., Dominguez, V. *et al*. (2009) First birth of an animal from an extinct subspecies (Capra pyrenaica pyrenaica) by cloning. *Theriogenology* 71, 1026–1034.

Food and Drug Administration (FDA) (2015) *Genetically Engineered Animals: General Q & A*. Available at: http://www.fda.gov/AnimalVeterinary/DevelopmentApprovalProcess/GeneticEngineering/GeneticallyEngineeredAnimals/ucm113605.htm (accessed 18 July 2016).

Gepts, P. (2002) A comparison between crop domestication, classical plant breeding, and genetic engineering. *Crop Science* 42, 1780–1790.

Golovan, S.P., Meidinger, R.G., Ajakaiye, A., Cottrill, M., Wiederkehr, M.Z. *et al*. (2001) Pigs expressing salivary phytase produce low-phosphorus manure. *Nature Biotechnology* 19, 741–745.

Gomez, M.C., Pope, C.E., Ricks, D.M. *et al*. (2009) Cloning endangered felids using heterospecific donor oocytes and interspecies embryo transfer. *Reproduction, Fertility and Development* 21, 76–82.

Gottleib, S. and Wheeler, M.B. (2011) *Genetically Engineered Animals and Public Health: Compelling Benefits for Health Care, Nutrition, the Environment, and Animal Welfare*. Available at: https://www.bio.org/sites/default/files/files/2011_ge%20animal_benefits_report.pdf (accessed 30 January 2018).

Hackett, P.B., Fahrenkrug, S.C. and Carlson, D. (2014) The promises and challenges of precision gene editing in animals of agricultural importance. Presented at: *New DNA-Editing Approaches: Methods, Applications and Policy for Agriculture*. Ithaca, New York. Available at: http://nabc.cals.cornell.edu/Publications/Reports/nabc_26/26_1_3_Hackett.pdf (accessed 29 July 2016).

Hammer, R.E., Pursel, V.G., Rexroad, C.E., Jr, Wall, R.J., Bolt, D.J., Ebert, K.M., Palmiter, R.D. and Brinster, R.L. (1985) Production of transgenic rabbits, sheep and pigs by microinjection. *Nature* 315, 680–683.

Hew, C.L., Fletcher, G.L. and Davies, P.L. (1995) Transgenic salmon: tailoring the genome for food production. *Journal of Fish Biology* 47(S), 1–19.

Holt, W.V., Pickard, A.R. and Prather, R.S. (2004) Wildlife conservation and reproductive cloning. *Reproduction* 127, 317–324.

Horton, H. (2016) First couple to clone dead pet dog pick up puppies from South Korea. *The Telegraph*. Available at: http://www.telegraph.co.uk/news/uknews/12133278/First-British-couple-to-clone-dead-pet-dog-pick-up-puppies-from-South-Korea.html (accessed 26 July 2016).

Hsu, P.D., Lander, E.S. and Zhang, F. (2014) Development and applications of CRISPR-Cas9 for genome editing. *Cell* 157, 1262–1278.

Jackson Laboratory (n.d.) Why mouse genetics? Available at: https://www.jax.org/personalized-medicine/why-mouse-genetics (accessed 30 January 2018).

Jones, W.P., Hansen, L.B. and Chester-Jones, H. (1994) Response of health care to selection for milk yield of dairy cattle. *Journal of Dairy Science* 77, 3137–3152.

Joung, J.K. and Sander, J.D. (2013) TALENs: a widely applicable technology for targeted genome editing. *Nature Reviews Molecular Cell Biology* 14, 49–55.

Kim, M.J., Oh, H.J., Kim, G.A., Park, J.E., Park, E.J. *et al.* (2012) Lessons learned from dog cloning. *Reproduction in Domestic Animals* 47, 115–119.

Lai, L., Kang, J.X., Li, R., Wang, J., Witt, W.T. (2006) Generation of cloned transgenic pigs rich in omega-3 fatty acids. *Nature Biotechnology* 24, 435–436.

Laible G. (2009) Enhancing livestock through genetic engineering – recent advances and future prospects. *Comparative Immunology and Microbiology* 32, 123–127.

Larson, C. and Schaffer, S. (2014) Genome editing: the ability to create primates with intentional mutations could provide powerful new ways to study complex and genetically baffling brain disorders. *MIT Technology Review*. Available at: https://www.technologyreview.com/s/526511/genome-editing/ (accessed 29 July 2016).

Laurencin, C.T. and El-Amin, S.F. (2008) Xenotransplantation in orthopedic surgery. *Journal of the American Academy of Orthopedic Surgery* 16, 4–8.

Ledford, H. (2015) Salmon approval heralds rethink of transgenic animals. *Nature News*. Available at: http://www.nature.com/news/salmon-approval-heralds-rethink-of-transgenic-animals-1.18867 (accessed 28 July 2016).

Lee, B.C., Kim, M.K., Jang, G., Oh, H.J., Yuda, F. (2005) Dogs cloned from adult somatic cells. *Nature* 436, 641.

Lescourret, F., Coulon, J.B. and Faye, B. (1995) Predictive model of mastitis occurrence in the dairy cow. *Journal of Dairy Science* 78, 2167–2177.

Lieschke, G.J. and Currie, P.D. (2007) Animal models of human disease: zebrafish swim into view. *Nature Reviews Genetics* 8, 353–367.

Macnaghten, P. (2001) Animal futures: public attitudes and sensibilities toward animals and biotechnology in contemporary Britain, IEPPP, Lancaster University, UK.

Macnaghten, P. (2004) Animals in their nature: a case study on public attitudes to animal, genetic modification and 'nature'. *Sociology* 38, 533–551.

Maga, E.A. and Murray, J.D. (2010) Welfare applications of genetically engineered animals for use in agriculture. *Journal of Animal Science* 88, 1588–1591.

Mäntysaari, E.A., Quass, R.L. and Gröhn, Y.T. (1991) Clinical ketosis, phenotypic and genetic correlations between occurrences and with milk yield. *Journal of Dairy Science* 74, 3985–3993.

Morrow, T. (2009) Transgenic goats are key to antithrombin production. *Management and Care* 18, 46–47.

Murray, J.D. and Maga, E.A. (2010) Is there a risk from not using GE animals? *Transgenic Research* 11, 9341–9345.

National Human Genome Research Institute (2016) *Cloning*. Available at: https://www.genome.gov/25020028/cloning-fact-sheet/ (accessed 28 July 2016).

Nature Biotechnology News (2014) Rabbit milk Ruconest for hereditary angioedema. *Nature Biotechnology* 32, 849.

Nebel, R.L. and McGilliard, M.L. (1993) Interactions of high milk yield and reproductive performance in dairy cows. *Journal of Dairy Science* 76, 3257–3268.

Niemann, H. and Kues, W.A. (2007) Transgenic farm animals: an update. *Reproduction, Fertility and Development* 19, 762–770.

Oltenacu, P.A. and Broom, D.M. (2010) The impact of genetic selection for increased milk yield on the welfare of dairy cows. *Animal Welfare* 19(S), 39–49.

Ormandy, E.H. and Schuppli, C.A. (2014) Public attitudes towards animal research: a review. *Animals* 4, 391–408.

Ormandy, E.H., Schuppli, C.A. and Weary, D.M. (2009) Worldwide trends in the use of animals in research: the contribution of genetically-modified animal models. *Alternatives to Laboratory Animals* 37, 63–68.

Ormandy, E.H., Dale, J. and Griffin, G. (2011) Genetic engineering of animals: ethical issues, including welfare concerns. *Canadian Veterinary Journal* 52, 1–6.

Ormandy, E.H., Schuppli, C.A. and Weary, D.M. (2012) Factors affecting people's acceptance of the use of zebrafish and mice in research. *Alternatives to Laboratory Animals* 40, 321–333.

Ormandy, E.H., Dale, J. and Griffin, G. (2013a) The use of genetically-engineered animals in science: perspectives of Canadian animal care committee members. *Alternatives to Laboratory Animals* 41, 1–8.

Ormandy, E.H., Schuppli, C.A. and Weary, D.M. (2013b) Public attitudes toward the use of animals in research: effects of invasiveness, genetic modification and regulation. *Anthrozoös* 26, 165–184.

Parker, M.H., Birck-Wilson, E., Allard, G., Masiello, N., Day, M. *et al.* (2004) Purification and characterization of a recombinant version of human alpha-fetoprotein in the milk of transgenic goats. *Protein Expression and Purification* 38, 177–183.

Phillips, C.J.C. (1997) Animal welfare considerations in future breeding programmes for farm livestock. *Animal Breeding Abstracts* 65, 645–654.

Pina-Aguilar, R.E., Lopez-Saucedo, J., Sheffield, R., Ruiz-Galaz, L.I., Barroso-Padilla, J. de. J., Gutierrez-Gutierrez, A. (2009) Revival of extinct species using nuclear transfer: hope for the mammoth, true for the Pyrenean ibex, but is it time for 'conservation cloning'? *Cloning and Stem Cells* 11, 341–346.

Pollock, D.P., Kutzko, J.P., Birk-Wilson, E., Williams, J.L., Echelard, Y. and Meade, H.M. (1999) Transgenic milk as a method for the production of recombinant antibodies. *Journal of Immunological Methods* 231, 147–157.

Porteus, M.H. and Carroll, D. (2005) Gene targeting using zinc-finger nucleases. *Nature Biotechnology* 23, 967–973.

Pryce, J.E., Nielsen, B.L., Veerkamp, R.F. and Simm, G. (1999) Genotype and feeding system effects and interactions for health and fertility traits in dairy cattle. *Livestock Production Science* 57, 193–201.

Rauw, W.M., Kanis, E., Noordhuizen-Stassen, E.N. and Grommers, F.J. (1998) Undesirable side effects of selection for high production efficiency in farm animals: a review. *Livestock Production Science* 56, 15–33.

Robinson, V., Morton, D.B., Anderson, D., Carver, J.F.A., Francis, R.J. *et al.*(2003) *Refinement and Reduction in the Production of Genetically Modified Mice*. Sixth report of the BVAFF/FRAME/RSPCA/UFAW Joint Working Group on Refinement. *Laboratory Animals* 37(S), 1–51.

Rooney, N. and Sargan, D. (2008) Pedigree dog breeding in the UK: a major welfare concern? An independent scientific report commissioned by the RSPCA. Available at: http://www.rspca.org.uk/adviceandwelfare/pets/dogs/health/pedigreedogs/report (accessed 29 July 2016).

Ryder, O.A. and Benirshke, K. (1997) The potential use of cloning in the 'conservation' effort. *Zoo Biology* 16, 295–300.

Sander, J.D. and Joung, J.K. (2014) CRISPR-Cas systems for editing, regulating and targeting genomes. *Nature Biotechnology* 32, 347–355.

Sandøe, P., Nielsen, B.L., Christiensen, L.G. and Sørensen, P. (1999) Staying good while playing God – the ethics of breeding farm animals. *Animal Welfare* 8, 313–328.

Schuppli, C.A., Fraser, D. and McDonald, M. (2004) Expanding the 3Rs to meet new challenges in humane animal experimentation. *Alternatives to Laboratory Animals* 32, 525–532.

Shen, H. (2013a) CRIPSR technology leaps from lab to industry. *Nature News*. Available at: http://www.nature.com/news/crispr-technology-leaps-from-lab-to-industry-1.14299 (accessed 24 July 2016).

Shen, H. (2013b) Precision gene editing paves way for transgenic monkeys. *Nature News*. Available at: http://www.nature.com/news/precision-gene-editing-paves-way-for-transgenic-monkeys-1.14098 (accessed 24 July 2016).

Shen, H. (2014) First monkeys with customized mutations born. *Nature News*. Available at: http://www.nature.com/news/first-monkeys-with-customized-mutations-born-1.14611 (accessed 24 July 2016).

Shin, T., Kraemer, D., Pryor, J., Liu, L., Ruglia, J. (2002) Cell biology: a cat cloned by nuclear transplantation. *Nature* 415, 859.

Shreeve, J. (2013) Species revival: Should we bring back extinct animals? *National Geographic News*. Available at: http://news.nationalgeographic.com/news/2013/03/130305-science-animals-extinct-species-revival-deextinction-debate-tedx/ (accessed 27 July 2016).

Sidman, R.L. and Green, M.C. (1965) Retinal degeneration in the mouse: location of the rd locus in linkage group. *Journal of Heredity* 56, 23–29.

Siedel, G.E. (1999) The future of transgenic farm animals. In: Murray, J.D., Anderson, G.B., Oberbauer, A.M. and McGloughlin, M.M (eds) *Genetically Engineered Animals in Agriculture*. CAB International, New York, pp. 269–283.

Simm, G. (1998) *Genetic Improvement of Cattle and Sheep*. Faring Press, Ipswich, UK.

Snow, A. (2003) Unnatural selection. *Nature* 424, 619.

Snow, A.A., Andow, D.A., Gepts, P., Hallerman, E.M., Power, A., Tiedje, J.M. and Wolfenbarger, L.L. (2005) Genetically engineered organisms and the environment: current status and recommendations. *Ecological Applications* 15, 377–404.

Stafford, K.J. and Mellow, D.J. (2005) Dehorning and disbudding distress and its alleviation in calves. *Veterinary Journal* 169, 337–349.

Stevens, J.C., Banks, G.T., Festing, M.F.W. and Fisher, E.M.C. (2007) Quiet mutations in inbred strains of mice. *Trends in Molecular Biology* 13(12), 512–519.

Sullivan, E.J., Pommer, J. and Robl, J.M. (2008) Commercializing genetically engineered animal biomedical products. *Reproduction Fertility and Development* 20, 61–66.

Summers, J.F., Diesel, G., Asher, L., McGreevy, P.D. and Collins, L.M. (2009) Inherited defects in pedigree dogs. Part 2: Disorders that are not related to breed standards. *The Veterinary Journal* 183, 39–45.

Tanooka, H., Sasaki, H., Shiroishi, T. and Moriwaki, K. (2001) p53 pseudogene dating: identification of the origin of laboratory mice. *Gene* 270, 153–159.

Van Eenennaam, A. (2015) Overview of the ethical issues of germ line modification in animals. Presentation for the ILAR roundtable workshop: *Gene Editing to Modify Animal Genomes for Research – Scientific and Ethical Considerations*. December, Washington DC. Available at: http://nas-sites.org/ilar-roundtable/files/2015/11/ALISON-VAN-EENENAAM.pdf (accessed 29 July 2016).

Vogel, G. (2015) E.U. Parliament votes to ban cloning of farm animals. *Science*. Available at: http://www.sciencemag.org/news/2015/09/eu-parliament-votes-ban-cloning-farm-animals (accessed 29 July 2016).

Von Keyserlingk, M.A.G., Rushen, J., de Passillé, A.M. and Weary, D.M. (2009) Invited review: the welfare of dairy cattle – key concepts and the role of science. *Journal of Dairy Science* 92, 4101–4111.

Weaver, S.A. and Morris, M.C. (2005) Risks associated with genetic modification: an annotated bibliography of peer-reviewed natural science publications. *Journal of Agricultural and Environmental Ethics* 18, 157–189.

Wells, D.N. (2000) Cloning for animal conservation. *Cloning* 2, 152–155.

Wells, D.N. (2005) Animal cloning: problems and prospects. *Scientific and Technical Review of the Office International des Epizooties* 24, 251–264.

Windig, J.J., Hoving-Bolink, R.A. and Veerkamp, R.F. (2015) Breeding for polledness in Holstein cattle. *Livestock Science* 179, 96–101.

Witmer, P.D., Doheny, K., Adams, M.K., Boehm, C.D., Dizon, J.S. *et al.* (2003) The development of a highly informative mouse simple sequence length polymorphism (SSLP) marker set and construction of a mouse family tree using parsimony analysis. *Genome Research* 13, 485–491.

Woestendiek, J. (2011) *Dog, Inc.: The Uncanny Inside Story of Cloning Man's Best Friend*. Avery Publishing Group, New York.

Yang, Y. and Santamaria, P. (2006) Lessons on autoimmune diabetes from animal models. *Clinical Science* 110, 627–639.

Yoshiki, A. and Moriwaki, K. (2006) Mouse phenome research: implications of genetic background. *ILAR* 47, 94–102.

Zheng, Q.Y., Johnson, K.R., Erway, L.C. (1999) Assessment of hearing in 80 inbred strains of mice by ABR threshold analyses. *Hearing Research* 130, 94–107.

11

From Bionic Cat to Superdog: Ethical Challenges of Advanced Prosthetic Technology in Veterinary Medicine

MANUEL MAGALHÃES-SANT'ANA*

Disciplinary Committee, Ordem dos Médicos Veterinários, Lisboa, Portugal; Faculdade Medicina Veterinária, Universidade de Lisboa, Portugal

'Four legs good, two legs bad'
(Snowball, in George Orwell's *Animal Farm*)

'Three legs good, four legs awesome'
(adapted from Kaufman, 2014)

Exploring the Issues

Disabled animals, i.e. animals suffering from congenital or acquired physical disabilities, bone cancers or other orthopaedic diseases, have benefited from recent advances in veterinary orthopaedics and traumatology. Veterinary orthotics and prosthetics (V-OP) have been used to manage pain and as a tool for rehabilitating disabled animals (Mich, 2014). Orthoses are external devices that are placed to protect and support complete limbs (Marcellin-Little *et al.*, 2015). Static exorthoses (also known as braces) have been used for centuries in humans and gradually adapted to suit quadruped animals. The last decade saw the development of modern exorthoses, which replicate articular motion and allow for dynamic biomechanical control (Fig. 11.1). Dynamic exorthoses are used in conjuction with surgery but can also replace orthopaedic surgery in humans and animals (Mich, 2014).

Prostheses are devices that are secured to incomplete limbs to enable locomotion (Marcellin-Little *et al.*, 2015). Endoprostheses are prosthetic devices that are internally anchored to the bone. Exoprostheses fit externally into a stump (socket prosthesis – Fig. 11.2) or into a previously fitted bone-anchored endoprosthesis. The pros and cons of these devices have been described before (Mich, 2014). Socket prostheses are relatively inexpensive, simple to apply and versatile. They may, however, cause sores due to soft tissue trauma. Osseointegrated endoprosthetic devices are much more expensive and invasive (they usually require several surgeries) but they cause little soft tissue trauma and better biomechanical support.

*E-mail: manuel.santana@omv.pt

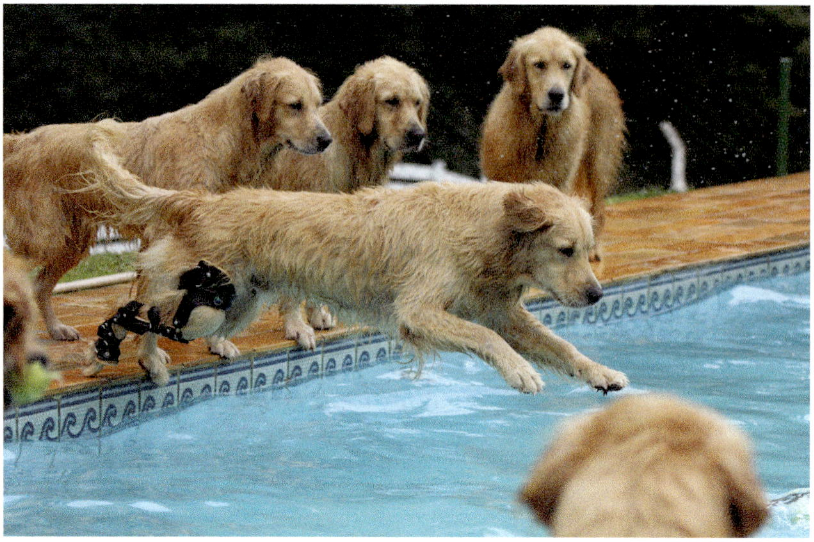

Fig. 11.1. Combined tarsal and stifle dynamic orthose (brace) in a retriever dog. (Photo: Copyright ©2013 Yara Quintanilha, OrthoPets Brazil. Used with permission).

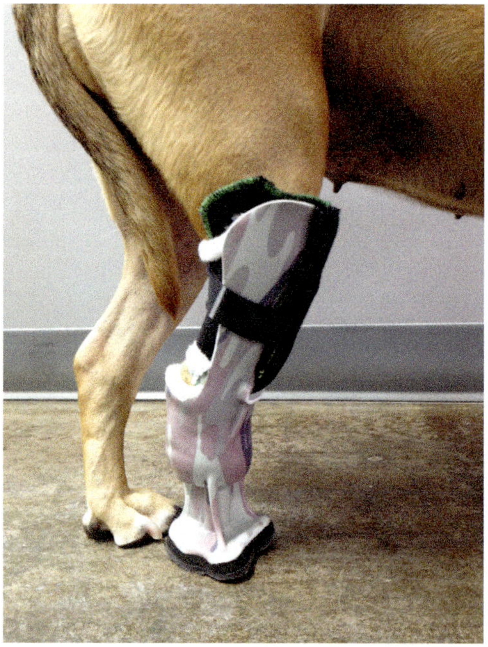

Fig. 11.2. Pelvic limb socket prosthesis in a dog. (Photo: Copyright ©2017 Amy Kaufmann OrthoPets LLC. Used with permission).

The use of orthopaedic biotechnologies in companion animals raises several ethical issues that require an applied contextual analysis. I have argued elsewhere that the application of advanced biotechnologies in companion animal practice does not necessarily present ethical issues that did not already exist (Magalhães-Sant'Ana, 2015). Nonetheless, increased technological sophistication has raised the complexity of ethical issues involved, namely in terms of well-being, autonomy and justice (Mepham, 2000; Sandøe *et al.*, 2016).

Arguably, the most renowned case of V-OP is that of the 'bionic cat' Oscar. In 2010, an amputated cat received intraosseous transcutaneous amputation prostheses (ITAP) – commonly known as bionic limbs – in his hind paws. This technology has since been successfully applied for limb salvage in dogs (Fitzpatrick *et al.*, 2011) and similar bone anchored limb prostheses have been applied to humans (Pitkin, 2013) and experimental cats (Farrell *et al.*, 2014). The ability of Noel Fitzpatrick – the veterinary surgeon responsible for Oscar's bionic implants – to save the life of a cat that was destined to be euthanized touched deeply the hearts and minds of animal lovers across the world (Fig. 11.3).

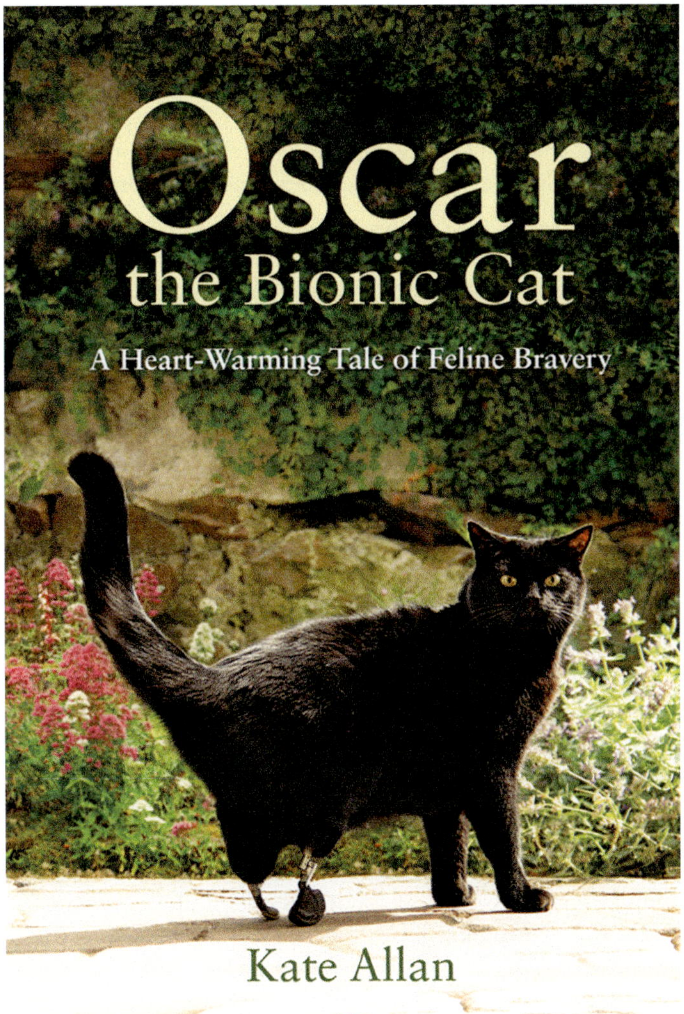

Fig. 11.3. Cover of Oscar the Bionic Cat: A Heart-Warming Tale of Feline Bravery, by Kate Allan (Summersdale, 2015; image © Michael Nolan. Used with permission). Oscar is now part of contemporary popular culture, featuring in the first episode of the BBC Series The Bionic Vet.

The use of experimental V-OP to treat physical disabilities in companion animals requires, however, a more detailed ethical scrutiny. In an article exploring the UK television documentary series *The Supervet* (Channel 4), featuring Noel Fitzpatrick and his team, Brett Mills (2016) described how the series legitimizes the dominance exerted by humans over other species and, by doing so, mostly fails to consider animals as moral subjects. Mills argues that:

> [T]here may be valuable activities humans can carry out in order to make the lives of animals longer and better; but it is to note that *The Supervet* fails to engage with debates about how appropriate it is to do so, nor does it explore the legitimacy of humans making such decisions. Fitzpatrick's genuine ethical concerns for his practice concern whether risks are justified – such as that of the potential shattering of Willow's bone during surgery – and not his own expertise or legitimacy (as a vet, or just as a human) in making such decisions.
>
> (Mills, 2016, pp. 248–249)

The above critique is directed at Noel Fitzpatrick, the TV star veterinarian, but can it be applied *mutatis mutandis* to Noel Fitzpatrick, the orthopaedic surgeon? Looking back at the literature on the ITAP technique (which was applied to four dogs with tumours in their limbs), Fitzpatrick and colleagues consider, in their ethics statement, that:

> It remains possible that the dogs reported here may have had adequate quality of life provided by full-limb amputation, but we submit that maintaining the function of all 4 limbs was warranted in light of the perceived risk of suboptimal outcomes in all 4 dogs. ITAP limb-salvage procedures should only be performed where the potential benefits gained by the procedure outweigh the potential risks and short-term disadvantages.
>
> (Fitzpatrick *et al.*, 2011, p. 923)

This segment provides a typical utilitarian cost–benefit justification for the ethical acceptability of the ITAP procedure: ethics is about weighing harms against benefits. Such arguments are commonly used in the field of animal ethics and ground much of the decision-making from ethics committees regarding animal experimentation. But however popular cost–benefit ethical analyses might be, their limitations should, nonetheless, be considered.

Probably the main difficulty with utilitarian ethical approaches lies in identifying who is to benefit – and to bear the cost – from the procedure. In the case of laboratory animal experimentation, for example, benefits are measured strictly from an anthropocentric standpoint, whereas costs are shared between the experimental animals (in terms of welfare) and society (in terms of resources). In the case of clinical research involving companion animals, however, zoocentric benefits will have to take precedence over anthropocentric ones. Likewise, primary consideration should be given to animals when considering costs. Additionally, benefits and costs are more difficult to assess in animals that live in dynamic family environments, such as companion animals, than in those living in more controlled environments under constant veterinary supervision, such as laboratory animals.

Another limitation from the aforementioned statement is that it diverts the ethical discussion from the motives of performing the ITAP technique to focus on its outcomes. In effect, the utilitarian rationale was presented as if the dogs in question were faced with only two alternatives: to live suboptimal lives with three limbs or to have an endoprosthesis implanted. But at least a third option, subtotal amputation followed by a custom-made socket exoprosthesis, would have been available. We can only conjecture why such alternative options were not considered for a cohort of senior dogs suffering from tumours (sarcomas) in their limbs. However, the seemingly straightforward decision for an invasive endoprosthesis warrants a range of ethical questions about the legitimacy of the procedure in face of arguably more conservative approaches. This reflection brings us to a similar argument to that made by Brett Mills about *The Supervet*: were the best interests of these animals taken into account?

In conclusion, cost–benefit analyses seem to leave some of the contentious issues arising from animal enhancement unexplored and are insufficient to consider the wide range of ethical implications on the use of therapeutic enhancement technologies in companion animals. Thus a more considered and structured approach is warranted. In this chapter, an ethical appraisal of the use of veterinary treatments to improve physical disabilities in companion animals is presented, using the 'ethical matrix', a decision support framework.

Extending the Boundaries of Animal Enhancement

A valuable approach to analyse the ethical implications of modern biotechnologies involves the use of the ethical matrix, developed by Professor Ben Mepham from the University of Nottingham, UK (Mepham, 2000; Mepham *et al.*, 2006). The ethical matrix is a moral reasoning tool that aims to facilitate decision making and ethical deliberation. It relies upon three core principles in normative ethics: the utilitarian principle of well-being; the deontological principle of autonomy; and the contractarian principle of justice; and translates them for several interest groups in a matrix. In the case of small animal biotechnologies, the main affected interest groups include the recipient animal, other animals, the veterinary profession, and clients and society. Several ethically relevant questions can be made regarding each of these stakeholders (Table 11.1). In this section, an answer to most of these questions will be sought in order to assess the ethical impact of V-OP.

Utilitarians consider animal biotechnologies per se as ethically neutral, and their ethical acceptability derives from the consequences of their use. The utilitarian principle of well-being aims to maximize happiness and minimize suffering for all those involved. From the animals' point of view, well-being is often expressed in terms of quality of life (QoL). Quality of life for the recipient animal should weigh short-term as well as long-term costs and benefits, and some of its implications have been explored above, when considering *The Supervet*.

Measuring QoL will have to take into consideration risk factors such as age, concomitant metabolic or orthopaedic diseases, the lesion severity, post-operative recovery care and life expectancy. Decisions regarding best treatment may change between an elderly dog and a young animal. For example, QoL of young animals with congenital orthopaedic defects can be greatly enhanced by bionic limbs to restore locomotion. Likewise, an osteosarcoma – a form of bone cancer with around one-year life expectancy – would probably be better dealt with a more conservative approach. On the other hand, QoL can be severely impaired if the owner is incompetent in maintaining good stump condition or if multiple surgeries are involved.

Concerns to other animals should also be part of the moral equation, particularly how animals might benefit or be harmed should these technologies become available in the foreseeable future. For well over a century, at least since the photographic

Table 11.1. The ethical matrix applied to the use of biotechnologies in companion animal practice. (Adapted from Magalhães-Sant'Ana, 2015)

Respect for	Well-being	Autonomy	Justice
Recipient animal	What is the animal's expected quality of life? Is prolonged/unjustified suffering involved? What are the short-/long-term benefits/risks?	Will the animal still *be* that animal (*Telos*)? Will the interests of the animal be respected?	Have alternatives been considered? Would the animal be better off with a more conservative approach?
Other animals	How will this technique benefit or damage other animals (presently or in the future)?	Does it require the use of donor animals or of additional experimental animals? Are the interests of other animals respected?	Will these techniques be widely available in the future (non-discrimination)? Are these animals fairly treated?
Veterinary profession	How can the technique affect vets' income and working environment? Is the reputation of the veterinary profession affected?	Are vets provided with the tools to make managerial decisions? How are individual choices affected?	How are other practices affected? Will other vets have access to the same expertise and resources?
Clients and society	What are the emotional and financial costs? How will the human–animal bond be affected? How will client/public trust be affected?	Was informed consent sought? Was the client informed of the alternatives? How will future clients' choices be affected?	Who will have access to these procedures (distributive justice)? Is responsible pet ownership promoted?

experiments of Eadweard Muybridge, it has been known that animal locomotion is much more than an aesthetic issue (Muybridge, 1957). As the biomechanical principles at play in quadruped animals are increasingly understood, our ability to prevent and treat injuries also increases. However, dogs and cats are still believed to 'do well' with three limbs, and anecdotal evidence suggests that they can thrive with only two. Dogs normally bear 30% of their body weight on each of the forelimbs and 20% on each of the hindlimbs. Forelimb amputees, however, bear 47.5% of their weight on the remaining forelimb (Cole and Millis, 2017), an increase of almost 60% in weight bearing. The resulting overload predisposes the contralateral thoracic limb to orthopaedic or neural disease. In addition, gait is significantly altered after amputation within all limbs, including ground reaction forces, impulses and stance durations (Jarvis *et al.*, 2013; Mich, 2014).

In the light of current scientific evidence, it could be argued that recommending a prosthetic device in detriment of full-limb amputation is, at least in some cases, the preferred approach in terms of welfare and probably a moral imperative from a deontological point of view (see below). As prosthetic options become increasingly available, primary care veterinary practitioners are required to seek advice from orthopaedic specialists and refer to better judgement, before they decide to amputate.

A similar line of argument can be used to decide between some forms of orthopaedic surgery and the alternative use of orthotic devices. For example, orthoses are already considered viable options to stabilize a cranial cruciate ligament-deficient canine stifle joint (Bertocci *et al.*, 2017).

From a deontological perspective, the principle of autonomy must be respected regardless of its consequences. The principle of autonomy, when applied to animals, refers not to their capacity of making autonomous decisions but to the moral right of having their interests defended. When applied to animal biotechnologies, these interests can include concepts such as integrity, *telos* and naturalness (Hauskeller, 2016). I will not attempt to define these concepts, but instead will rely upon the concept of *telos* provided by American philosopher Bernard Rollin: 'the unique, evolutionarily determined, genetically encoded, environmentally shaped set of needs and interests that characterize the animal in question' (Rollin, 1989, p. 146). Therefore, *telos* is the intrinsic and species-specific nature of an animal (the 'pigness' of the pig, the 'dogness' of the dog). In order to thrive, animals should not be prevented from fulfilling their *teloi*.

The use of examples can help to explore the argument of animal *telos*. Imagine fitting racing greyhounds with prosthetic limbs. These bionic racing dogs would be not only capable of running longer and faster but also would be immune to foot injuries, such as fractures, toe avulsion or paw sores. From a mere welfare perspective, their lives as racing dogs would, arguably, improve since they could enjoy running longer and faster and suffer from fewer injuries. Another, perhaps less futile, example is to devise more resilient bionic search and rescue dogs, fit to operate in any terrain, and able to resist, for example, frost burns. Notwithstanding the hypothetical benefits brought by these technological undertakings, our moral intuition prevents us from seriously considering them. One possible reason is that they would be perceived as an unacceptable violation of the *telos* of these animals. In this regard, endoprosthesis can be seen as a form of *overtreatment* in which the procedure has been performed against the best interests of the animal (Sandøe *et al.*, 2016).

The previous examples allude to the concept of animal enhancement and should make us reflect on whether or not it is admissible to create a 'superdog' or 'supercat'. Animal enhancement can be defined as a novel function, an increase or improvement of a natural function, or one that enables greater fulfilment of the animal's own interests (Chan, 2009). Farm animals have been routinely enhanced in order to meet human needs (Twine, 2010), and that has often been achieved at the expense of their *teloi*. However, the social moral consensus regarding how companion animals can and should be treated has prevented the development of much of the enhancement biotechnologies often used in farm animals. As of this writing, prosthetic devices have been used to restore normal function and not to improve animals' natural abilities or to provide them with novel features that they did not already possess (Fig. 11.4). From a contractarian point of view, aiming for the morally fuzzy concept of 'superdog' seems unjustified and in breach of the tacit moral contract between humans and companion animals.

A similar debate has been under way regarding pedigree dog breeding (Nicholas, 2011). Some musculoskeletal pathologies are not incidental but the result of sustained and negligent breeding practices. These can include hip and elbow dysplasia in large and giant breeds, and odontoid process dysplasia, shoulder dysplasia and patellar luxation in small breeds (Asher *et al.*, 2009). Simply providing a technological solution to an otherwise breeding problem, fails to address the underlying cause and transfers the

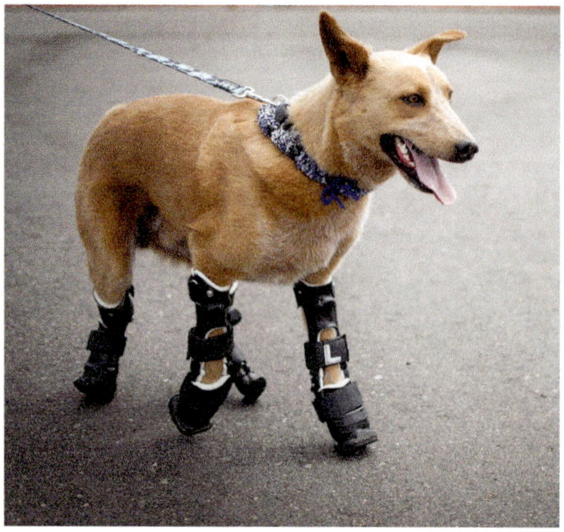

Fig. 11.4. A disabled dog fitted with four prosthetic devices. But what if current prosthetic technology was used to create 'superdog'? (Photo: Amy Kaufmann, Orthopets LLC. Used with permission).

societal responsibility to address it to the veterinary profession. On the contrary, a compelling argument towards the use of experimental V-OP is that bionic pets help to raise awareness of conformational related disorders in pedigree breeds and are a source of inspiration for other pet keepers who might have lost hope of improving the lives of their animals. For these reasons, veterinarians have a role in educating clients to responsible pet ownership and in promoting animal welfare-friendly changes to breed standards.

The contractarian principle of justice requires that all those involved are treated with fairness. Norms and regulations are usually the means by which society ensures fair treatment, non-discrimination and distributive justice. However, the regulatory landscape provides little guidance on the acceptable limits for small animal biotechnologies. The Royal College of Veterinary Surgeons (RCVS) Code of Professional Conduct provides specific guidance on canine surgical artificial insemination and feline renal transplantation but fails to address other forms of veterinary enhancement (Magalhães-Sant'Ana *et al.*, 2015). This is further complicated whenever V-OP are applied in a clinical setting but on an experimental level, as one would expect to occur in the development process of cutting-edge technologies. By not being contextualized as experiments, such interventions are excluded from the level of regulation and scrutiny of similar experiments carried out in the same species in laboratories.

In the absence of specific legislation regulating clinical experiments, veterinary surgeons in the UK rely on the Veterinary Surgeon's Act 1966 and are exempt from formal ethical review, which is in contrast with the statutory requirements put in place to regulate clinical research in human patients (Fordyce and Mullan, 2017). Veterinary clinical researchers face a dilemma between the need to build robust evidence for the advancement of science and their responsibility to provide animals with the best possible care. This generates a source of potential reputational damage for the veterinary profession in addition to welfare concerns. Not surprisingly, a recent survey reports lack of governance of veterinary clinical research in the private sector in the UK, including lack of records on the actual number of animals involved, the nature of the research, and provisions in place in terms of ethical reviewing (Fordyce and Mullan, 2017).

A set of key principles to assist veterinary surgeons in their ethical decision making regarding advanced treatments has recently been suggested (Yeates, 2016). According to the principle of justice, veterinary surgeons who wish to perform advanced surgeries or other biotechnological procedures in companion animals are required to adopt standard experimental protocols and abide by animal research reporting guidelines, such as the ARRIVE guidelines (Kilkenny *et al.*, 2010). Moreover, conflicts often arise because the ethical review process is external to the experimental design, which renders veterinary researchers particularly vulnerable to criticism. In effect,

> In reviewing manuscripts submitted for publication, most journals continue merely to require a statement affirming that the research complies with official recommendations, or relevant legislation, or an ethics committee's decision (local, regional or national), rather than encouraging, or requiring, those involved in the peer-review procedure to seriously consider whether the submitted study was indeed carried out with the smallest achievable negative impact on the animals.
>
> (Magalhães-Sant'Ana *et al.*, 2009, p. 59)

In this regard, rather than requesting from authors a statement that often reflects the view of a third party on what is considered appropriate ethical standards, journals should ask authors to describe the ethical rationale that justifies the study, which merits would be assessed by the scientific community. Alternative methods to gauge the animal research policies of biomedical journals have been suggested, such as the EXEMPLAR (Excellence in Mandatory Policies on Animal Research) scale (Martins and Franco, 2015).

The work of multidisciplinary ethics committees is required to effectively tackle the complex combination of technological, scientific, legal and moral issues that animal biotechnologies usually entail. The establishment of the RCVS Ethics Review Panel in 2016, responsible for the voluntary ethical reviewing of veterinary practice-based research in the UK, is a step in that direction. The above discussion also highlights the need for a debate within the veterinary community on the accepted limits in terms of enhancement of companion animals. In particular, an agreement should be reached regarding the risk factors that may determine under what circumstances animals are poor candidates for receiving invasive technologies, such as bionic limbs. Other issues that require reflection include experimental protocols, ethical decision making, humane endpoints, informed consent and the regulatory framework.

From a human perspective, ethical decision making will have to take into consideration the emotional costs of treatment. Oncological diseases, in particular, can be particularly challenging for pet-keepers and are known to interfere with the human–animal relationship. Finally, from the viewpoint of clients and society, justice requires that costs should be considered. On the one hand, it would be unethical to enforce on financially stranded clients an expensive operation that could jeopardize the livelihood of their children. On the other hand, prosthetic technologies should be made available to animals in need, and social awareness may help to safeguard that these technologies become available to owners of limited means. With regard to the principle of autonomy, clients – including the less well-off – should not be prevented from accessing the full range of treatment options that will allow them to make conscientious and informed decisions.

Recommendations

This chapter aimed at providing a value-based reflection on the use of veterinary orthopaedic treatments to improve physical disabilities in companion animals. In addition to utilitarian cost–benefit analysis, advanced treatment should take into account deontological principles such as autonomy and justice, and the ethical matrix was applied in this regard. It concludes that the use of osseointegrated prostheses and other invasive experimental orthopaedic technologies should not be used as a substitute for responsible breeding practices and/or pet ownership. Moreover, surgical decisions should take into account the integrity of animals, and procedures that compromise the animals' *telos*, such as the ability to design 'superdog', are ethically questionable. As prosthetic options become increasingly available, primary care veterinary practitioners are required to seek advice from orthopaedic specialists or refer to better judgement. Veterinarians have a role in educating clients towards responsible pet ownership and in promoting animal welfare-friendly changes to breed standards. In turn, veterinary clinical researchers are required to seek permission from an ethics committee, such as the RCVS Ethics Review Panel, before engaging in experimental surgical technologies. A debate within the veterinary community on the accepted limits in terms of enhancement of companion animals should be promoted. In particular, an agreement should be reached regarding which risk factors render animals as poor candidates for receiving invasive technologies.

Acknowledgements

I wish to express my gratitude to Dr Nuno Henrique Franco (I3S – Instituto de Investigação e Inovação em Saúde, Universidade do Porto, Porto, Portugal) for his diligence, insight and patience in reviewing a previous version of this manuscript. The author is in receipt of a post-doctoral fellowship from Fundação para a Ciência e a Tecnologia (FCT) (*VETHICS-2022 – A Structured Approach to Describing and Addressing the Ethical Challenges of the Veterinary Profession in Portugal* (FCT ref. SFRH/BPD/117693/2016)). I thank FCT for their financial support.

References

Asher, L., Diesel, G., Summers, J.F., McGreevy, P.D. and Collins, L.M. (2009) Inherited defects in pedigree dogs. Part 1: Disorders related to breed standards. *The Veterinary Journal* 182(3), 402–411.

Bertocci, G.E., Brown, N.P. and Mich, P.M. (2017) Biomechanics of an orthosis-managed cranial cruciate ligament-deficient canine stifle joint predicted by use of a computer model. *American Journal of Veterinary Research* 78(1), 27–35.

Chan, S. (2009) Should we enhance animals? *Journal of Medical Ethics* 35(11), 678–683.

Cole, G.L. and Millis, D.L. (2017) The effect of limb amputation on standing weight distribution in the remaining three limbs in dogs. *Veterinary and Comparative Orthopaedics and Traumatology (VCOT)* 30(1), 59–61.

Farrell, B.J., Prilutsky, B.I., Kistenberg, R.S., Dalton IV, J.F. and Pitkin, M. (2014) An animal model to evaluate skin–implant–bone integration and gait with a prosthesis directly attached to the residual limb. *Clinical Biomechanics* 29(3), 336–349.

Fitzpatrick, N., Smith, T.J., Pendegrass, C.J., Yeadon, R., Ring, M., Goodship, A.E. and Blunn, G.W. (2011) Intraosseous transcutaneous amputation prosthesis (ITAP) for limb salvage in 4 dogs. *Veterinary Surgery* 40(8), 909–925.

Fordyce, P. and Mullan, S. (2017) Nature and governance of veterinary clinical research conducted in the UK. *Veterinary Record* 180(3), 69.

Hauskeller, M. (2016) *Biotechnology and the Integrity of Life: Taking Public Fears Seriously*. Routledge, Abingdon, UK.

Jarvis, S.L., Worley, D.R., Hogy, S.M., Hill, A.E., Haussler, K.K. and Reiser, R.F. (2013) Kinematic and kinetic analysis of dogs during trotting after amputation of a thoracic limb. *American Journal of Veterinary Research* 74(9), 1155–1163.

Kaufman, F. (2014) *My Bionic Pet*. Nature TV series. Thirteen Productions LLC.

Kilkenny, C., Browne, W.J., Cuthill, I.C., Emerson, M. and Altman, D.G. (2010) Improving bioscience research reporting: the ARRIVE guidelines for reporting animal research. *PLOS Biology* 8(6), e1000412.

Magalhães-Sant'Ana, M. (2015) New technologies, old dilemmas – the ethics of using biotechnologies in companion animal practice. *Veterinary Ireland Journal* 5(8), 369–372.

Magalhães-Sant'Ana, M., Sandøe, P. and las Olsson, P. (2009) Painful dilemmas: the ethics of animal-based pain research. *Animal Welfare* 18(1), 49–63.

Magalhães-Sant'Ana, M., More, S.J., Morton, D.B., Osborne, M. and Hanlon, A. (2015) What do European veterinary codes of conduct actually say and mean? A case study approach. *Veterinary Record* 176, 654.

Marcellin-Little, D.J., Drum, M.G., Levine, D. and McDonald, S.S. (2015) Orthoses and exoprostheses for companion animals. *Veterinary Clinics of North America: Small Animal Practice, Rehabilitation and Physical Therapy* 45(1), 167–183.

Martins, A.R. and Franco, N.H. (2015) A critical look at biomedical journals' policies on animal research by use of a novel tool: the EXEMPLAR scale. *Animals* 5(2), 315–331.

Mepham, B. (2000) A framework for the ethical analysis of novel foods: the ethical matrix. *Journal of Agricultural & Environmental Ethics* 12(2), 165–176.

Mepham, B., Kaiser, M., Thorstensen, E. *et al.* (2006) *Ethical Matrix Manual*. LEI, The Hague, The Netherlands.

Mich, P.M. (2014) The emerging role of veterinary orthotics and prosthetics (V-OP) in small animal rehabilitation and pain management. *Topics in Companion Animal Medicine, Advances in Rehabilitation* 29(1), 10–19.

Mills, B. (2016) 'If This Was a Human…': pets, vets and medicine. *Critical Studies in Television: The International Journal of Television Studies* 11(2), 244–256.

Muybridge, E. (1957) *Animals in Motion*. Dover Publications Inc., New York.

Nicholas, F.W. (2011) Response to the documentary *Pedigree Dogs Exposed*: three reports and their recommendations. *The Veterinary Journal*, Special Issue: *Canine Genetics* 189(2), 126–128.

Pitkin, M. (2013) Design features of implants for direct skeletal attachment of limb prostheses. *Journal of Biomedical Materials Research Part A* 101(11), 3339–3348.

Rollin, B.E. (1989) *The Unheeded Cry: Animal Consciousness, Animal Pain and Science*. Vol. xviii. Studies in Bioethics. Oxford University Press, New York.

Sandøe, P., Corr, S. and Palmer, C. (2016) *Companion Animal Ethics*. UFAW Animal Welfare Series. Wiley-Blackwell, Chichester, UK.

Twine, R. (2010) *Animals as Biotechnology: Ethics, Sustainability and Critical Animal Studies*. Earthscan, London.

Yeates, J.W. (2016) Ethical principles for novel therapies in veterinary practice. *Journal of Small Animal Practice* 57(2), 67–73.

12 Animal Welfare and the Brave New World of Modifying Animals

Donald M. Broom*

Centre for Animal Welfare and Anthrozoology, Department of Veterinary Medicine, University of Cambridge, Cambridge, UK

Introduction

Conventional breeding can have extreme negative effects on the welfare of animals; for example the breeding of dogs for cosmetic features and of broiler chickens and dairy cows for high levels of production. Any breeding that can be predicted to result in poor welfare should be illegal. Biotechnology can lead to much faster and greater change in the animals than can conventional breeding, so needs special legislation. Ethical consequences of the work should be considered whenever research in biotechnology is carried out. Genetic modification of animals and, to a lesser extent, cloning can have some positive effects on animal welfare. However, cloning procedures for farm animals have negative effects that are so great that current methodologies are never likely to be acceptable. Given the developments in the scientific assessment of animal welfare, the consequences of genetic modification can be evaluated. A checklist for animal welfare should take account of current scientific knowledge about assessing animal welfare and should be further developed for evaluating all genetically modified animals. When sold, every GM product for use with animals should have details of properly tested effects on animal welfare.

Domestication and Conventional Breeding of Animals

Animals kept and used by people have always been modified from their wild state, because only some of those that are kept survive, and hence this selection results in some genetic change in the population kept. In addition, people deliberately selected animals with certain characteristics. A definition of domestication (Broom and Fraser, 2015, modified after Price, 2002) is: the process, occurring over generations, by which a population of animals becomes adapted to man and to the captive environment by some combination of genetic changes and environmentally induced developmental events. The animals that have been domesticated, or, one might say, the animals that have allowed themselves to be domesticated or which have domesticated humans, are mainly social species with high levels of cognitive ability.

Selection of farm animals was initially limited to docility and manageability, but in the last 60 years, breeding programmes have focused on the genetic improvement of production traits, such as milk yield, growth rate and number of eggs, and were

*E-mail: dmb16@cam.ac.uk

based on animals' phenotypes. A major advance in selection practice occurred in the mid-20th century with the advent of quantitative genetics based on principles of heredity and modern statistical theory (Hazel, 1943). The method is still based on phenotypic selection but more easily identifies variation at loci. Essentially, the statistical genetics method calculates an average of all genetic loci contributing to a trait as transmitted by the individual, and reports it as an estimated breeding value (EBV) (Lynch and Walsh, 1998). As a result, the animal production industry has undergone dramatic change during the last century (Ensminger and Parry, 1996).

Conventional breeding methods need not affect welfare but can change animals in such a way that they have more difficulty in coping or are more likely to fail to cope (Broom, 1995; 2008). One example of such an effect is the sensory, neurological or orthopaedic defects found commonly in certain breeds of dog. Others are the effects of the genes promoting obesity in mice, double muscling linked to parturition problems in cattle, and many examples of selection promoting fast growth and large muscles in farm animals. Modern strains of pigs have relatively larger muscle blocks, more anaerobic fibres and smaller hearts than their ancestral strains (Dämmrich, 1987). They are more likely to die or to become distressed during any vigorous activity, for example during transport. Modern broiler strains grow to a weight of 2–2.5 kg in 35 days, as compared with 12 weeks 30 years ago. Their muscles and guts grow very fast but the skeleton and cardiovascular system do not. Hence many of the birds have leg problems, such as tibial dyschondroplasia or femoral head necrosis, or cardiovascular malfunction, often giving rise to ascites (Bradshaw *et al.*, 2002). Genetic selection of dairy cows for high milk production has led to increased leg disorders, mastitis and reproductive disorders, all of which are major welfare problems (Oltenacu and Broom, 2010). Any breeding that can be predicted to result in poor welfare should be illegal.

Biotechnology Definitions and Methods

Those aspects of modern biotechnology that are having, or are likely to have, the greatest impact on animal welfare are the use of genetically modified animals (GM animals) and cloning by nuclear transfer. The term 'GM animals' is used here to refer to animals whose genetic material has been altered using a method that does not occur naturally, but excluding chemical or physical mutagenesis. Cloning is not genetic modification but it means producing more than one genetically identical individual. Cloned amphibians were produced by Gurdon and collaborators in the 1970s (see review by Gurdon and Byrne, 2003), and many mammals have now been cloned. The first GM animal, a mouse, was made in the early 1980s (Gordon *et al.*, 1980; Palmiter, 1986) and this technology has been successfully applied to most mammals including cattle, pigs and sheep (Hammer *et al.*,1985; Simons *et al.*, 1988), and to poultry (Love *et al.*, 1994) and fish (Devlin *et al.*, 2001).

Microinjection was the earliest method of making GM animals. Electroporation has also been used. Both of these lead to mosaics, i.e. genetic variability in the cells of the animal. Sperm mediated gene transfer (SMGT) is the injection of a transgene vector, often viral, for GM. Androgenesis, gynogenesis and embryonic cell nuclear transplantation (ECNT) are used for cloning. Somatic cell nuclear transfer (SCNT) is used for cloning or for GM.

Effects of Biotechnology Procedures on Animal Welfare

Animal welfare varies from very good to very poor and can be evaluated scientifically using a wide range of measures (Broom and Fraser, 2015). The effects of biotechnology procedures on animal welfare might be: (i) to improve it; (ii) to have no effect on it; or (iii) to make it poorer. Members of the public express positive and negative views about GM and cloning. Some of the issues raised by scientific studies and public comments are listed in Boxes 12.1 and 12.2.

Examples of benefits from the effects of genetic modifications of animals are: to benefit the animals by conferring disease resistance (Behboodi *et al.*, 2005); to help to treat human disease by producing a blood clotting factor in sheep's milk (Houdebine, 2005); to develop new products for other purposes (Niemann and Kues, 2003); and to increase efficiency of animal production (Wheeler, 2003). Some people would find none of these to be acceptable whilst others might accept them all. Many people would accept some with qualifications, and a major reason for rejection is that animal welfare may be poorer in the modified animals than in those that are not modified. A major problem in relation to GM research is the complete failure of the community of researchers in this area to investigate the welfare of the animals produced. In a

Box 12.1. Possible negative effects of cloning and GM.

1. Welfare problems – effects of the procedure, e.g. SCNT can lead to placental or foetal abnormality.
2. Welfare problems – effects of the transgene, e.g. insertion of the human growth hormone gene into pigs has caused major growth abnormalities.
3. Genetic uniformity in the population produced could increase the risk of disease epidemics.
4. There could be effects on the safety of transgenic animal products for human consumption.
5. There could be effects of transgenic animals on wild animal populations, for example those of fish that escape from captivity.
6. Ethical issues and societal issues such as equity of access to products by consumers, or freedom to make ethical consumption choices.

(modified after Broom, 2014)

Box 12.2. Possible positive effects of cloning and GM.

1. Improved welfare for the transgenic animals, for example due to deliberately enhanced disease resistance.
2. Reduction in the number of animals required for breeding programmes – cloning allows copying of individuals so fewer are needed.
3. GM change could enhance the nutritional value of animal products.
4. Decreased pollution if GM increases animal digestion ability.
5. Reduced cost of food, increased production of food.
6. Engineering of animals suited to arid or other harsh environments.

(modified after Broom, 2014)

recent review of developments in transgenic animal production, Murray and Mega (2016) wondered why no transgenic animal had been taken up for animal production, but at no point in their paper did they mention the welfare of the animals produced.

Effects of Cloning Procedures on Animal Welfare

There are effects of cloning procedures on animal welfare. Cloned common carp and rainbow trout are more variable and some do not survive well. A proportion of the cloned fish offspring are haploid and non-viable whilst diploid hatchlings appear to have normal survival. Birds cannot be fully cloned at present but there has been primordial germ cell transplantation, involving some cloned cells, in domestic chicks. The hatching rate of these birds was reduced by about 60% and survival of hatched to adulthood was reduced by 20%. Bovine clones have a high level of mortality, particularly *in utero*, where only 27% of pregnancies survive to term (e.g. Chavatte-Palmer *et al.*, 2012). There is also increased mortality in early life, and cloned cattle often show developmental problems such as the large offspring syndrome. Cloned pigs show some increased early mortality, and in the few animals studied, the life expectancy was reduced. When sheep clones were produced, only 42% of pregnancies were maintained and only 50% of live-born lambs survived to weaning. For goat clones, 31% of pregnancies were maintained but 80% of live-born kids survived to weaning. In three studies of horses, 2%, 3% and 26%, respectively, resulted in a birth (Campbell, 2016).

Many of these problems are a result of epigenetic abnormalities. If the clones survive the juvenile period there are usually no further welfare problems. For example, Sinclair *et al.* (2016) found that the osteoarthritis described in the SCNT-produced, cloned sheep Dolly was not present in 12 other similar cloned sheep. Neither were there metabolic or other joint disorders. The severe welfare problems are during the production of the cloned animals rather than in those that survive.

In general, mortality is too high and problems are too frequent with SCNT. Chavatte-Palmer *et al.* (2012) report that after cloning using SCNT, placentomegaly and foetal overgrowth are commonly observed; placental vascularization is modified; steroidogenesis is perturbed so there is lack of preparation for parturition; production of glycoproteins in the mother and production and transport of sugars in the young animals is modified. Gene expression analyses of the SCNT placenta show that multiple pathways and functions are affected. There have been some attempts to improve methodology but Rodrigues Sangalli *et al.* (2014) found that treatment of cloned cattle cells with valproic acid did not improve survival. For farm animals, cloning procedures are very negative for welfare and are not likely to be acceptable to the public or legislators, or to be commercially viable except in experimental situations.

Effects of Genetic Modification Procedures on Animal Welfare

The following are some effects of genetic modification procedures on animal welfare. Most GM work is part of biomedical research with a small amount of work involving farm animals. However, most of the examples given here are for farm animals:

1. The production of the DNA often involves no animal welfare considerations because the source is tissue culture, human cells or animals that are killed humanely.

However, if embryos or tissues must be removed from living animals in order to obtain the DNA, effects on welfare must be considered.

2. The production of an embryo for the insertion of DNA involves procedures used in producing lines of GM animals that may have negative welfare consequences for the donor animals: (a) The donor female may be injected with hormones to produce large numbers of oocytes; (b) In large animals, artificial insemination may be used, sometimes using laparoscopy or laparotomy to fertilize the oocytes; (c) Embryo collection may involve killing the female or procedures such as oviduct flushing during laparotomic surgery.

3. During microinjection of DNA into the embryo, there is evidence that microinjection of the transgene itself can lead to increased foetal loss. Many embryos injected with DNA die. However, this occurs at an early stage of development so is not a significant welfare problem for the foetus.

4. When there is production of GM offspring, the insertion of the DNA construct within the genome can cause disruption of genes at that site, or there may be effects of the inserted gene. These effects may be apparent at birth, or may only become apparent at a later point in the animal's development, or when it is put under some kind of stress or put into a particular type of environment. The survival of transgenic, cloned offspring after SCNT in cattle is similar to or better than that of non-GM cloned animals. However, in pigs, survival is somewhat worse. There are alternatives to SCNT and these can result in fewer problems.

5. When GM animals are fostered onto normal females, the welfare of the fostered pups may be poor. Also, normal pups of the foster mother may have been killed to allow fostering of GM pups and the method of killing could affect welfare.

6. The consequence of the genetic change for the GM animals is a major animal welfare issue for laboratory animals because many of the GM animals are produced in order that they will be susceptible to developing pathological conditions. For example, GM mice are produced that are likely to develop a tumour in order that anti-cancer treatments can be tested on them. Most people would say either that this should never be done or that the tumour development should never be allowed to reach the point where the animal would suffer. Some genetic modifications lead to an unexpected malfunction.

It is clearly necessary to use good quality animal welfare science measures to check each GM line that might be continued in order that they will not be continued if problems exist. No problems were revealed in a study of the behaviour of sheep genetically modified to produce human alpha-l-antitrypsin, which is used for treatment of human emphysema, in their milk (Hughes *et al.*, 1996). However, the sheep did not live long. Salmon and other fish transgenic for a growth hormone gene have been produced. Many of these have an enlarged head and a bulging operculum. The problems become worse with increasing age.

Other positive and negative examples of genetic change effects are that GM catfish with a gene for cecropin are more resistant to enteric septicaemia. GM grass carp transgenic for human lactoferrin are resistant to haemorrhagic virus and *Aeromonas hydrophila* infection. Transgenic chickens that can synthesize RNA that interferes with influenza virus replication and packaging are less likely to suffer from or transmit the disease (Lyall *et al.*, 2011). Some other GM chickens had positive and negative anti-disease consequences. As mentioned above, pigs transgenic for human growth hormone have many negative effects. However, Huber *et al.* (2012) assessed the welfare of a large number of pigs transgenic for the green fluorescent protein gene and found no deleterious effects.

An alternative to transgenesis is the direct administration of transgenes to the tissues of adult animals, resulting in a transient transgene expression in these tissues. Han *et al.* (2007) infused a vector carrying the bovine lactoferrin gene into the mammary glands of goats via the teat canal. Lactoferrin was expressed in the milk for up to about a week, with the potential to protect against mastitis. As in most GM studies, the consequences have not been evaluated using a range of welfare indicators.

Genetic Modification, Cloning, Public Attitudes and Laws

Biotechnology can lead to much faster and greater change in the animals than can conventional breeding, so needs special legislation. The production of GM or cloned animals is allowed only in specified circumstances by the law in the UK and several other countries. The creation or duplication of favourite pets, or of animals intended as toys or fashion accessories would not be permitted. Box 12.3 summarizes the views of government committees, such as the UK Animal Procedures Committee, and of the public in the EU about what is not acceptable in GM animal production.

Use of GM Products and Animal Welfare

Whilst the majority of this section refers to genetic modification and cloning of animals, it is also necessary to consider carefully any proposed use of genetically modified materials that would change an animal in some way. An example is the injection of a form of the hormone bovine somatotrophin (BST) produced by genetically modified bacteria. Although BST is a naturally occurring hormone, the GM form is slightly different,

Box 12.3. What are publicly unacceptable consequences of genetic modification?

1. Animals should not be produced if they would be subject to harm of a degree and kind that ought not, under any circumstances, to be inflicted upon an animal; for example, GM animals that would suffer severe or lasting distress, including animals to be created as disease models, unless there is clear evidence that the problems could be handled humanely.
2. The production of GM animals should not occur if such work is likely to strip animals of their biological integrity or render them incurably insentient.
3. There should not be production of chimaeras, especially human–animal chimaeras, or of hybrids that involve a significant degree of hybridization between animals of very dissimilar kinds.

(after Broom, 2014)

chemically, and the amounts that can be given to cows to increase milk production are much greater than those that would normally be present in the animals. The question considered by two EU scientific committees was whether or not there was scientific information about the consequences of the use of BST that would allow a decision about permission for its use in the EU. One report concerned animal welfare, the other human consumer health. A later report concerned dairy cow welfare in general.

An assessment of the risk to consumers if dairy cows are regularly injected with recombinant BST was conducted (European Union Scientific Committee on Public Health, 1999). This identified a very small increased risk because there is increased concentration of insulin-like growth factor (IGF-1) in milk and IGF-1 can make existing tumours grow faster. However, a much bigger effect on animal welfare was found (European Union Scientific Committee on Animal Health and Animal Welfare, 1999). There was an increase of about 35% in the risk of clinical mastitis above the risk in non-treated cows, as demonstrated using meta-analyses or large datasets. BST increased the incidence of foot disorders by 2.2 times, with 2.1 times more days affected. The pregnancy rate dropped from 82% to 73% in multiparous cows and from 90% to 63% in primiparous cows, and multiple births were substantially increased. There were severe reactions at the injection site in at least 4% of cows. These comparisons were made between untreated cows and BST-treated cows with a much greater milk yield. The extra milk yield is a key factor as the highest-producing cows have greater incidences of lameness, mastitis and reproductive disorders, whatever the means of pushing the cows metabolically to high production (EFSA, 2009; Oltenacu and Broom, 2010). A recent paper by American animal scientists using data on use of a dose of 500 mg for 14 days found no adverse effects of BST usage on some reproductive problems, lameness or mastitis (St Pierre *et al*., 2014). However, the quality of some of the measures of welfare was not clear, and any comparison of BST-treated and other high-producing cows is subject to the problem described above. As a result of the publications and the reports summarizing this information, the use of bovine somatotrophin was banned in the EU and in most other countries. Although low-producing cows, caused to produce at a somewhat higher rate by BST, may not have worse welfare as a consequence, many producers use BST to make fairly high-producing cows very high-producing. This will always cause poor welfare, and, if BST use is legal, some producers will use it to push cows to very high levels of milk production. In order to prevent poor welfare of cows, EFSA recommended that producers who have more than 10% of their cows lame should be penalized and that the ban on BST should be continued. Both of these measures would improve welfare, and the number of cows dying or culled early would be reduced, so there is also an economic advantage.

Conclusions

Some conclusions can be drawn as a result of information like that described above.

1. Moral issues associated with biotechnology will be considered by the public and should be taken into account at an early stage in any biotechnology research.
2. One of the possible consequences of the use of GM products or GM animals is on animal welfare. Many different systems for coping with the environment should be considered when assessing welfare. These systems interact, and health is an important part of welfare in such assessments.

3. A checklist for animal welfare should take account of current scientific knowledge about assessing animal welfare and should be further developed for general cage-side use in the case of GM animals.
4. When sold, every GM product for use with animals should have details of properly tested effects on animal welfare.

Acknowledgements

I thank Dr Richard Kirkden and Dr Toni Oltenacu for collection of data and helpful discussion.

References

Behboodi, E., Ayres, S.L., Memili, E., O'Coin, M., Chen, L.H. *et al.* (2005) Health and reproductive profiles of malaria antigen-producing transgenic goats derived by somatic cell nuclear transfer. *Cloning Stem Cells* 7, 107–118.

Bradshaw, R.H., Kirkden, R.D. and Broom, D.M. (2002) A review of the aetiology and pathology of leg weakness in broilers in relation to their welfare. *Avian Poultry Biology Reviews.* 13, 45–103.

Broom, D.M. (1995) Measuring the effects of management methods, systems, high production efficiency and biotechnology on farm animal welfare. In: Mepham, T.B., Tucker, G.A. and Wiseman, J. (eds) *Issues in Agricultural Bioethics*, pp. 319–334.

Broom, D.M. (2008) Consequences of biological engineering for resource allocation and welfare. In: Rauw, W.M. (ed.) *Resource Allocation Theory Applied to Farm Animal Production*. CAB International, Wallingford, UK, pp. 261–275.

Broom, D.M. (2014) *Sentience and Animal Welfare*. CAB International, Wallingford, UK.

Broom, D.M. and Fraser, A.F. (2015) *Domestic Animal Behaviour and Welfare* (5th edn). CAB International, Wallingford, UK.

Campbell, M.L.H. (2016) Is cloning horses ethical? *Equine Veterinary Education.* DOI: 10.1111/eve.12566.

Chavette-Palmer, P., Camous, S., Jammes, H., Le Cleac'h, N., Guillomot, M. and Lee, R.S. (2012) Review – placental perturbations induce the developmental abnormalities often observed in bovine somatic cell nuclear transfer. *Placenta* 33, S99–S104.

Dämmrich, K. (1987) Organ change and damage during stress: morphological diagnosis. In: Wiepkema, P.R. and van Adrichem, P.W.M. (eds) *Biology of Stress in Farm Animals: An Integrated Approach*. Martinus Nijhoff, Dordrecht, The Netherlands, pp. 71–81.

Devlin, R.H., Biagi, C.A., Yesaki, T.Y., Smailus, D.E. and Byatt, J.C. (2001) Growth of domesticated transgenic fish. *Nature* 409, 781–782.

EFSA (European Food Safety Authority) (2009) Scientific opinions and report on the effects of farming systems on dairy cow welfare and disease. *Annex to the EFSA Journal* 1143, 1–38.

Ensminger, M.E. and Parry, R.C. (1996) *Beef Cattle Science*. The Interstate Printers and Publishers, Danville, Illinois.

European Union Scientific Committee on Animal Health and Animal Welfare (1999) *Report on Animal Welfare Aspects of the Use of Bovine Somatotrophin*. Available at: ec.europa.eu/food/fs/sc/scah/out21_en.pdf.

European Union Scientific Committee on Public Health (1999) Report on public health aspects of the use of bovine somatotrophin. Available at: https://ec.europa.eu/food/sites/food/files/safety/docs/sci-com_scv_out19_en.pdf (accessed 1 February 2018).

Gordon, J.W., Scangos, G.A., Plotkin, D.J., Barbosa, J.A. and Ruddle, F.H. (1980) Genetic transformation of mouse embryos by microinjection of purified DNA. *Proceedings of the National Academy of Sciences U.S.A.* 77, 7380–7384.

Gurdon, J.B. and Byrne, J.A. (2003) The first half-century of nuclear transplantation. *Proceedings of the National Academy of Sciences U.S.A.* 100, 1048–1052.

Hammer, R.E., Pursel, V.G., Rexroad Jr, C.E., Wall, R.J., Bolt, D.J., Ebert, K.M., Palmiter, R.D. and Brinster, R.L. (1985) Production of transgenic rabbits, sheep and pigs by microinjection. *Nature* 315, 680–683.

Han, Z.S., Li, Q.W., Zhang, Z.Y., Xiao, B. and Gao, D.W. (2007) High-level expression of human lactoferrin and underlying mechanisms: a review of experimental and clinical studies. *Protein Expression and Purification* 53, 225–231.

Hazel, L.N. (1943) The genetic basis for constructing selection indexes. *Genetics* 28, 476–490.

Houdebine, L.M. (2005) Use of transgenic animals to improve human health and animal production. *Reproduction in Domestic Anim*als 40, 269–281.

Huber, R.C., Remuge, L., Carlisle, A., Lillico, S., Sandøe, P., Sørensen, D.B., Whitelaw, C.B.A. and Olsson, I.A.S. (2012) Welfare assessment in transgenic pigs expressing green fluorescent protein (GFP). *Transgenic Research* 21, 773–784.

Hughes, B.O., Hughes, G.S., Waddington, D. and Appleby, M.C. (1996) Behavioural comparison of transgenic and control sheep: movement order, behaviour on pasture and in covered pens. *Animal Science* 63, 91–101.

Love, J., Gribbin, C., Mather, C. and Sang, H. (1994) Transgenic birds by DNA microinjection. *Biotechnology* 12, 60–63.

Lyall, J., Irvine, R.M., Sherman, A., Mckinley, T.I., Núñez, A. *et al.* (2011) Suppression of avian influenza transmission in genetically modified chickens. *Science* 331, 223–226.

Lynch, M. and Walsh, B. (1998) *Genetic Analysis of Quantitative Traits*. Sinauer Associates, Sunderland, Massachusetts.

Murray, J.D. and Maga, E.A. (2016) Genetically engineered livestock for agriculture: a generation after the first transgenic animal research conference. *Transgenic Research* 25, 321–327.

Niemann, H. and Kues, W.A. (2003) Application of transgenesis in livestock for agriculture and biomedicine. *Animal Reproduction Sci*ence 79, 291–317.

Oltenacu, P.A. and Broom, D.M. (2010) The impact of genetic selection for increased milk yield on the welfare of dairy cows. *Animal Welfare* 19(S), 39–49.

Palmiter, R.D. (1986) Germline transformation of mice. *Annual Review of Genetics* 20, 465–499.

Price, E.O. (2002) *Animal Domestication and Behaviour*. CAB International, Wallingford, UK.

Rodrigues Sangalli, J., Chiaratti, M.R., Camara De Bem, T.H., Roldi de Araújo, R., Fernandes Bressan, F. *et al.* (2014) Development to term of cloned cattle derived from donor cells treated with valproic acid. *PLOS ONE* 9(6), e101022. DOI:10.1371/journal.pone.0101022.

Simons, J.P., Wilmut, I., Clark, A.J., Archibald, A.L., Bishop, J.O. and Lathe, R. (1988) Gene transfer into sheep. *Biotechnology* 6, 179–183.

Sinclair, K.D., Corr, S.A., Gutierrez, P.A., Lee, J.-H., Rathbone, A.J. *et al.* (2016) Healthy ageing of cloned sheep. *Nature Communications* 7, 12359.

St. Pierre, N.R., Milliken, G.A., Bauman, D.E., Collier, R.J., Hogan, J.S. *et al.* (2014) Meta-analysis of the effects of sometribove-zinc suspension on production and health of dairy cows. *Journal of the American Veterinary Medical Association* 245, 550–564.

Wheeler, M.B. (2003) Production of transgenic livestock: promise fulfilled. *Journal of Animal Sci*ence 81, Suppl 3, 32–37.

13 A Duty to the Enhanced, not a Duty to Enhance: Welfare Responsibilities Associated with Domestication

Stephen May*

Royal Veterinary College, University of London

Introduction

The human race has been 'enhancing' animals for thousands of years (Roots, 2007). By selective breeding, wild species have been domesticated for human purposes, including food production, work, and as companions in the home. The changes from the wild have been of two main types: physical, involving changes in size and shape; and psychological, involving selection of animals with temperaments to suit different living arrangements and relationships with human beings. However, these enhancements have not, on the whole, been undertaken for the benefit of the animals themselves (Burgat, 2015). The enlarged udder of the dairy cow provides large amounts of milk for human consumption, not for the animal's calves. The size and temperament of the heavy horse were selected to provide an animal that was strong and safe for its handlers. Various breeds of dog were developed to point at and retrieve game during hunts, as well as to live, apparently contentedly, with their human owners and their families.

The questioning of the human race's practice of modifying other species is a relatively recent phenomenon (Ferrari, 2015), stimulated by the advent of much more powerful techniques for enhancement and a modern concern for animals for their own sakes. In the past there were limits on what could be done to animals, linked to the reality that, in a pre-antibiotic world, animal health was linked to animal welfare (Rollin, 2006), and, in the age that preceded genetic engineering, modification was a relatively slow process linked to within-species selective breeding practices. Even where hybrids such as mules (donkey male × horse female) could be produced to suit human requirements, such cross-species selective breeding resulted in offspring that were essentially infertile (Short, 1997). However, the greater use of therapeutic agents to maintain animals has allowed the extremes of animal form to be extended – the dairy cow with the larger udder that is prone to mastitis, controlled by antibiotics, for example. In addition, genetic engineering techniques have opened potential avenues for the transfer of genes across species to create hybrids that are impossible to produce by within-species, male–female fertilization methods. This makes it timely to consider

*E-mail: smay@rvc.ac.uk

two issues relating to enhancement of animals: (i) the extent to which it is acceptable, and even our duty, to enhance; and (ii) our duties to animals that have been enhanced.

Defining Enhancement

Various authors have attempted to define and distinguish different categories of enhancement for the purpose of ethical discussion. These include the functional focus of enhancement, the motivation behind enhancement, the degree of enhancement and the mechanism of enhancement. Regarding the functional focus, the process of domestication has, to a variable extent, embraced all aspects of biological systems including the physical (both appearance and production capacity) and psychological (the animals' acceptance and apparent enjoyment of human contact), according to the intended purpose of a species by its human owners (Roots, 2007). Historically, the motivation for this animal modification was entirely based on human interests; however, a zoocentric ethical perspective (Verhoog, 2000), focused on animal welfare and quality of life (Sandoe *et al*., 1999), would support enhancement focused on an animal's interests, which could include an increase in some natural function or even the introduction of a novel function (Chan, 2009). This leads to a consideration of the degree of change an intervention causes in an animal. This can be regarded as a spectrum from the elimination of a disability (abnormal rendered normal), through improvement within the range of natural variation (lower functional societal member converted to more highly functional), to 'true' enhancement beyond normal functioning (Bostrom and Savulescu, 2008). This is helpful in distinguishing medical therapies from enhancement (Sandel, 2004). Some have argued that the distinction is not clear and even unhelpful (Kamm, 2005). However, correcting a physical disability returns an animal to a known normal state in which, for instance, if an abnormal gene is replaced by its normal counterpart, the animal's body can be expected to achieve an understood equilibrium. In contrast, enhancement that goes beyond the normal takes an animal from a known, stable biological state to one that is unknown, and potentially unstable, leading to a significant risk, and associated consequences, of failure (Kamm, 2005; Borenstein, 2009). Finally, the mechanism of enhancement may be by breeding, including *in vitro* methods, relying on concentration of desired genetic characteristics and selection of propitious random mutations, or more targeted interventions such as administration of pharmacological agents that change physical and psychological characteristics (Bateman *et al*., 2015) or incorporation of a specific gene, either present within the gene pool of that species (e.g. functional counterpart of defective gene) or a foreign gene from another species (Wells, 2000; Ormandy *et al*., 2011). Consideration of how all these different facets of treatment, improvement and enhancement apply to animals is beyond the scope of this chapter. Its main focus is around human motivations and duties to animals, although other aspects will become relevant as different interests, animal and human, are considered.

The Ethics of Human–Animal Interactions

Early bioethical theories were essentially 'anthropocentric', and legal systems were established based on animals as possessions. In the 19th century, ethical theories became more pathocentric, with the recognition that particularly higher sentient creatures could feel pain, and most of the progress made in animal welfare in the 19th and 20th centuries focused on the physical state of animals and the pain and suffering they experienced as a result of human interactions (Sandoe and Jensen, 2013). The latter half of the 20th century saw a questioning of the adequacy of the pathocentric focus, and zoocentric theories came to prominence that considered the *telos* of animals (its species-specific nature) and the contribution of their psychological needs to their quality of life (Rollin, 2003; 2013). These three perspectives – anthropocentric, pathocentric and zoocentric – can be seen as particularly relevant to domesticated species and have progressively framed legislation (property law and increasingly sophisticated animal welfare law) that protects human and, increasingly, animal interests (Hepple and Gibbens, 2013). More problematic is our relationship with the wild animals with which we share this planet. Bioethical theories that embrace all living things have a biocentric focus that is concerned with the 'naturalness' of animals and their ability to express their wild *telos*, or an ecocentric focus that is concerned with larger ecosystems. These five distinct sets of bioethical theories, moving from emphasis on human to non-human interests, and from individual animal, or group of domestic animals, to all animals, are important in helping with both the ethical context for a consideration of animal enhancement and insight into how different considerations can be balanced, based on normative principles.

It is worth considering at this point to what extent non-human animals should matter to humans. One group of ethical theories would argue that animals have rights, and some have argued that these rights cannot be distinguished from those of humans (Singer, 1975; Regan, 1983). This debate will not be pursued here; rather the position adopted will be based on the modern contractarian approach of Gauthier (1986; 2014). Human interactions with others lead to an interdependency, to a degree that is linked to the intensity of those interactions. This leads to 'social contracts' that variously place duties on 'masters' (those in power) and 'subjects'. However, this ethical argument has been developed for human–human interactions in which both parties are equal. Humans cannot be obligated to animals (Kant, 1996). However, the human race's treatment of its domestic animals is a reflection of its humanity. In acknowledging animals as 'analogues of humanity', society has recognized that their presence should not disrupt the very order that contractarian approaches have created (Korsgaard, 2011). Brutalization of the animals that it has domesticated leads to humankind's own brutalization (Kant, 1996) and the possibility that the way animals are treated today is a reflection of how people may treat one another tomorrow (Becker and French, 2004). Therefore, humans choose to make themselves obligated to animals through the rational legislation to protect society's values, which incorporates animal keepers' duties to them (Larrère and Larrère, 2000).

The Acceptability of Animal Enhancement

The arguments around the acceptability of animal enhancement have never been more polarized, with some arguing that domestication is an indefensible process (Francione and Charlton, 2015) and others that humans have a duty to enhance the other species with which they share the planet (Chan, 2009). For over 40 years, those in the former camp have been prone to releasing animals from captivity, often to the detriment of the individual animals concerned (Mann, 2007). Some have also advocated a cessation of breeding that would lead to domesticated species becoming extinct once the current generations have died of old age (Milligan, 2015). Their argument would appear to be that domesticated species have all been enhanced out of human interest, so there can be no justification in their retention. Such arguments fail to recognize the world as it is for these altered species. Through selection, for instance of dogs, breeds have emerged that are clearly dependent on and enjoy the relationship they have with humans, and there are numerous reports of animals protecting people and apparently suffering when deprived of their human companions (e.g. Roper, 2012; Ascher-Walsh, 2013). Their *telos* is not now that of their wild ancestors but rather that of the domesticated species that has been created, and zoocentric theories would support attention to this new species' needs (Rollin, 2003) rather than a mistaken nostalgia for its wild-type, and acceptance of a single perceived 'right not to be treated as someone's property', which could lead to animal suffering and species extinction (Milligan, 2015). This has meant that many who accept domestication see an appropriate focus of their concerns related to enhancement as being the welfare of the animals that are domesticated, rather than a question about domestication itself. The issue is whether the physical adaptations, or any lack of psychological adaptation, mean that animals suffer when housed for food production, work or human companionship. In zoos that house wild animals (in some cases tamed), where the animals have not been domesticated, this has led to much public concern about the psychological suffering caused, and this has led to individual zoological collections examining whether they should hold certain species, such as polar bears (Bostock, 1993) and elephants (Rees, 2009), as well as the development of 'safari parks', in countries such as the UK, for grazing and other animals adapted to extensive environments (Flack, 2016).

The extreme that argues a duty to enhance animals does so on the basis that it is not just an obligation to recognize animal interests in terms of the base position that is a consequence of evolutionary natural selection, or selective breeding associated with domestication, but additionally 'to use enhancement technologies on animals when it is in those animals' interests' (Chan, 2009). The problem of determining the interests of another species is acknowledged, but assumptions such as 'any creature that has an interest in continued life will presumably benefit from an increase in length of life' are then used as justifications for potential enhancement. The problems here are that it is hard to know that such a concern for life extension is anything other than a human preoccupation; and even in humans life extension for its own sake is increasingly seen as undesirable in situations where poor health and old age compromise the quality of life (Gawande, 2014). An argument has also been made for cognitive enhancement, based on the correlation in humans of intelligence with socioeconomic success, health and longevity (Chan and Harris, 2006; Chan, 2009), but this is dangerously anthropomorphic as it assumes that the type of life a cognitively enhanced chimpanzee might achieve would be a life that it recognized as superior to the life that an unenhanced chimpanzee enjoyed.

A clear ethical issue with such arguments for humanization of chimpanzees and other species, based on human perceptions of what constitutes a fulfilled life, is that in its extreme form it leads to the conclusion that all life should be enhanced to the point of it being human! This anthropomorphic, zoocentric perspective fails to incorporate any biocentric or ecocentric perspectives. This extreme outcome would result in massively reduced diversity in animal species and major changes to long-established ecosystems. It is recognized that the biosphere is fragile and it is argued that the disappearance of the pollinating insects would result in significant reductions in food production (Losey and Vaughan, 2006; Gallai *et al.*, 2009), which cannot be fully restored by managed pollination (Garibaldi *et al.*, 2013). So while it might be argued that enhancement would be in the interests of an individual representative of a species, or even a single species, widespread enhancement and humanization of multiple species could have widespread effects on plant productivity and the food chain, hardly in the ultimate interests of either individual animals or species.

Although superficially it might seem that ethical theories focused on the individual are in conflict with those focused on large groups, in fact both deontological and utilitarian theories converge in the sense that it cannot be acceptable for an individual to undergo an enhancement that could not be extended to all.

The Duty to the Enhanced

The ethics of animal welfare dictate that humans have a duty towards animals that they have 'enhanced' as a part of the domestication process. The dairy cow with the oversized udder for milk production for human consumption, the thoroughbred racehorse with its poor hoof conformation, and the various breeds of short-nosed dogs that struggle to breathe and give birth naturally are all examples of animals that depend on human keepers to take care of their welfare interests (Grandin and Deesing, 2014). In contrast to wild species that have evolved to suit their natural habitats, and which form part of biosystems when it comes to structures such as food chains – for which, arguably, the human race has no responsibility other than to preserve wild habitats – the domestic animal is adapted, both physically and psychologically to an environment that is man-made. This adaptation includes the selection that has been permitted through surgical and medical therapies and maintenance of individuals as breeding stock that would previously have died or been killed in early life. At the very least, these individuals deserve 'a life worth living' (Wathes, 2010), and a humane end when this cannot be maintained for economic or other reasons. Even those who feel that the maintenance of domestic animals is an unacceptable practice recognize this duty to the existing members of domestic species (Francione and Charlton, 2015). Others see the obligation of humans as much more far-reaching. In arguing a right to life for such animals, they argue a duty to preserve life, even if this may be against economic and other interests of human keepers (Yeates, 2010). This has led to 'no-kill charities' (Kass *et al.*, 2001) and some veterinary surgeons who see it as a duty of animal ownership that keepers accept all the costs of treatment and care until their animal dies of natural causes, or its life becomes undeniably compromised in terms of suffering.

While the 'right to life' can be debated, a zoocentric perspective based on contractarian principles means that, if the choice is to keep animals alive, as already argued, they must be treated well and, as far as possible, given a 'life worth living', or, ideally, a good life (Wathes, 2010). This will include attention to both their physical and psychological needs. This means the provision, as far as possible, of an environment that matches their domesticated *telos*, or it may, in some cases, with our greater enlightenment, support engagement in further enhancement so that their *telos* can better match the compromise associated with human-mandated confinement (Rollin, 2003). Controversially, it has been suggested that this might involve modification of certain senses to prevent stereotypical behaviours that are a consequence of confinement (Sandoe *et al*., 1999). However, the limits of this, as in all enhancement, must be dictated by society taking seriously its contractarian responsibilities and considering the consequences of intervention on the way we think of ourselves as human beings.

Achievement of the Duty to the Enhanced

The way society agrees a common framework for human behaviours, including the duty to the enhanced, is through a legal system that holds individuals accountable for their actions. Laws are devised based on the normative presuppositions of the polity, which in modern society embraces a diversity of views of what is good and right (Rosenfeld, 1998). Historically, anthropocentric perspectives led to laws protecting animals for their value as property (Hepple and Gibbens, 2013) and interesting legal cases with this focus – such as whether a horse could develop a catastrophic long-bone fracture several days after being hit by a stone, and the perpetrator thus held responsible for the economic loss (Mayer, 1838) (the judge ruled that the owner did not have a case as a tibial fracture should have been evident immediately, not recognizing that fissure fractures, caused by trauma, can predispose to subsequent complete fractures). In passing, it is worth observing that, in a variety of circumstances, society places obligations of care on owners of property (Milligan, 2015). This includes historic buildings and works of art, as well as animals. The value that society places on these special types of property renders their owners more akin to custodians, and means that they cannot mutilate or destroy such properties without being held accountable for unacceptable actions.

The distinctive challenge related to animals is that, as a variety of pathocentric and zoocentric perspectives have emerged, law has had to be developed that maintains a balance between plurality in normative ethical positions, as well as incorporating firmly embedded cultural and religious beliefs about the use of animals, and unity in required behaviours, enforced through a legal definition of right and wrong (Rosenfeld, 1998). In the UK, this led to the Prevention of Cruelty to Animals Act 1849, the first legislation describing a welfare outcome, the Cruelty to Animals Act 1876, specifically dealing with animal experimentation, and most recently the Animal Welfare Act 2006, which imposed a duty of care on animal owners (Hepple and Gibbens, 2013). The latter, in section 9, extended UK law to ensure that persons responsible for animals not only protected them from 'pain, suffering, injury and disease', and took care of their physical requirements, but also recognized the 'need to be able to exhibit normal behaviour patterns'.

Analogies have been drawn between the development of society's attitudes to slavery and human rights legislation and the evolution of its attitudes to animals and animal welfare legislation (Milligan, 2015). However, unlike human rights, where the enlightenment view has always been that 'all men are created equal', these parallels fail to take account of two fundamentally different beliefs regarding the status of animals: on the one hand, the human race is distinctive and, within limits, is able to use animals in its own interests; and on the other, that all sentient creatures are equal and should be dealt with by society on that basis (Singer, 1975). These competing philosophies, and the spectrum of views on the balance between animal interests and human interests to which they give rise, means that there are those who feel badly treated by zealous interpretations of animal welfare law (e.g. Derbyshire, 2008; Copping, 2009) and those who feel society has not gone far enough in its protection of the rights of animals (Singer, 1975; Regan, 1983). For instance, tolerance of extreme conformations in some breeds of dogs means that many members of those breeds still undergo surgery to give birth, and are at risk of producing offspring with respiratory difficulties (Packer *et al.*, 2012; 2015). Domestic animals are still kept for food production for meat eaters, and respect for religious beliefs means that non-stun slaughter is still practised in the UK. As in other areas of social policy, principled individuals, who accept the right of other citizens within a plural society to hold contrary views, will assume behaviours that align with ethical positions that go beyond the foundations of current law. In contrast, some who seek to impose their ethical positions and beliefs on others may adopt violent approaches to make their point (Mann, 2007), not always respecting the interests of the individual animals that are targeted in such demonstrations.

Conclusions

This chapter has explored different ethical positions and views on our duties to enhance animals and to care for those that have been enhanced. Such enhancement is of two types: that associated with domestication, largely in the interests of the human keepers of animals; and that (still largely theoretical) seen as in the interests of the animals themselves. A consequence of the domestication changes, often physical, driven by human interests, has been psychological changes that have made animals easier to keep by helping them accept being housed in human environments. This has led to changed species that seek human company rather than avoiding it, and which often have a preference for being housed rather than being free to roam, particularly under adverse weather conditions. Both the physical changes and the need for treatment to prevent or minimize the welfare consequences of modified physiques, and the psychological adaptation to man-made environments, mean that human keepers have a duty to these domesticated species that they do not have for wild animals. These duties are defined in law, although the presence of a plurality of normative ethical positions means that, in modern society, a variety of stances may be taken on individual duties to domestic species, leading on occasion to violent confrontations between some who advocate very different attitudes to animal keeping and those who 'only' meet their current legal obligations.

In contrast, the question of a duty to enhance all animal species in their interests is much more challenging. A justification for enhancement that modifies a domesticated animal's *telos* to help it enjoy its life alongside humans can be made, but the ethical imperative to enhance wild animal species is unclear. Both deontological and utilitarian arguments break down when considerations beyond individuals and single-species groups are considered, and, in addition, it is virtually impossible to define animal interests as other than those related to the lives to which they are adapted (whether wild or domesticated). Life is complex and precarious. As human beings, we will inevitably intervene to reduce individual suffering. That defines our humanity (Schantz, 2007). However, the extension of individual attention to large groups is much more problematic, with biocentric and ecocentric theories favouring respect of animal species as they are. Ultimately, these broader considerations of animal enhancement coalesce around one of the big challenges of our age, the preservation of all life on the planet.

References

Animal Welfare Act 2006, c. 45. Available at: http://www.legislation.gov.uk/ukpga/2006/45/pdfs/ukpga_20060045_en.pdf (accessed 5 April 2017).

Ascher-Walsh, R. (2013) *Devoted*. National Geographic, Washington, DC.

Bateman, S., Gayon, J., Allouche, S., Goffette, J. and Marzano, M. (2015) Introduction. In: *Inquiring into Animal Enhancement*. Palgrave Macmillan, Basingstoke, UK, pp. 13–33.

Becker, F. and French, L. (2004) Making the links: child abuse, animal cruelty and domestic violence. *Child Abuse Review* 13, 399–414.

Borenstein, J. (2009) The wisdom of caution: genetic enhancement and future children. *Science and Engineering Ethics* 15, 517–530.

Bostock, S. St C. (1993) *Zoos and Animal Rights: The Ethics of Keeping Animals*. Routledge, London, p. 90.

Bostrum, N. and Savulescu, J. (2008) Human enhancement ethics: the state of the debate. In: Savulescu, J. and Bostrum, N. (eds) *Human Enhancement*. Oxford University Press, Oxford, UK, pp. 1–22.

Burgat, F. (2015) Improving animals, improving humans: transpositions and comparisons. In: Bateman, S., Allouche, S., Gayon, J., Marzano, M. and Goffette, J. (eds) *Inquiring into Animal Enhancement*. Palgrave Macmillan, Basingstoke, UK, pp. 34–48.

Chan, S. (2009) Should we enhance animals? *Journal of Medical Ethics* 35, 678–683.

Chan, S. and Harris, J. (2006) Cognitive regeneration or enhancement: the ethical issues. *Regenerative Medicine* 1, 361–366.

Copping, J. (2009) Fat dogs seized by RSPCA. *The Telegraph*. Available at: http://www.telegraph.co.uk/news/uknews/4331467/Fat-dogs-seized-by-RSPCA.html (accessed 6 April 2017).

Derbyshire, D. (2008) Barking mad: owners of obese dogs and fat cats could face jail under controversial new rules. *Mail Online*. Available at: http://www.dailymail.co.uk/news/article-1083010/Barking-mad-Owners-obese-dogs-fat-cats-face-jail-controversial-new-rules.html (accessed 6 April 2017).

Ferrari, A. (2015) Technovisionary paternalism and the colonisation of nature. In: Bateman, S., Allouche, S., Gayon, J., Marzano, M. and Goffette, J. (eds) *Inquiring into Animal Enhancement*. Palgrave Macmillan, Basingstoke, UK, pp. 13–33.

Flack, A.J.P. (2016) Lions loose on a gentleman's lawn: animality, authenticity and automobility in the emergence of the English safari park. *Journal of Historical Geography* 54, 38–49.

Francione, G.L. and Charlton, A. (2015) *Animal Rights: The Abolitionist Approach*. Exempla Press.

Gallai, N., Salles, J.-M., Settele, J. and Vaissière, B.E. (2009) Economic valuation of the vulnerability of world agriculture confronted with pollinator decline. *Ecological Economics* 68, 810–821.

Garibaldi, L.A., Steffan-Dewenter, I., Winfree, R. *et al.* (2013) Wild pollinators enhance fruit set of crops regardless of honey bee abundance. *Science* 339, 1608–1611.

Gauthier, D. (1986) *Morals by Agreement*. Oxford University Press, Oxford, UK.

Gauthier, D. (2014) Twenty-five on. *Ethics* 123, 601–624.

Gawande, A. (2014) *The Problem of Hubris*. The Reith Lectures, no. 3. Available at: http://downloads.bbc.co.uk/radio4/open-book/2014_reith_lecture3_edinburgh.pdf (accessed 2 February 2018).

Grandin, T. and Deesing, M.J. (2014) Genetics and animal welfare. In: Grandin, T. and Deesing, M.J. (eds) *Genetics and the Behavior of Domestic Animals* (2nd edn). Elsevier, Amsterdam, pp. 455–456.

Hepple, S. and Gibbens, N. (2013) Animal ethics and the government's policy: 'To guard and to protect'. In: Wathes, C.M., Corr, S.A., May, S.A., McCulloch, S.P. and Whiting, M.C. (eds) *Veterinary and Animal Ethics*. Wiley-Blackwell, Oxford, pp. 229–244.

Kamm, F.M. (2005) Is there a problem with enhancement? *The American Journal of Bioethics* 5(3), 5–14.
Kant, I. (1996) *The Metaphysics of Morals* (trans. M. J. Gregor). Cambridge University Press, 6: 443, pp. 192–193.
Kass, P.H., New, J.C., Scarlett, J.M. and Salman, M.D. (2001) Understanding animal companion surplus in the United States: relinquishment of non-adoptables to animal shelters for euthanasia. *Journal of Applied Animal Welfare Science* 4, 237–248.
Korsgaard, C.M. (2011) Interacting with animals: a Kantian account. In: Beauchamp, T.L. and Frey, R.G. (eds) *The Oxford Handbook of Animal Ethics*. Oxford University Press, Oxford, UK, pp. 91–118.
Larrère, C. and Larrère, R. (2000) Animal rearing as a contract? *Journal of Agricultural and Environmental Ethics* 12, 51–58.
Losey, J.E. and Vaughan, M. (2006) The economic value of ecological services provided by insects. *Bioscience* 56, 311–323.
Mann, K. (2007) *From Dusk 'til Dawn: An Insider's View of the Growth of the Animal Liberation Movement*. Puppy Pincher Press, London.
Mayer, T.W. (1838) On fractures of the extremities in the horse. *The Veterinarian* 11, 144–146.
Milligan, T. (2015) *Animal Ethics: The Basics*. Routledge, Abingdon, UK, pp. 132–133.
Ormandy, E.H., Dale, J. and Griffin, G. (2011) Genetic engineering of animals: ethical issues including welfare concerns. *Canadian Veterinary Journal* 52, 544–550.
Packer, R.M.A., Hendricks, A. and Burn, C.C. (2012) Do dog owners perceive the clinical signs related to conformational inherited disorders as 'normal' for the breed? A potential constraint to improving canine welfare. *Animal Welfare* 21(S1), 81–93.
Packer, R.M.A., Hendricks, A., Tivers, M.S. and Burn, C.C. (2015) Impact of facial conformation on canine health: brachycephalic obstructive airway syndrome. *PLOS ONE*. DOI:10.1371/journal.pone.0137496.
Rees, P.A. (2009) The sizes of elephant groups in zoos: implications for elephant welfare. *Journal of Applied Animal Welfare Science* 12, 44–60.
Regan, T. (1983) *The Case for Animal Rights*. University of California Press, Berkeley, California.
Rollin, B.E. (2003) On telos and genetic engineering. In: Armstrong, S.J. and Botzler, R.G. (eds) *The Animal Ethics Reader*. Routledge, London, p. 346.
Rollin, B.E. (2006) *An Introduction to Veterinary Medical Ethics* (2nd edn). Blackwell Publishing, Oxford, UK, pp. 29–30.
Rollin, B.E. (2013) Telos. In: Wathes, C.M., Corr, S.A., May, S.A., McCulloch, S.P. and Whiting, M.C. (eds) *Veterinary and Animal Ethics*. Wiley-Blackwell, Oxford, UK, pp. 75–83.
Roots, C. (2007) *Domestication*. Greenwood Press, London.
Roper, M. (2012) Loyal dog ran away from home to find his dead master's grave – and has stayed by its side for six years. *Mail Online*. Available at: http://www.dailymail.co.uk/news/article-2202509/Loyal-dog-ran-away-home-dead-masters-grave--stayed-years.html (accessed 12 January 2017).
Rosenfeld, M. (1998) *Just Interpretations: Law between Ethics and Politics*. University of California Press, Berkeley, California, pp. 1–9.
Sandel, M. (2004) The case against perfection. *The Atlantic Monthly* 293(3), 51–62.
Sandoe, P. and Jensen, K.K. (2013) The idea of animal welfare – developments and tensions. In: Wathes, C.M., Corr, S.A., May, S.A., McCulloch, S.P. and Whiting, M.C. (eds) *Veterinary and Animal Ethics*. Wiley-Blackwell, Oxford, pp. 19–31.
Sandoe, P., Nielsen, B.L., Christensen, L.G. and Sorensen, P. (1999) Staying good while playing God – the ethics of breeding farm animals. *Animal Welfare* 8, 313–328.
Schantz, M.L. (2007) Compassion: a concept analysis. *Nursing Forum* 42, 48–55.
Short, R.V. (1997) An introduction to mammalian interspecific hybrids. *Journal of Heredity* 88, 355–357.

Singer, P. (1975) *Animal Liberation: A New Ethics for Our Treatment of Animals*. New York Review, New York.

Verhoog, H. (2000) Defining positive welfare and animal integrity. In: M. Hovi and R. Garcia Trujillo (eds) *Diversity of Livestock Systems and Definition of Animal Welfare*. University of Reading, Reading, pp. 108–118.

Wathes, C. (2010) Lives worth living? *Veterinary Record* 166, 468–469.

Wells, K.D. (2000) Genome modification for meat science: techniques and applications. *Proceedings of the Annual Reciprocal Meat Conference of the American Meat Science Association* 53, 87–93.

Yeates, J.W. (2010) Death is a welfare issue. *Journal of Agricultural and Environmental Ethics* 23, 229–241.

14 Pressing Animals Beyond Their Biological Limits

Bernard Rollin*

Colorado State University, Fort Collins, Colorado, USA

Throughout my academic career as a philosopher specializing in animal ethics, I have avoided making predictions about the future. After all, if the CIA, equipped with cameras in space that could photograph a pack of cigarettes in the shirt pocket of Russian soldiers, were caught completely unaware by the collapse of the Soviet Union, what chance did I have at accurate foretelling? Eventually, however, I realized that, at least in the biblical sense, prophecy did not mean gazing into a crystal ball, functioning as a TV set pointing into the future; rather, the prophets of the Old Testament were adroit at identifying the likely implications of current tendencies, as was the case when Jeremiah prophesied the defeat and exile of the Hebrews if they continued to vex the Babylonians.

If, then, we are to assay this weaker sense of prophecy, it is obligatory to look to where we have been in order to anticipate where we are likely or possibly going. And thus it is reasonable to begin with the advent of domestication of animals more than 12,000 years ago. Archaeological, anthropological and various other forms of evidence have helped show that domestication was a plausible and rational successor to an earlier period of hunting and gathering. Hunting and gathering was inherently unpredictable, dependent on the vagaries of weather, animal reproductive success and forage. This in turn created instability in communities, given the need for constantly following the food supply. Such a situation created a roadblock to the stability and predictability presuppositional to the development of culture and civilization.

The Importance of Husbandry

It was therefore inevitable that, by way of natural selection, animals congenial (or at least not inimical) to the company of humans created a state of symbiotic mutual benefit for humans as well as for the animals possessed of these traits. As Darwin pointed out, this was gradually augmented by artificial selection, further refining the traits of animals amenable by nature to domestication.

The key point regarding the beginnings of domestication is that it would at that stage in history not even occur to humans to push the animals beyond their biological limits. At the most, they would, by selective breeding, attempt to modify biological limits in relatively minor ways, for example by selecting for such traits as docility, diminished flightiness, increased musculature and success in reproduction. And in the

*E-mail: bernard.rollin@colostate.edu

event that someone was thoughtless enough to try to exceed biological limits, the process would self-correct by virtue of the animals' self-destruction by sickness or death.

As approaches to domesticated animal agriculture grew more rational, its basis in *good husbandry* became firmly established as well as becoming both a prudential and an ethical imperative. 'Husbandry' is derived from the old Norse phrase *hus bond*, meaning bonded to the household. Husbandry has been termed 'the ancient contract with animals', where, as in any fair contract, both parties benefit from the relationship. Virtually until the 20th century, husbandry was the key concept in animal agriculture. Even today, among western ranchers, one of the last major groups of husbandry agriculturalists remaining, one can intone the phrase 'we take care of the animals', and the audience will reply 'and they take care of us'.

By definition, then, husbandry agriculture could not push animals beyond their biological limits. The essence of husbandry was, in fact, care. Humans put animals into the most optimal environment congenial to the animals not only surviving but thriving, the environment for which they had evolved and been selected. The better the animals did, the better farmers did. Sanctioned by their own self-interest, humans provided farm animals with sustenance, water, shelter, protection from predation, such medical attention as was available, help in birthing, food during famine, water during drought, safe surroundings and comfortable appointments.

The singular beauty of husbandry is that it was at once an ethical and prudential doctrine. It was prudential in that failure to observe husbandry inexorably led to ruination of the person keeping animals. Failure to feed, water, protect from predators, respect the animals' physical, biological, physiological needs and natures – what Aristotle called their *telos* (the 'cowness of the cow', the 'sheepness of the sheep') – meant your animals did not survive and thrive, and thus neither did you. Failure to know and respect the animals' needs and natures had the same effect. Indeed, even Aristotle, whose world-view was fully hierarchical, with humans at the top, implicitly recognized the contractual nature of husbandry when he off-handedly affirmed that, although the natural role of animals is to serve man, domestic animals are 'preserved' through so doing. The ultimate sanction of failing at husbandry – erosion of self-interest – obviated the need for any detailed ethical exposition of moral or legal rules for husbandry: anyone unmoved by self-interest is unlikely to be moved by moral or legal injunctions! Therefore, one finds little written about animal ethics and little codification of that ethic in law before the 20th century, with the bulk of what is articulated aimed at identifying overt, deliberate, sadistic cruelty, hurting an animal for no purpose or for perverse pleasure, or such outrageous neglect as not providing food or water. Until recently, pushing domestic animals beyond their biological limit was not an issue for almost all of civilization (Rollin, 2015).

Judeo-Christian Teachings on Animal Treatment

The Noah story is emblematic of this 'ancient contract'. In the Noah story, we learn that even as God preserves humans, humans preserve animals. The ethic of husbandry is, in fact, taught throughout the Bible: the animals must rest on the Sabbath even as we do; one is not to seethe a calf in its mother's milk (so we do not grow insensitive to animal needs and natures); we can violate the Sabbath to save an animal. Proverbs tells us that 'the wise man cares for his animals'. The Old Testament is replete with injunctions against inflicting unnecessary pain and suffering on animals, as exemplified in the strange story of Balaam, who beats his ass and is reprimanded by the animal, speaking through the grace of God.

The full force of the husbandry ethic is best expressed in the 23rd Psalm. There, in searching for an apt metaphor for God's ideal relationship to humans, the Psalmist invokes the good shepherd: 'The Lord is My shepherd; I shall not want. He maketh me to lie down in green pastures: he leadeth me beside the still waters. He restoreth my soul.' We want no more from God than the equivalent of what the good shepherd provides to his animals. Without a shepherd, the animal would not easily find forage or water, would not survive the multitude of predators the Bible tells us prowled the land. In return for comfort and security, the animals provide their products and sometimes their lives. Significantly, Jesus is depicted both as shepherd and lamb, from the origin of Christianity until the present, in paintings, literature, song, statuary and poetry, as well as in sermons. To this day, ministers are called shepherds of their congregation.

Islamic Teachings on Animal Treatment

Quran and subsequent Muslim writings, for example, repeatedly stress the need for avoiding the infliction of unnecessary suffering on animals. Like the Judeo-Christian Bible, Muslim theology stresses that while humans have been given domination over animals and the right to use them for food and work, causing unnecessary suffering or inflicting pain for no reason are strictly forbidden. For example, directly paralleling kosher slaughter, Islam dictates rules for Halal slaughter, which was meant to limit animal suffering. In support of this claim, Muslim religious authorities today have allowed for the modern practice of animal stunning to mitigate suffering (Nakyinsige *et al.*, 2013; Fuseini, *et al.*, 2017; http://edenkeeper.org/2014/08/14/animal-rights-islam-part-care-sustainability/).

Gharebaghi *et al.* (2007), in Iran, have reviewed Islamic prohibitions that forbid separating baby birds or animals from their mother. There are also many passages in the Quran that state that sustenance and water must be provided to working animals (https://www.islamreligion.com/articles/185/humane-treatment-of-animals/). Rahman and Aidaros (2012), members of the World Organization for Animal Health (OIE) animal welfare working group, cite many Quranic passages that clearly emphasize kindness to animals. Rahman (2017) also quotes many passages from Islamic writings and the Quran that teach concern for the welfare of animals.

Taoist Confucianism and Buddhist Teachings

Taoism, too, explicitly expresses moral concern for animals, albeit without enjoining husbandry. Taoist texts stress the fact that, from a moral perspective, domestication of animals is a form of oppression, and that the ideal human attitude towards animals is to leave them alone to live the life they were created for (http://advocacy.britannica.com/blog/advocacy/2011/09/daoism-and-animals/).

Confucianism, in turn, expresses little concern for the treatment of animals, perhaps accounting for the traditional prevalence in China of what the West would consider animal cruelty (http://uselesstree.typepad.com/useless_tree/2007/03/humane_treatmen.html).

In fact, only recently has animal welfare become a prominent concern in China as a result of the influx of western ideas, and the globalization of trade. Evidence for this claim is provided by the fact that the Chinese ambassador explicitly stated in a speech that China needed to begin taking cognizance of animal welfare. In 2014, the concept of animal welfare was introduced into Chinese law regulating wildlife, a first in Chinese legal history (http://www.scmp.com/news/china/article/1663199/china-write-animal-welfare-law-first-time).

Given its commitment to a belief in reincarnation, Buddhism also expressed moral concern for animals, resulting in a strong but not universal commitment to vegetarianism. Buddhism condemns the infliction of suffering on animals (www.bbc.com/religion/religions/buddhism/buddhistethics/animals.shtml). A similar ethic can be found in Hinduism. Again, animal cruelty is condemned (http://www.humanesociety.org/assets/pdfs/faith/hinduism_and_the_ethical.pdf). Little is said in these traditions regarding husbandry, just as little is said about vegetarianism in western religions.

Sustainability Issues

Not only was traditional husbandry agriculture largely ethical in terms of animal treatment, but it also met what, as we shall see, has become a major concern today in that it was *sustainable*, i.e. it was 'a balanced aquarium' requiring very minimal additional inputs. Pasture fed the animals; the animals also ate the weeds, thereby minimizing the need for herbicides; animal manure nourished the ground, with no petrochemical material incorporated into the soil. We shall return to this point.

We have thus argued that the development of animal agriculture based in husbandry is presuppositional to the development of western civilization and culture, which is itself presuppositional to the development of industry and technology. And in this surely resides one of the most profound ironies in human history. For it is the very fact of husbandry undergirding civilization that created the possibility of the undoing of husbandry based agriculture! As Thomas Hobbes once remarked, 'leisure is the mother of philosophy' (i.e. intellectual activity, including science and technology) in the broadest sense of the term. And surely a secure food supply provided by a portion of the population is a presupposition of leisure.

Agricultural Industrial Revolution

In any case, the 18th century witnessed an industrial revolution in both plant and animal agriculture that greatly increased productivity. It has been said that this created a mindset oriented towards business, or capitalism, rather than one aimed primarily at feeding the population. As Mark Overton (1996) has pointed out in his classic book *Agricultural Revolution in England: Transformation of the Agrarian Economy 1500–1850*, the industrialization of agriculture in essence created room for capitalism in agriculture. Agriculture could now be done for profit, not just for sustenance. Animal producers no longer viewed themselves as constrained by the animals' nature and thus by their biological limits. No longer were breeding and good husbandry the limiting factors for animal productivity. The animal welfare that was assured by the need to put square pegs into square holes and round pegs into round holes was rendered obsolete by newly emerging 'technological sanders' that allowed producers to force square pegs into round holes and round pegs into square ones – animals into environments congenial to profit, but radically inimical to the animals' biological natures.

In essence, new technology radically severed the connection traditionally existing between productivity and animal welfare. Under technological agriculture, animals were ripped from the pastoral environments they were evolved to live in, and crowded into abrasive and alien confinement situations where they were totally unable to express their *telos,* i.e. their inherent psychological and biological natures (Rollin, 2017). If husbandry-era producers had attempted to raise, for example, hundreds of thousands of chickens in cages for egg production, the animals would be dead within months, the flocks decimated by disease that could take hold and spread like wildfire. Under an agriculture based in husbandry, animals were slaughtered, processed and consumed within a relatively short distance of where they were reared. Today, animals are shipped hundreds and even thousands of miles under conditions highly erosive of their health and well-being, and sold to consumers oblivious of how they came to be.

Cattle, for example, evolved to live as grazing animals, subsisting on a diet of plant life achieved by foraging and grazing, with small amounts of grain occasionally consumed. Today, the majority of US cattle (over 80%) are 'finished' under concentrated conditions in 'feed yards' with the majority of their diet constituted by grain. This is a result of the significant increase in grain production accomplished by the technology of the 'green revolution' after World War II. Feed lots added vast amounts of value to abundant grain by putting it through cattle and selling it as beef. For a certain percentage of animals, the very high calorie diet creates health problems, specifically ruminal and liver abscesses, representing both an economic loss and a welfare problem. But the enormous amount of weight gain in the majority of cattle more than compensates for the lost carcasses. And, most significantly, the loss of welfare is not of concern to producers, because *productivity has been severed from welfare.* The health and well-being of individual animals as a primary agricultural value has become radically supplanted by the economic values of efficiency and productivity of an entire operation.

In addition, the *sustainability* inherent in pastoral agriculture has been eroded. Feed lots, and the industrial production of grain that fuels them, depend on cheap oil to drive the machinery and create chemical fertilizer (rather than manure to fertilize pasture), as well as to transport the beef over great distances. Cheap energy is not naturally sustainable and can be eroded by political and societal considerations.

The full panoply of costs arising from industrialized, non-husbandry based confinement agriculture was described only in 2008, when the report of the Pew Commission on Industrial Farm Animal Production was released. A joint effort of the Pew Charitable Trusts and the Johns Hopkins Bloomberg School of Public Health, as well as a significant group of experts on public health, food production, animal welfare and environmental despoliation, the Commission was created when Johns Hopkins researchers found the cutting-edge antibiotic vancomycin in groundwater in the Delaware-Maryland-Virginia poultry production area. It turned out that these antibiotics were necessary to keep the chickens alive in huge pathogenic confinement operations. Such essentially frivolous use created resistance in pathogenic bacteria, compromising human (and animal) health.

Other issues described by the Commission included animal welfare (a major priority); environmental despoliation; loss of small farmers (who Thomas Jefferson argued were the backbone of democracy); loss of rural communities; domination of agriculture by huge corporations; loss of sustainability; creation of new diseases in animals by virtue of crowding under pathogenic conditions; dangers to human health by way of zoonoses and erosion of air and water quality; loss of 'local agricultural wisdom'; problems of food safety; and development of antibiotic resistance.

Now that we have traced the trajectory of agriculture from its rational and sustainable basis in husbandry, working within the animals' biological limits, to the unfortunate effects of industrialization, which has created the currently dominant values of efficiency and productivity and led to pushing the animals beyond their biological limits, regardless of the consequences, we can make an attempt at 'prophecy' in the sense described.

Threshold of Biotechnology Revolution

We are at the threshold of a new industrial revolution based in genetics and biology, aptly termed 'biotechnology', wherein instead of technological sanders roughly grinding square pegs to fit into round holes, we can now rapidly restructure the pegs themselves. In a sense, this is not new; both natural and artificial selection have done this throughout history; but it occurred in a self-correcting way with negative consequences selected out. New methods allow for biological change 'in the fast lane', with the real possibility of extremely pernicious consequences downstream.

More to the point, we have no reason to believe that the same human mindset that was driven by greed to abandon husbandry will not prevail with regard to this new technology. In fact, there is already evidence of this dominant motivation.

Let us stress from the outset that, contrary to many religious authorities and alarmists, there is nothing intrinsically wrong with genetic engineering per se; any wrongness arises from pernicious uses to which it is put. Such claims as 'genetic engineering violates God's will' or '...desacralizes Nature', have no genuine moral content, but play to the emotions. One genuine moral issue would arise from utilizing genetic engineering to create suffering animals whose *telos* and welfare are compromised by that engineering. If on the one hand one utilizes genetic engineering to preclude genetic diseases that afflict the animal, such use is not morally problematic. On the other hand, given the history of what we have called 'technological sanders', their use has been to circumvent welfare constraints on productivity. There is no reason to believe that similar use would not prominently dominate biotechnology. The mindset, as we remarked earlier, is oriented towards efficiency and productivity, not animal welfare. It will most likely and inevitably be used to exceed biological limits.

In agriculture, attempts to genetically engineer animals have instantiated this mindset. It is clear that any pain, suffering, distress or disease that does not interfere with profit and resulting from genetic engineering is likely to be ignored, just as production diseases are currently ignored; and, in fact, early attempts to genetically engineer farm animals have generated serious welfare problems. For example, early attempts to increase the growth rate and efficiency of pigs and sheep by insertion of modified genes to control growth, while achieving that result, engendered catastrophic consequences for the health and welfare of the animals. Pigs suffered from kidney and liver problems, lethargy, lameness, gait issues, bulging eyes, thickening of the skin, gastric ulcers, severe synovitis, degenerative joint diseases, heart disease, nephritis and pneumonia (Pursel, *et al.*, 1989).

One major lesson learned from such experiments is that it is impossible to effect one-to-one correspondence between genes and desired phenotypic traits. Genes have multiple effects; phenotypic traits are often controlled by multiple genes. Another example from my own institution grew out of an attempt to genetically engineer cattle for double muscling. Though the calf was born normal, within a month it was unable to stand up on its own for reasons that were unknown. In short, genetic manipulation, from a functional point of view, is better described as genetic 'tinkering' than as genetic engineering.

Principle of Conservation of Welfare

One can thus be morally certain that biotechnology utilized to push animals beyond their biological limit will be deployed with primary emphasis on increasing profit, productivity and efficiency with little regard for animal welfare, animal suffering or sustainability notions that were effectively built into traditional husbandry agriculture. For this reason, I have proposed a guiding principle for regulating genetic engineering of agricultural animals as a mandated constraint on genetic engineering, which I have called the *Principle of Conservation of Welfare.* This principle affirms that *genetically engineered animals should be no worse off than the parent stock would be were they not so engineered, and ideally should be better off.* Engineering satisfying this principle can be found in genetically creating resistance to disease in animals, assuming such resistance carries with it no hidden deleterious effects. It is very interesting that when I suggested this at a USDA symposium on genetic engineering, virtually everyone in the audience was in agreement with the principle.

In addition, biotechnology threatens genetic diversity. If a given animal is seen to be superior, for example a dairy cow or laying hen, it will come to dominate commercial production, as in fact has occurred already with chickens. Thus certain breeds will be allowed to die out, or preserved only by hobby fanciers. Yet we can be wrong about what is needed from an animal, for example if environmental conditions rapidly change. Further, what was considered the exemplary bull from which subsequent dairy Holsteins were propagated turned out to be carrying a genetic defect that later compromised the breed.

As the old commonsense cliché affirms, 'there is no free lunch'. Raising animals with respect for their biological limitations is not a rule that is easily overridden. In today's world, where concern for animal welfare has reached unprecedented heights in society, it is extremely unlikely that society will tolerate new sources of infliction of suffering on animals. Agriculture would do far better to return to a more husbandry based approach that does not attempt to exceed biological limits in a manner resulting in new sources of suffering.

References

Fuseini, A., Wotton, S.B., Hadley, P.J. and Knowles, T.G. (2017) The perception and acceptability of pre-slaughter and post slaughter stunning for halal production: the views of UK Islamic scholars and halal consumers. *Meat Science* 123, 145–150.

Gharebaghi, R., Reza Vaez Mahdavi, M., Ghasemi, H., Dibaei, A. and Heidary, F. (2007) Animal rights in Islam. In: *Proceedings of the Sixth World Congress in Alternatives and Animal Use in the Life Sciences*, 21–25 August, Tokyo, pp. 61–63.

Nakyinsige, K., Che Man, Y.B., Aghwan, Z.A., Zulkifili, I., Goh, Y.M., Baker, F.A., Al-Kahtani, H.A. and Sazili, A.Q. (2013) Stunning and animal welfare from an Islamic and scientific perspective. *Meat Science* 95, 352–361.

Overton, M. (1996) *Agricultural Revolution in England: Transformation of the Agrarian Economy 1500–1850*. Cambridge University Press, Cambridge, UK.

Pew Commission (2008) Putting meat on the table: industrial farm production in America. Pew Commission on Industrial Farm Animal Production in America. Available at: http://www.ncifap.org/_images/pcifapfin.pdf (accessed 13 April 2015).

Pursel, V.G., Pinkert, C.A., Miller, K.F., Bolt, D.J., Campbell, R.G., Palmiter, R.D., Brinster, R.L. and Hammer, R.E. (1989) Genetic engineering of livestock. *Science* 244, 1281–1288.

Rahman, S.A. (2017) Religion and animal welfare: an Islamic perspective. *Animals* 7(2). DOI: 10.3390/ani7020011.

Rahman, S.A. and Aidaros, H. (2012) Islam and animal welfare with special reference to cruelty to animals during transport and slaughter. Available at: http://kb.rspca.org.au/what-is-halal-slaughter-in-australia_116.html (accessed 5 February 2018).

Rollin, B. (2015) Why is agricultural animal welfare important? The social and ethical context. In: Grandin, T. (ed.) *Improving Animal Welfare: A Practical Approach* (2nd edn) CAB International, Wallingford, UK.

Rollin, B. (2017) *A New Basis of Animal Ethics: Telos and Common Sense*. University of Missouri Press, Columbia, Missouri.

15 Concluding: Pushing Animals to Their Limits

Martin Whiting*

Royal Veterinary College, UK

Introduction

At the outset of this book Andrew Gardiner introduced the spectrum of modification, improvement and enhancement (Chapter 2); from the mutually beneficial modification by domestication of the wolf, which symbiotically enhanced the lives of those wolves and humans living together (Harraway, 2003), to the grossly distorted enforced conformational changes of the modern domestic dog resulting in human pleasure at considerable cost to the welfare of the animal (Asher *et al.*, 2009). The spectrum of intervention on animals is substantial and decisions around planned modifications do not always require a demonstrable benefit to the animal within a regulatory framework. In most countries, there is almost no regulation or legislation controlling selective breeding to specify a consideration to be granted to the enhanced welfare of the offspring (LOC, 2014).

One consideration of the ethics of animal modification, or animal enhancement, may be achieved once it is understood what the purpose of the modification is, and the associated cost–benefit analysis. But such a basic analysis disrespects an element of the naturalness of the animals involved (Rollin, 1986; Verhoog, 1992) and potentially demonstrates a level of anthropocentricism which is not consistent with modern welfare science. Moreover, we run a great risk of normalizing the abnormal, a concept called 'normalcy', where things become 'socially normal' because of their common occurrence (Wellman, 1958). The development of normalcy associated with the modification of animals can lead to blinding ourselves as to the negative consequences that have arisen. When normalcy occurs, and is combined with cognitive dissonance, substantial welfare compromise can arise and yet pass by completely undetected (Packer *et al.*, 2012). That is one purpose of this book – to explore how the abnormal has become normal, or standard practice, and how those animals may be affected by their change. However, detection of this detrimental normalcy and defining it for animal modification is surprisingly culturally taxing; for example, castration of dogs in the UK is considered 'good husbandry' but in other countries it is an unacceptable mutilation (Palmer *et al.*, 2012). So how does one determine the compromise associated with change? Does restoration of health to the unhealthy constitute an appropriate endeavour, but adapting an otherwise healthy individual to one that has excellent traits for one aspect of its life combined with detrimental aspects to another is then rendered ethically compromised?

*E-mail: martinwhiting@mac.com

Defining the Modification

Chan (Chapter 3) refines the definition of modification and enhancement as it may apply to animals and provides a structure for moral relevance of its consideration. The concept of enhancement as applied to humans is one where the intervention that is applied does generally, or specifically, increase that individual's general abilities, or allows them to flourish (Chan, 2008). This definition is constrained by the individual's interests and so changing an individual to one with greater abilities, which were not in their interest, or perhaps the sequela of these modifications were not in their interests, falls short of the definition of enhancement (Harris, 2007). If this is transposed to animals, then modifications of animals that improve our interests but which are harmful to their interests are perhaps more appropriately called 'animal de-hancements'. Examples of these de-hancement modifications occupy the majority of Chapters 4 to 12 and lead to the moral questions of where human duties reside with these de-hanced individuals. For example, is there an obligation to rectify or correct their negative welfare? Such post hoc correction can occur in two ways: to adapt the animal to the environment or to adapt the environment to the animal. However, it is not that simple; for the blind chicken who flourishes in the battery farm to a greater extent than the sighted chicken, the *mutation* is the advantage for the chicken when placed in that environment, and the correction of the chicken, or the environment, in isolation, will yield a worse outcome for all; an outcome that also negatively impacts the productivity and efficiency of the farming system.

Understanding the Limits

The example above of the blind chicken typifies one aspect of animals being pushed to their limits. Animal production systems, such as farming, or animal 'refinement breeding', such as pedigree dogs, have taken species that were evolutionarily adapted to their environment and asked more from them. By asking for more 'beauty' from the dog, we have simultaneously reduced its ability to breathe, reproduce and survive without assistance (Packer *et al*., 2015). By asking for a more efficient growth rate to slaughter weight from the chicken, we have simultaneously created a chicken with persistent hunger (De Jong and Guémené, 2011). It is disingenuous to say that these animals have been enhanced, in the sense of that term's common understanding, but it is fair to assert that their biology (and by that we mean their genetics, morphology and behaviour) has been deviated from the wild type in a way that has an advantage for an external party but a disadvantage for them. But what does it mean to be pushed *to their limits*? Within the context of these de-hanced animals, the limit that may be imposed is one of the limitation of their biological function. For example, there may be a maximum growth rate that it is possible for a chicken to achieve through selective breeding, husbandry modification, drug enhancement and dietary change. When there are no more genetic changes, nor more interventions or technology available to modify an animal to 'push it more', then it could be said to be at its limit. Such a limitation, may not be morally relevant if the animal's welfare is not compromised. Additionally, its *telos* may have changed so much from the original wild type, that a new *telos* has to be defined (Rollin, 1995).

The second type of limit that animals may be pushed to is that of welfare compromise, and this is where a moral value can be found. To determine what is meant by this limit, there are two subcategories to explore. First, it is necessary to question how far *should* we distort or deviate an animal from its evolutionary functional type for human benefit, when that animal will experience more negative welfare as a consequence? This question is asking what level of welfare compromise a society is willing to impose on an animal for that society's benefit. Second, what is our duty of care to the dis-hanced? To those animals that are now experiencing a compromise in welfare, does the society that created them have a duty of care to ameliorate their welfare compromise, and if they fail to do so, should some penalty be imposed on them? This second aspect, impacts greatly on the first. For if a society distorts an animal beyond what is a socially acceptable level of suffering, and then actively reduces that suffering, are we still able to say that the animal has been pushed to its limit, or may we push it further?

To explore this interplay, the racehorse becomes a suitable example. Selective breeding and training regimes over the centuries have allowed for the successful creation of faster thoroughbred horses to be used in racing. This is an advantage to the society that created them, in having an increased entertainment value and economic value. However, if there were no negative consequences to the horse in this breeding, then this could be a true enhancement, as those horses, if left wild, may be better able to outrun predators than were their predecessors. Therefore society would have created a fitter, faster horse. This would be the first type of limitation expressed above; the only limit to that animal's speed would be how fast it can choose to run. There may be a biological limit or top speed that is achievable for a horse, and eventually it may be possible to reach that limit. There may not be a morally relevant concern with this hypothetical situation.

However, it is known that the reality of that hypothetic situation and breeding programme is, in fact, a de-hancement. Although there are benefits to human society, and maybe some for the horse, in racing breeding regime, the horse does experience welfare compromises. As explained by May (Chapter 13), these modified horses are more prone to injury and poor hoof conformation, which may require the use of a corrective shoe. Thus, when we push these horses to their limit, we are doing so in the second definition of limit, that of a 'societally limited acceptable welfare compromise'. The first aspect of this 'welfare limitation' above could be that the rules of horse racing do not permit the use of a shoe or any form of coercion or encouragement to the horse, therefore horses may only be pushed as far as they are willing to run, as the pain of their own compromise will be their own limiter. We can see that an alternative society that is willing to compromise welfare to a greater extent, may wish to allow the use of tools, such as the whip, to encourage the horse to run faster still, despite their welfare compromise. Lameness becomes a major limiter, and there will be a point where the pain associated with the lameness cannot be overcome by the use of any tool, coercion or encourager.

If we were to say we have a duty of care to these animals, as a 'duty to the enhanced' (or more accurately a duty to the de-hanced), then we should step in and ameliorate or mitigate that welfare compromise. This could be done by using analgesic drugs, for example, or a surgical neurectomy to prevent the sensation of pain (Jackman *et al.*, 1993). In doing so, we may have met our duty of care to these horses. At this point, the interplay within the welfare limit definition arises. Now that the welfare compromise from lameness has been removed, this welfare limiter has been removed, too; we cycle back to being able to push the horse further again. By meeting our duty of care to the de-hanced, we remove welfare limits and provide scope for that animal to be pushed further. The limit that these horses can be pushed to is yet to be defined.

The situation of the horse above, as an example, is easily rectified; there is an international agreement for racing horses which is that neurectomies and drug doping are not permitted and these horses are not allowed to compete (see articles 1034 and 1055 of FEI, 2017). However, the principle explained here remains relevant. In the category of sporting animals, we may define the notion of limitation and prohibit abuses of it, namely once an animal's welfare is compromised to a certain degree and it becomes necessary to alleviate that compromise, that animal is then unable to be pushed further. This principle does not extend to all other situations considered in this book. Different limits and their acceptability seem to apply according to the different types of animal use.

All Animals Are not Equal

The social rules established for the racing horse above, which prohibit some abuses of the welfare limit do not extend to all animal species or animal uses. Generating generalized moral principles of the limits that animals may be pushed to seems an impossible task when almost all countries place great variety in the standards they apply to different species or to different uses of animals. For example, in Chapters 9 and 10, multiple animal modifications are highlighted where animals are being pushed to their limits of ill health or welfare for the purpose of scientific discovery or drug development. The types and severity of harms issued to those animals are typically justified by a utilitarian cost–benefit analysis (Graham and Prescott, 2015) and yet it is rare to find any benefit to the individual animals involved in those modifications. The extent and severity of the harm caused to these animals are largely unmatched by any harm caused to companion or farming animals through their selective breeding programmes. The benefits to society of pushing these laboratory animals to their biological limits is for human (and occasionally animal) improved health and welfare. With this as the objective, the end justifies the means (although this is disputed, e.g. Knight, 2014). Thus the permitted harms to the laboratory animals is greater than the permitted harms to those animals that are used for entertainment (such as the racing horse above). This does not seem to be species-specific, as although the majority of laboratory animals are rodents and fish, it is not exclusively their domain, and cats, dogs, primates and ruminants are also used in harmful research; although in almost all counties the 'higher' the species, the more justification is needed in order to cause harm to it.

If it is not exclusively 'species' that determines the level of permissible harm, and it is not exclusively 'animal use' that is the determinate, then may be it is a combination of both. The sociozoological scale, proposed by Arluke and Saunders (1996), suggests that an animal's moral status, and therefore the willingness of society to allow harm to come to it or to protect it from harm, is formulated by the combination of species and animal use together. The sociozoological scale generates a hierarchy that describes a pet rat as more socially protected than a vermin rat, and a pet dog more protected than a laboratory dog. This theoretical scale has been used to explain the global community's approach to animal protectionism (or approach to varying permitted harms) in many contexts (Sandøe and Christiansen, 2008; Olsson and Sandøe, 2011; Whiting, 2012; Gross and Tolba, 2015). Permissibility of animal modification, and the consequential welfare compromise to the de-hanced, seems to similarly fall into the broad framework of this sociozoological scale. Aesthetic changes to animals (pedigree dog conformational concerns, cosmetic surgery and drug enhancements) may attract greater criticism than other changes, which may, at face value, appear to have more direct benefit to human society (e.g. animal farming where increased productivity and decreased costs are the output).

Setting the Boundary

While the sociozoological scale may go some way to explain how previous animal de-hancements have occurred, it does not go so far as to explain our duty to those animals that have been pushed towards their limit. If we are morally responsible and have a duty to those animals we have modified, we should seriously consider the extent to which we should rectify these concerns. Either we ameliorate them, slowly breed them out of future generations, or immediately stop them. The severity and immediacy of response to our duty of care to the de-hanced will be equally impacted by societal demands for the sociozoological scale, the arguments of economics and the arguments of tradition. One area where we can set a definite boundary is that proposed by Rollin (Chapter 14). Although there is often a primary emphasis on increasing profit, productivity and efficiency (to this I might also add aesthetic and entertainment traits, too, in order to include companion and sporting animals), we should apply the Principle of Conservation of Welfare. Originally proposed exclusively for genetically engineered animals, it has scope to be applied in the consideration of any new or proposed method of modifying an animal, namely that those animals being modified (or their offspring) should be no worse off than the parent stock, and should, ideally, be better off.

The application of such a principle can easily occur retrospectively to certain modifications undertaken by veterinarians such as those described by Magalhães-Sant'Ana (Chapter 11). Cosmetic surgery, like tail docking and ear cropping, could not be argued to leave the recipients in an improved condition. Modifications such as de-voicing dogs or de-clawing cats may similarly fall foul of the cost–benefit analysis where an animal's *telos* ought not to be compromised as it remains a 'sacred thing'. Even common practices in many countries like neutering, or increasingly common procedures like limb prosthesis, may need to be re-evaluated for their impact. The reach of our duty to the de-hanced is apparently substantial.

Moral Framework

While long-term solutions to system problems of animal modification, such as the blind chicken example earlier, may be far beyond our current technological, economic or social capabilities, our duty to those animals is not diminished. It is possible to address the moral duty of humans to the de-hanced animals by a revised moral framework. It could be a framework of interspecies justice, as eluded to by Chan (Chapter 3). In this framework, it becomes relevant if the harm and benefit of animals and humans are unjustly or disproportionately distributed; correction of this unjust distribution becomes as important a mission today as other injustices have been in the past. To formulate a framework of interspecies justice, it may be necessary to revisit the theory of social contractarianism as Chan, May (Chapter 13) and others (Gabardi, 2017) have suggested, to more fully recognize animals as active and participatory members of human society (Donaldson and Kymlicka, 2011).

Even without this revised framework, our duty of care to those animals to whom we have caused physical or psychological harm remains. The urgency of our response is directly proportional to the amount of harm caused. The triviality of the modification should also factor into the urgency of the rectification, with those harmful modifications that are done seemingly on a whim of personal preference attended to first. The magnitude of the task of rectifying or redressing those animals pushed to the limits in systems so ingrained in society (such as farming or sporting animals) should not deter us from attempting a solution. It seems that that Principle of Conservation of Welfare could be implemented internationally for many, if not all, types of animal use and represents a starting point of our 'taking care of animals so they can take care of us'.

Conclusion

The authors and editors have not sought to impose a moral standard of acceptable types of animal use within this book. While we appreciate that many people do not accept the use of animals as food sources, experimental tools or for entertainment value, we also accept that animals are currently used in these forms internationally and therefore need to be considered, and their welfare improved, where possible. Those who object to the forms of animal use within this book are at liberty to do so, but our aim is to provide evidence in order to improve the welfare of those animals so used. Not all forms of animal use described in this book are purely for human pleasure, and Upjohn (Chapter 4) has detailed the plight of a very different category of animal pushed to their limits; where the human–animal relationship is fundamental to both their survival.

Over 100 million working equids found worldwide are pushed to, and often far beyond, their biological limit in serving the human community around them. They do this to provide the very basics of food and water, and to provide transport of the raw materials needed for building shelters. They are pushed to work hard and for long hours with little rest, in harsh environmental conditions, and often have the same limited access to food and water as their owners. Their owners, and the local community, have very limited financial resources to care for their welfare to a substantial degree. In fact, the welfare of these animals is often impacted very severely, with many dying directly as a result of their working conditions and husbandry. The situation of these animals differs greatly to that described in the other chapters, as these animals are pushed to their limits for reasons of human survival. They are not manipulated or pushed for reasons of improved economics, efficiency or aesthetics. It may be that with these animals the greatest harms are found and the greatest need for improvement recognized, but where there is the least amount of money and resources available to rectify these issues. When dealing with the concept of interspecies justice, it is important to determine if the harms arise to the animals out of human extravagance or just survival.

This book has described and evaluated many forms of animal manipulations in use in the world today. It has, through the expertise of internationally renowned scientists and philosophers, detailed the ways in which mankind has dominated the animal kingdom and manipulated it for its own gains. In doing so, the animals affected have been distorted and deviated far from their wild types, and while they may now possess traits that would seem alien to their ancestors, we have not always done this for the animals' benefit. The welfare compromises described throughout this book, as well as the reasons and causes for them, serve as a starting point for rectification. Without first defining the problem, it is impossible to reach a resolution. The duty of care of all humans to all the animals worldwide affected by being pushed to their biological limit is not optional. With the power to dominate the animal kingdom comes the responsibility to take care of its welfare. Whether we are directly responsible, or not, there is always something that can be done to improve their lot.

References

Arluke, A. and Sanders, C.R. (1996) *Regarding Animals*. Temple University Press, Philadelphia, Pennsylvania.

Asher, L., Diesel, G., Summers, J.F., McGreevy, P.D. and Collins, L.M. (2009) Inherited defects in pedigree dogs. Part 1: disorders related to breed standards. *Veterinary Journal* 182, 402–411.

Chan, S. (2008) Humanity 2.0? Enhancement, evolution and the possible futures of humanity. *EMBO Reports* 9(Suppl 1), S70–74.

De Jong, I.C. and Guémené, D. (2011) Major welfare issues in broiler breeders. *World's Poultry Science Journal* 67, 73–82.

Donaldson, S. and Kymlicka, W. (2011) *Zoopolis: A Political Theory of Animal Rights*. Oxford University Press, Oxford, UK.

FEI (2017) Veterinary regulations. *Federation Equestre Internationale*. Lausanne, Switzerland.

Gabardi, W. (2017) *The Next Social Contract : Animals, the Anthropocene, and Biopolitics*. Temple University Press, Philadelphia, Pennsylvania.

Graham, M.L. and Prescott, M.J. (2015) The multifactorial role of the 3Rs in shifting the harm–benefit analysis in animal models of disease. *European Journal of Pharmacology* 759, 19–29.

Gross, D. and Tolba, R. (2015) Ethics in animal-based research. *European Surgical Research* 55, 43–57.

Harraway, D. (2003) The companion species manifesto. *Dogs, People and Significant Otherness*. Prickly Paradigm Press, Chicago, Illinois.

Harris, J. (2007) *Enhancing Evolution: The Ethical Case for Making Better People*. Princeton University Press, Princeton, New Jersey.

Jackman, B.R., Baxter, G.M., Doran, R.E., Allen, D. and Parks, A.H. (1993) Palmar digital neurectomy in horses: 57 cases (1984–1990). *Veterinary Surgery* 22, 285–288.

Knight, A. (2014) Weighing the harms and benefits: invasive animal research. *The Biochemist* 36, 30–33.

LOC (2014) *Restrictions on Genetically Modified Organisms: International Protocols*. The Law Library of Congress, Global Legal Research Center. Available at: http://www.loc.gov/law/help/restrictions-on-gmos/restrictions-on-gmos.pdf (accessed 5 February 2018).

Olsson, I.A.S. and Sandøe, P. (2011) Animal models of dementia: ethical considerations. *Neuromethods* 48, 15–33.

Packer, R.M.A., Hendricks, A. and Burn, C.C. (2012) Do dog owners perceive the clinical signs related to conformational inherited disorders as 'normal' for the breed? A potential constraint to improving canine welfare. *Animal Welfare* 21, 81–93.

Packer, R.M.A., Hendricks, A., Tivers, M.S. and Burn, C.C. (2015) Impact of facial conformation on canine health: brachycephalic obstructive airway syndrome. *PLOS ONE* 10.

Palmer, C., Corr, S. and Sandøe, P. (2012) Inconvenient desires: Should we routinely neuter companion animals? *Anthrozoos: A Multidisciplinary Journal of the Interactions of People & Animals* 25, 153–172.

Rollin, B.E. (1986) 'The Frankenstein thing': the moral impact of genetic engineering of agricultural animals on society and future science. In: Evans, J.W. and Hollaender, A. (eds) *Genetic Engineering of Animals*. Springer, Boston, Massachusetts, pp. 285–297.

Rollin, B.E. (1995) *The Frankenstein Syndrome: Ethical and Social Issues in the Genetic Engineering of Animals*. Cambridge University Press, Cambridge, UK.

Sandøe, P. and Christiansen, S.B. (2008) *Ethics of Animal Use*. Wiley-Blackwell, Oxford, UK.

Verhoog, H. (1992) The concept of intrinsic value and transgenic animals. *Journal of Agricultural and Environmental Ethics* 5, 147–160.

Wellman, M. (1958) The concept of normal in medicine. *Canadian Medical Association Journal* 79, 43–44.

Whiting, M.C. (2012) Justice of animal use in the veterinary profession. In: Wathes, C.M., Corr, S., May, S.A., McCulloch, S. and Whiting, M.C. (eds) *Veterinary and Animal Ethics*. UFAW, Wiley-Blackwell, Oxford, UK.

Index

Note: Page numbers in **bold** type refer to figures
Page numbers in *italic* type refer to tables

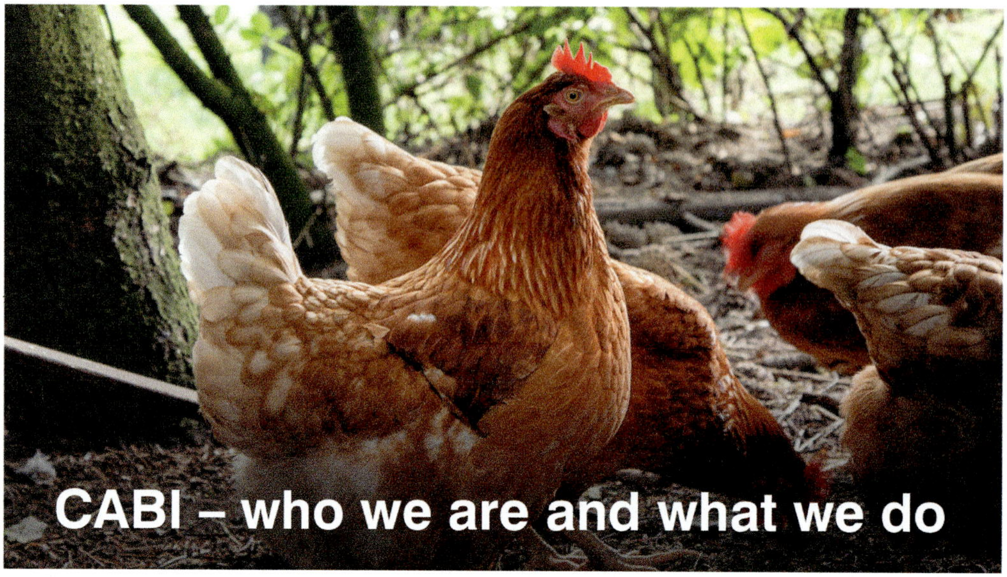

CABI – who we are and what we do

This book is published by **CABI**, an international not-for-profit organisation that improves people's lives worldwide by providing information and applying scientific expertise to solve problems in agriculture and the environment.

CABI is also a global publisher producing key scientific publications, including world renowned databases, as well as compendia, books, ebooks and full text electronic resources. We publish content in a wide range of subject areas including: agriculture and crop science / animal and veterinary sciences / ecology and conservation / environmental science / horticulture and plant sciences / human health, food science and nutrition / international development / leisure and tourism.

The profits from CABI's publishing activities enable us to work with farming communities around the world, supporting them as they battle with poor soil, invasive species and pests and diseases, to improve their livelihoods and help provide food for an ever growing population.

CABI is an international intergovernmental organisation, and we gratefully acknowledge the core financial support from our member countries (and lead agencies) including:

UKaid from the British people

Ministry of Agriculture People's Republic of China

Australian Government Australian Centre for International Agricultural Research

Agriculture and Agri-Food Canada

Ministry of Foreign Affairs of the Netherlands

Schweizerische Eidgenossenschaft Confédération suisse Confederazione Svizzera Confederaziun svizra Swiss Agency for Development and Cooperation SDC

Discover more

To read more about CABI's work, please visit: **www.cabi.org**

Browse our books at: **www.cabi.org/bookshop**,
or explore our online products at: **www.cabi.org/publishing-products**

Interested in writing for CABI? Find our author guidelines here:
www.cabi.org/publishing-products/information-for-authors/